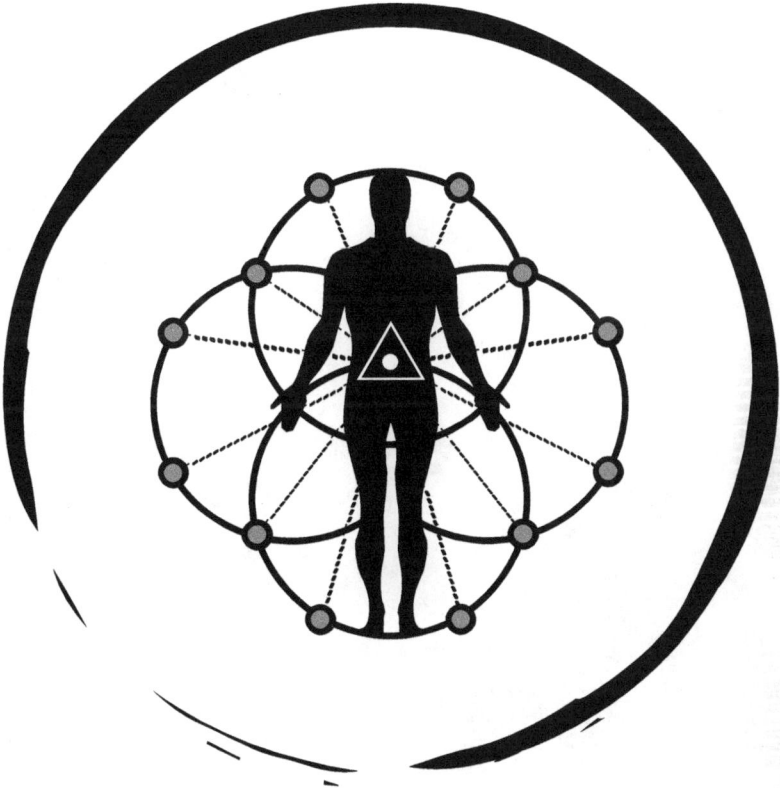

SELF

HEALTH CARE

INCLUDES BONUS INTERACTIVE BOOK

RORY CALLAGHAN

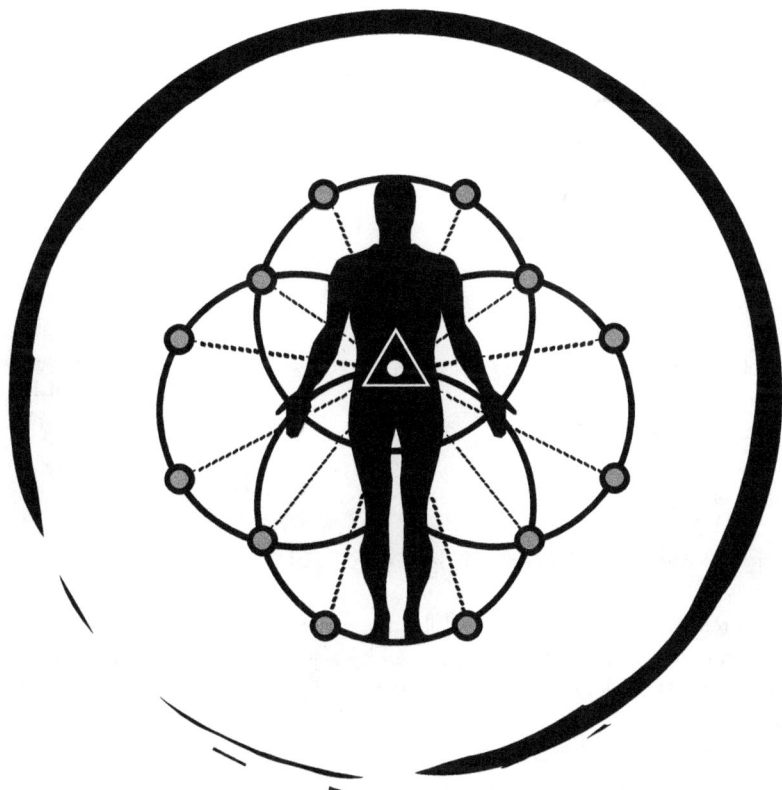

SELF

HEALTH CARE

Lifestyle Medicine for the People

First published in 2021 by Dean Publishing
PO Box 119
Mt. Macedon, Victoria, 3441
Australia
deanpublishing.com

DEAN PUBLISHING

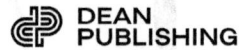

Cataloguing-in-Publication Data
National Library of Australia
Title: SELFCARE: Lifestyle Medicine for the People
Edition: 1st edn
ISBN: 978-1-925452-41-9
Category: Health/Alternative health

EVERY TIME SOMEONE BUYS THIS BOOK WE PLANT A TREE!

"The one who plants trees, knowing that he will never sit in their shade, has at least started to understand the meaning of life."
— Rabindranath Tagore —

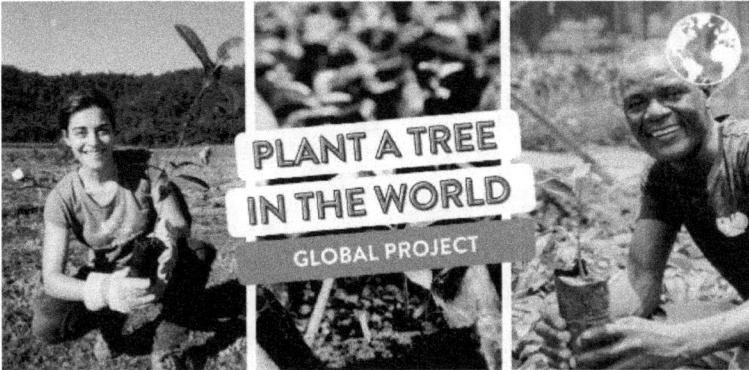

PLANT A TREE IN THE WORLD
GLOBAL PROJECT

Trees clean the air we breathe and serve as an important carbon sink for our emissions. A fully grown tree can absorb up to 21kg of carbon dioxide per year. Your support through this project help to plant tree saplings throughout the world which will eventually become fully-grown at a success rate of up to 85%, and in some cases also provide income for the local community.

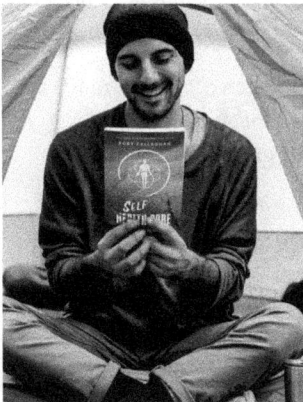

2X YOUR IMPACT!
AND HELP US REACH MORE PEOPLE

If you would like to create another impact and plant another tree. Take a lifestyle photo with the *SelfCare* book so we can see the shores we reach! Share a lesson and tag **selfcare. global** on socials. Each month we will choose the most creative photo and send that person a special gift.

Selfcare.global

This is more than just a book!

Rory has created an online SelfCare ecosystem and community that you can engage and interact with as you read this book.

He envisioned everyone, anywhere with Wi-Fi, having access to empowering SelfCare education, tools, resources, mentors and a real community with real people on a similar journey together.

Behind the scenes: **deanpublishing.com/selfcare**

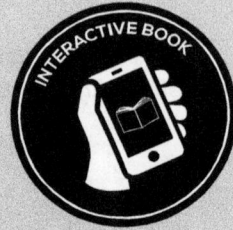

INTERACTIVE BOOK

5 AGREEMENTS & 7 ACKNOWLEDGMENTS BEFORE WE BEGIN

This book is a conversation, a framework, an adaptable matrix that will evolve over time just as we do. It's something set to challenge our underlying belief systems, reinforce thoughts and inspire embodied daily action. It is designed to show you where to look, to curate ancient wisdom and modern science, simply—but never tell you what to see or do; that is up to you.

On Reality: *"fundamental conclusion of the new physics also acknowledges that the observer creates the reality. As observers, we are personally involved with the creation of our own reality. Physicists are being forced to admit that the universe is a 'mental' construction."* — **R.C. Henry, Professor at Johns Hopkins University**

On Evidence and unknowns: *"The absence of evidence is not evidence of absence, or vice versa."* — **Donald Rumsfeld**

On Shared wisdom: *"All truly wise thoughts have been thought already thousands of times; but to make them truly ours, we must think them over again honestly, until they take root in our personal experience."* — **Johann Wolfgang von Goethe**

On Collaboration: *"We are like dwarfs sitting on the shoulders of giants. We see more, and things that are more distant than they did, not because our sight is superior or because we are taller than they, but because they raise us up, and by their great stature add to ours."* — ***Metalogicon* by John of Salisbury, 1159**

On Collective impact: *"We live by each other and for each other. Alone we can do so little. Together we can do so much."* — **Helen Keller**

DEDICATION

This is for all of us.

This curation of consciousness is for all the people who:
...are sick and tired of being sick and tired,
...are seeking simplicity in a sea of complexity,
...know that deep down they do not need to be fixed,
simply nourished,
...want to ignite their human potential through their
bodies' innate wisdom,
...want to live in their highest vibration so that they can
serve from abundant overflow,
...are driven to optimize their performance in this once-in-
a-lifetime human experience,
...are inspired to live their legacy, not just leave one,
...are empathetic and compassionate souls serving from
an empty cup,
...want to help everyone else, before helping themselves.

This is for you and everyone you care about.

Initially, I wrote this for my patients and my mum. But,
then I realized that I was writing it for me. My imperfect
perfect, self. I needed to learn and embody this message
and vision before sharing it with you. **Which means, we**
are all doing this together.

This is for my family, friends, my local community and our
global family. Mum, this is for you. You are the hero of
this story. To my dad, and my extended family that goes
beyond blood, thank you for your support, challenging
questions and guidance in the darkest of times.

This is a dedication to all the lightworkers, working
behind the scenes, illuminating the darkness.
You too are the heroes of this story. I see you.

This book is simply a reminder of what you already
know and feel to be true.

The keys are in your hands. The universe is conspiring in
your favor.

It's time to trust your innate wisdom and tune
into the source of it all. From my heart to yours.
Big love and thank you.

ONE SIMPLE REMINDER

If you take away just ONE thing, may you remember this: You have never needed to be fixed,simply nourished, supported and empowered by enabling environments.

THE SELFCARE SEVENTEEN

1. Nature is our primary life support system
2. Connection and community is the elixir to longevity
3. Self-care is not selfish; learn to take care of yourself so that others may never have to

Be courageous to go first. You will learn how to:
4. Ignite your untapped human potential
5. Optimize your human performance for any desired vision
6. Live a life by your own design, believing that anything is possible from here!
7. Make the most of this once-in-a-lifetime human experience; without comparison.
8. Live a meaningful life full of fulfillment, driven by your own unique standards
9. Live a life with no regrets, knowing tomorrow is not guaranteed for any of us
10. Thrive, not just survive. So that you can build longer tables, not just higher fences
11. Be a high-impact human and serve from abundant overflow
12. Live a legacy in real time, planting seeds today for trees that we may never sit under
13. Create ripple effects of positive change in this generation for the next
15. Understand that true purpose is human, connected innately with nature and the cosmos
16. Treat others (animals and nature too) in the same way that you would like to be treated
17. Feel more, knowing that empathy and compassion are the solutions we all seek

Lastly, remember that none of us are meant to go this journey alone; seek mentors who show you where to look, not gurus who tell you what to see. Trust your inner guru, you are your best SelfCare Doctor.

CONTENTS

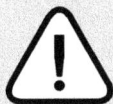

WARNING:

READING THIS COULD RISK
YOUR CURRENT HEALTH

This book is a book of choices. If you make a positive lifestyle choice or change—your life will also change. If you are suffering with fatigue, burnout, poor health and vitality, I warn you that reading this could risk your current state of poor health. If you are seeking the secrets hidden in plain sight to ignite your human potential, optimize your performance and live your ultimate experience, then you will find that here too, within the fields of ancient wisdom and evidence-based science.

Live fast and die young; enjoy healthy moderation; or live to longevity—the choice is yours! This is a supportive and non-judgmental community of people simply doing their best!

I intend for this book to be a positive disruption in your life and in the lives of those you care about. Naturally, like many new changes, it may seem strange at first, or even a little uncomfortable or inconvenient—but one thing I can assure you is that your life will change for the better!

It's time to live as an empowered driver in your life, not the passive passenger.

We do not need to be fixed, we simply need to make better daily choices and aim to create happy and healthy communities that enable us all to thrive.

So, I repeat—if you make a positive lifestyle change—your life will change; don't say I didn't warn you.

You may even do more of this 😊

FOREWORD

Sometimes, you meet people who "hit" you right away. Not a "hit" in a slap-your-face or punch kind of way, but "hit" as in impact. Pow!

Rory Callaghan does that. From the first moment you meet him it's clear; that he is a person with purpose, on purpose and committed to making something great happen. And you also get that, in the words of Imagine Dragon's 2018 hit song, he will do "whatever it takes" to make it happen.

He is positive, hopeful and a born optimist, determined to show that we can all thrive in harmony together. He lives what he believes in, which is, that one person can make a difference and together we can make the world work for all of us, not just for some of us.

He perseveres. He checks and double-checks. When others (like me, for example) would tend to say, "Okay...Let's get it out," Rory would go back and ensure that all the pieces are in place first, as if he energetically knows when the time is right to give this to the world.

Rory wants to ensure that no reader is left up in the air not knowing what to do next or where to go to in order to be empowered to follow their ideal path. And as you'll discover, he's done that magnificently.

We're surrounded by increasing levels of disease—almost 100% of it caused by the lifestyle choices we make individually and collectively. Rory gives us new paths to follow; paths grounded in the wonder of wisdom. As he'll show you, our bodies can do amazing things when we give them precisely the right building blocks and environments in which to thrive.

SelfCare shows everyone the path to better living, but it's also clear that it depends on...you...on self.

This book is a critical reminder, it gives you back the keys and empowers you to be the driver of your own human experience.

Go for it! Just take one simple step, then another. Rory's done some great work to show you the way. And you'll be doing some great and important work when you follow it too.

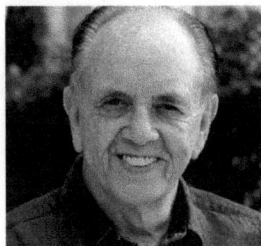

Paul Dunn, Chairman of B1G1.com
Creating a world full of giving—220 million impacts and counting—"for us, for us, for us."

Selfcare.global/Impact

THE MEANING AND THE MISSION

A number of great minds, from Albert Einstein to Dikran Marsupial and even Richard Freyman said a similar thing—"If you can't explain it simply enough to a six-year-old, then the truth is that you don't yet know it well enough yourself." So, here's our six-year-old version of truth.

OUR INTENTION—"EMPOWER & ENABLE"

Our intention is to empower you on your own personal journey, merging ancient wisdom with a modern existence so that you too can be happy, healthy, connected and living towards a unified and sustainable existence for all. Together as one global community on this fragile blue planet.

OUR VISION—"THE RISING BILLIONS"

We believe that good health and wellbeing is a human right for all people, of all ages, regardless of geography, race, religion or luck of birthright. It is a human right for all of us, not just for some us.

OUR MISSION—"1 IN 8 PEOPLE"

To empower good health and wellbeing by enabling personalized, integrated and holistic approaches to health, happiness and connection in a unified and sustainable world. All while reducing the burden of chronic preventable disease in this generation and future generations. If we influence 1 in every 8 people, we will create a ripple effect of positive change: one person, family and community at a time.

My personal mission is to promote health happiness and connection in a unified and sustainable world. SelfCare is about empowering each of us (me included) to look after ourselves so that others may never need to. It is a human-centric, natural, energetic and spiritual approach that unlocks our human potential and empowers each of us to optimize our human experience in our own unique way. This enables each individual to have an impact and create an intergenerational ripple effect of positive change. This is a natural outcome when we each learn to fill our own cup daily and serve from overflow. The future is abundant. There is enough for all of us. Let's learn to thrive together as one, sharing and circulating life's abundance so that we create a world that is a win for all.

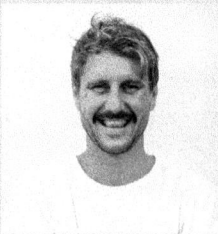

— Rory Callaghan

(rorycallaghan.com)

OUR SHARED GOAL—"THE RISING BILLIONS"

It all starts by having the courage to go first. Without comparison, judgment and the limiting beliefs that may have got you here in the first place. We share the same goal: to ignite our own human potential and take radical responsibility for our own health and wellbeing. Why this is important and meaningful to you right now, might be different to what it represents for me, or anyone else. But that is okay. This is a personal journey. We use an "inside-out approach," helping you master what is within your control, so that you can manifest and consciously engineer anything into your external reality. Living with a belief that "anything is possible from here!" Learn to trust your innate wisdom, connect to the universal source, knowing that the universe has your back. One person, just like you can make a difference. It is the only thing that ever has. If you can't yet do this for yourself, do it for others, or do it in the service of something greater!

HOW TO POSITIVELY IMPACT THE WORLD
IN 4 STEPS

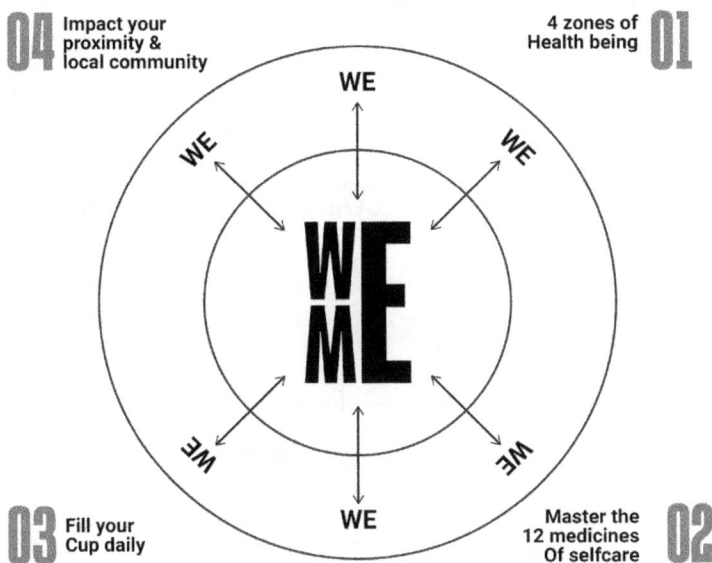

04 Impact your proximity & local community

01 4 zones of Health being

WE

WE

WE

WE ME

WE

WE

03 Fill your Cup daily

WE

02 Master the 12 medicines Of selfcare

5 CURIOUS QUESTIONS TO SELF

"Start with a heart-centered WHY. Create a meaningful WHAT by WHEN, and find the WHO that knows the HOW."

Throughout this book we will address 5 core areas and questions: WHY are you here, and why is this important for you right now and into the future? WHAT is a meaningful goal in the context of your unique life right now? WHEN would you like to embody, achieve and live these meaningful goals? WHO do you know right now that could help support you on this part of the journey? Mentors that show you where to look but not what to see. And communities that support you over the duration of this courageous journey. HOW do you take the first step and every step thereafter? How do you remain persistent, and grow consistently by 1% each day?

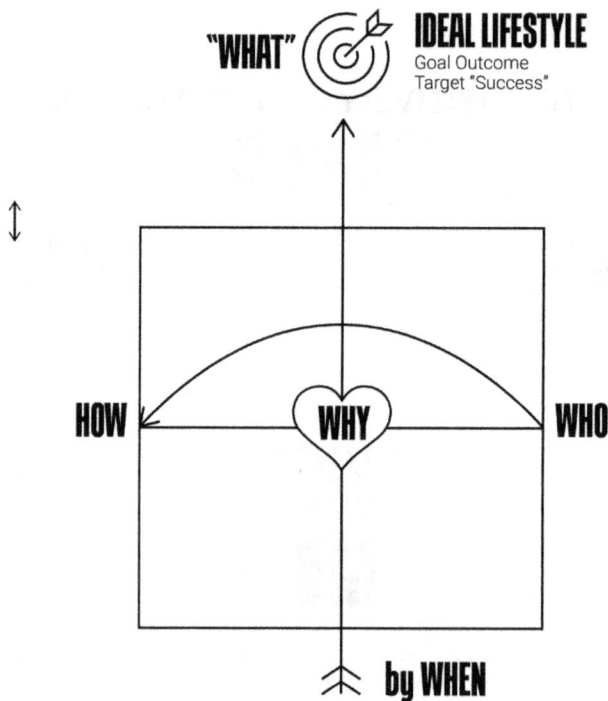

"WHAT" — IDEAL LIFESTYLE
Goal Outcome
Target "Success"

HOW   WHY   WHO

by WHEN

I hope this book serves as a daily reminder that "you have never needed to be fixed, simply nourished and supported." And that your human nature has an innate wisdom and untapped potential that can enable you to achieve anything your heart desires; especially when connected with nature and others. If we can travel into outer space in a metal object, then anything is truly possible. You can achieve anything that you believe, especially with a focused mind and embodied daily actions.

Enjoy this conscious creation and the SelfCare Matrix, I hope it helps you ignite your own SelfCare revolution. Together, we can create a ripple effect of positive global change that starts at our front doorstep. Let's unite in creating global Blue Zone communities where every person has the ability to live in good health, as well-beings on this beautiful and fragile blue planet. Let's live this shared message, mission and vision today.

One last message: before trying to save the world, put your own oxygen mask on first, fill your own cup each day so you can serve from abundant overflow.

ONE PERSON CAN MAKE A DIFFERENCE

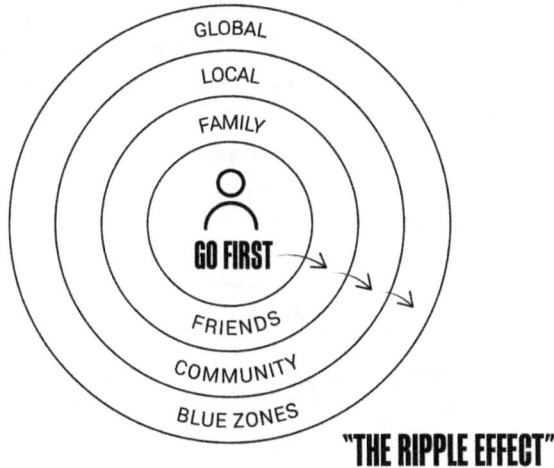

"THE RIPPLE EFFECT"

Former director of Yale University's Yale-Griffin Prevention Research Center and President and Founder of the non-profit True Health Initiative, David Katz, MD and his coalition of world experts declare that, "In today's society, a multitude of competing agendas and motivations obscure the fundamental, simple truths of healthy living. If we don't create enduring, sustainable change, we submit to a world where chronic disease and premature death are the norm, not the exception. There's a better way."[1]

DO IT YOURSELF (LEARN ~ ASSESS)

Our hope is to sift through all the noise, misinformation, misdiagnoses, BS, fake news, and hidden agendas so that you can embody healthy lifestyle choices today, with a deep sense of trust to share it with the people you care about. We hope to share multiple perspectives and truths so that you can come to your own realizations in your own time, from mentors who show you where to look but never tell you what to see. We simply want to remind you that you have never needed to be fixed, simply nourished, supported, and connected on your own unique path.

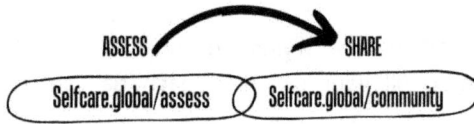

ASSESS → SHARE

Selfcare.global/assess ~ Selfcare.global/community

DO IT WITH US (DO ~ SHARE)

Dr. David Katz draws upon the latest scientific evidence and decades of clinical experience to explain how we can slash our risk of every major chronic disease—heart disease, cancer, stroke, diabetes, dementia, and obesity—by an astounding 80%.[2] By simply making better daily lifestyle choices, living in nourishing natural environments and being part of empowering communities. Share any tools that help you too and we will share them.

If you live a busy lifestyle and love simplicity, we have created simple courses and a structure to support and guide your journey. All the energy exchanged here will help us have a bigger impact.

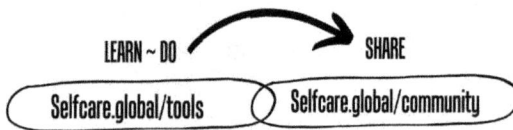

LEARN ~ DO → SHARE

Selfcare.global/tools ~ Selfcare.global/community

DO IT TOGETHER (EMBODY ~ BE)

Throughout this book I will often reference "the ripple effect." As some of you may know, this quote has been attributed to Mother Teresa: "I alone cannot change the world, but I can cast a stone across the waters to create many ripples." Although no one really knows if she did say it (there is a divide in the research)—what we do know is that this specific quote has had many ripples itself. The quote has impacted many just by its existence. This book recognizes ripples—and you're one of them.

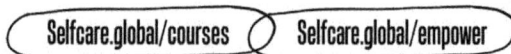

Selfcare.global/courses ~ Selfcare.global/empower

(WE / ME)

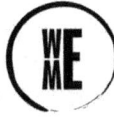

INTRODUCTION

WE AS ONE

"We are here to awaken from our illusion of separateness. True self is non-self, the awareness that the self is made only of non-self elements. There's no separation between self and other, and everything is interconnected. Once you are aware of that you are no longer caught in the idea that you are a separate entity."
— *Thich Nhat Hanh* —

"ME" — ARE YOU PART OF THE UPPER 8 PERCENT?

Simply by having access to this book to read, you belong to a minority group. In fact, if you can read you are luckier than over one-billion people who cannot read at all.

If you woke up this morning with more health than illness, then you are luckier than the million who will not survive this week. Luckier than the 4 billion people living with a chronic preventable non-communicable disease, and even luckier because you have a provincial healthcare card that guarantees you will have care in case of illness.

If you have never experienced the danger of battle, the loneliness of imprisonment, the agony of torture, or the pangs of starvation...then you are ahead of 500 million people in the world.

If you can attend any meeting you want—political, religious, social...then you are luckier than 3 billion people in the world.

If you have food in the refrigerator, clothes on your back, a roof over your head and a place to sleep...then you are more abundant than 75 percent of this world.

If you have money in the bank, in your wallet, and spare change in a dish some place...then you are among the top eight percent of the world's abundant population.[1] With this in mind, let's begin with a grateful heart.

YOU HAVE ALREADY HAD AN IMPACT!

By purchasing this book, you are part of the top 8 percent of the world. I personally thank you. I believe that it is our duty to go first, to take advantage of the abundant opportunities in front of us so that we can reach out and support the 92% who may never have access to this same opportunity.

I believe in circular and shared economies, and as a result of you purchasing this book, you have already created a ripple effect of change for people in the world who do not share this luxury.

We have created a giving impact on your behalf. To see our collective **IMPACT METER** and help us stay accountable to our *why*. Go to:

Selfcare.global/Impact

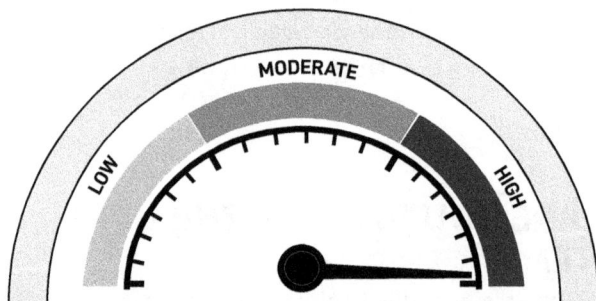

HELP US IMPACT 1 BILLION LIVES!

You made a choice to purchase this book and here is the ripple effect you created. 11% of the gross profits from each book go to:
- 5%—Local community projects
- 6%— National & Global community projects

The other 89% will help us continue to build the lifestyle Medicine Revolution, reminding people that SelfCare is not selfish. All whilst co-creating global Blue Zone communities, starting where we each stand. We can all start local and impact global, together!

IMPACT SCALE

10,000 +	GLOBAL COMMUNITY
1000	NATIONAL COMMUNITY
100	LOCAL COMMUNITY
10	FAMILY COMMUNITY
1	YOU, GO FIRST

IF WE ALL DID JUST THIS! TOGETHER WE COULD MAKE THE WORLD WORK FOR ALL OF US!

ONE TO MANY

FILL YOUR OWN CUP FIRST

Alhough the royalties of this book are essentially for others, it's important to state before reading this that **self-care is *not* selfish**. Filling your own cup, putting your oxygen mask on first is necessary in order to create lasting global change. You'll see this "Fill Your Own Cup" theme pop up throughout the book as a pleasant reminder that you matter. It's only if you take care of yourself first that you can take care of others.

Now, I know this can be a big pivot for some people, many mothers for example. But if you keep pouring and pouring—eventually you end up empty, with no vitality. As the saying goes, "You can't pour from an empty cup."

Let's use the simple diagram of a cup to get the picture (you being the cup of course).

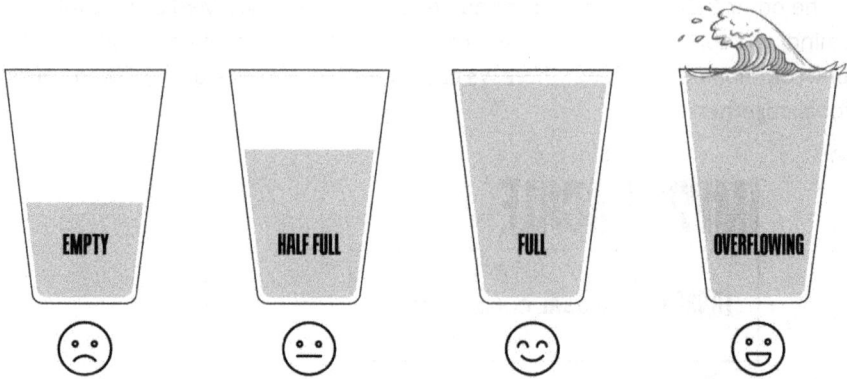

SERVE FROM ABUNDANT OVERFLOW

Our aim in this book is to get you here!

Full but with overflow. If you're full of life and vitality and joy, then this naturally brims over and allows you to serve others from your overflow. Make sense? Good!

GLOBAL IMPACT REQUIRES MORE CUPS IN OVERFLOW

This SelfCare Revolution will continue to focus on YOU and filling your cup, and also using the overflow in three key areas; the ones we believe will solve many future challenges. These are: **Education, Women and Children.**

The Clinton Global Initiative (CGI), along with the United Nations shows that around the world, girls and women continue to suffer from a lack of economic opportunity, inadequate healthcare and education, early marriage, sexual violence, and discrimination. But the great news is that empowering girls and women yields life-affirming returns for everyone. Educating young women increases a country's gross national product—and the benefits are shared by boys and men. CGI reports that, "when women work, they invest 90 percent of their income back into their families, compared with 35 percent for men."[2] We know that by taking care of women, they'll take care of many others.

We aim to help more women, girls and children have an overflowing cup. Imagine the world then. It's time to move from a masculine energy to a more inclusive feminine energy, one that empowers more nurturers to co-create nourishing communities and protect Mother Earth.

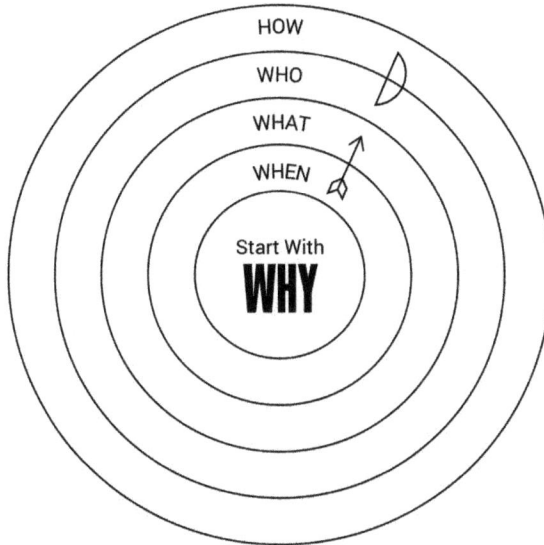

THIS IS OUR WHY

This is WHY we are truly here. Simon Sinek shares that "true purpose is human" and inspires every human being and conscious enterprise to "start with why," not the what and the how. Helping you go first and helping the people you care about is our why. Imagine a world where everyone lives in abundant overflow, looking after their families, friends and communities. If we all did just this ONE thing, together we can positively impact the narrative for future generations through our actions, not just through words and policies. Imagine a world where we all thrive together co-creating nourishing environments, supported by communities of high-vibing humans with one common goal. One person can make a difference!

If we ever meet in person one day, you can ask me why this work is important to me, and I will openly share what led me to this point. Let's uncover your why and maybe you can share that with me one day too! And if by chance, we share a similar mission, let's work together!

Selfcare.global/about

WHAT IS YOUR WHY?

....

....

....

....

....

....

....

....

6 STEPS TO HELP YOU UNCOVER YOUR UNIQUE WHY

Before we go deeper, let us remember that true purpose is human; bliss moments are our greatest guide, happiness is the purpose of life and you will know you have found your why when it ignites an emotion. You will probably cry. That's when you know your why.

1. Why do you get out of bed each morning?
2. Why should people care, why do you care?
3. What moments made time stand still? Why were you doing them?
4. What past experiences created a feeling of bliss and inner peace? Why were those moments important to you?
5. What past experiences created pain, trauma and challenged your shadows? Why do you want to share these lessons with others? Why is this a driver for you?
6. What are people naturally attracted to you for? And why do they feel that you are the go-to person to solve that problem?

If you find an answer, try this:

Go deeper and ask yourself—"Why is that important to me?" Do this 12 times and keep digging deeper. If you get stuck, try adding "so that" to keep the thoughts and feelings flowing. Once the answer creates an emotion (e.g. you cry), you will know your why. Once you have found it, use that to guide your decisions and expressions.

CALL TO COURAGE

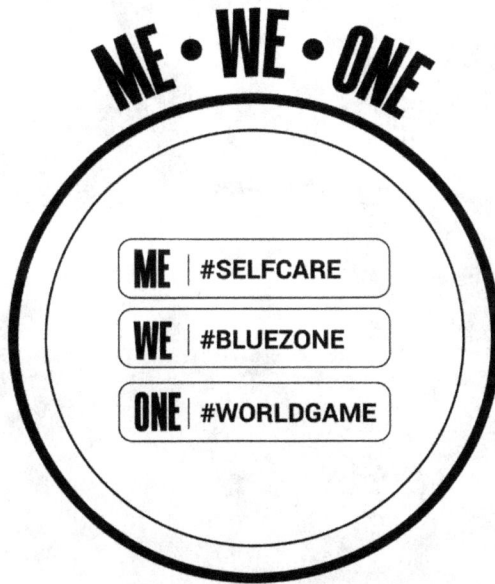

ME • WE • ONE

ME	#SELFCARE
WE	#BLUEZONE
ONE	#WORLDGAME

JOIN THE MOVEMENT

Want to Join Us?

Join Your Global Community Now @

Selfcare.global/community

As you read this book and take inspired action:
share learnings, share stories, tools and resources to help others.

LEARN – DO – EMBODY – SHARE

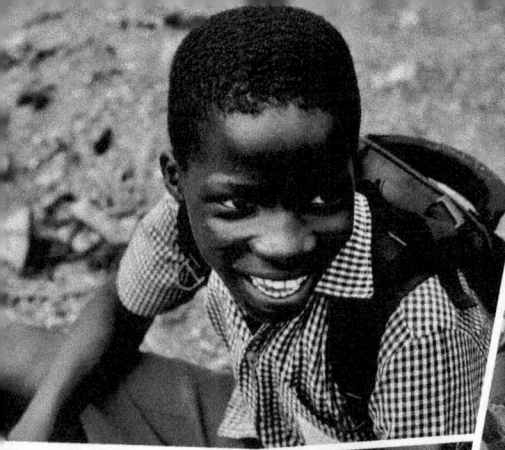

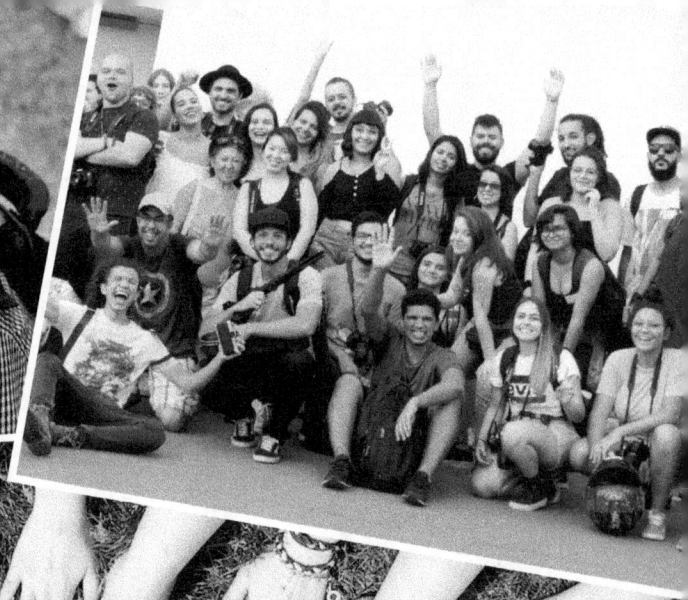

HELP US:

✓ Go first and create ripple effects that positively empower over 1 billion+ people together.

✓ Co-create global Blue Zone communities, where the burden of chronic preventable disease is a thing of the past, and living towards longevity is the new normal.

✓ Unlock the human potential available in ALL of us and live your ultimate human experience and life.

✓ Learn to feel happy, be healthy and connected right now, not tomorrow. Filling cups all over the world!

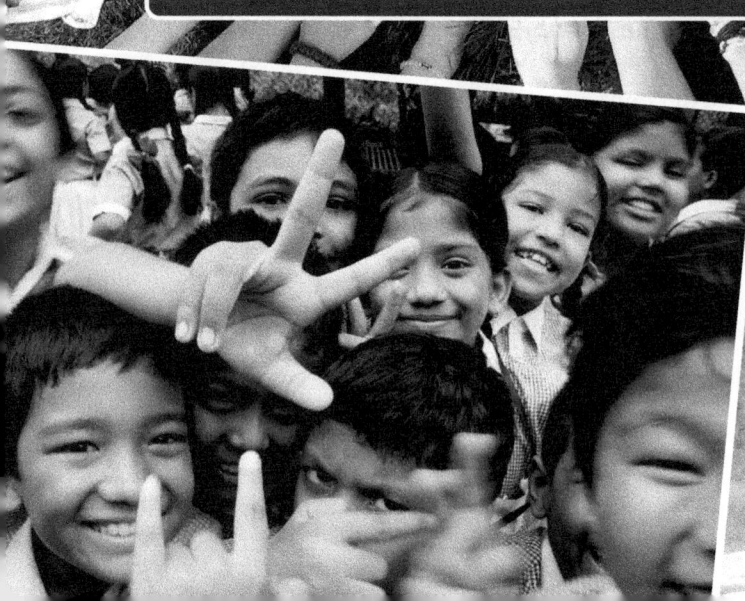

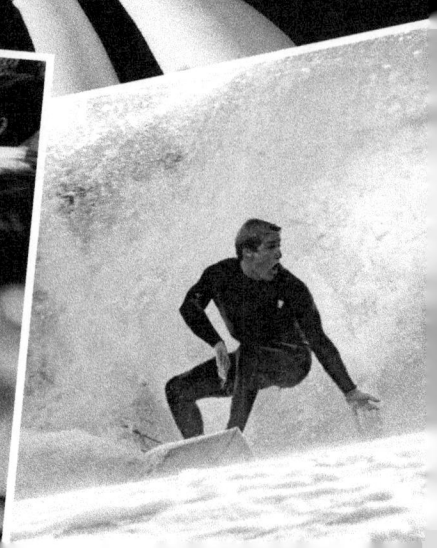

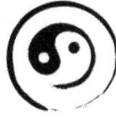

CHAPTER 1

PAIN TO PURPOSE

*"The journey of the hero is about the courage to seek the depths;
the image of creative rebirth; the eternal cycle of change within us;
the uncanny discovery that the seeker is the mystery which the
seeker seeks to know. The hero journey is a symbol that binds,
in the original sense of the word, two distant ideas, the spiritual
quest of the ancients with the modern search for identity,
always the one, shape-shifting yet marvelously
constant story that we find."[1]*
— Joseph Campbell, The Hero's Journey —

HEALTH PROFESSIONAL WHO LOST HIS HEALTH

One day, at 26 years of age, I woke up as health professional who had lost his health.

All the accolades, continued learning, bachelors and master's degree couldn't save me from how I felt in this moment. My knowledge had failed me, and I had failed to listen to my body's innate wisdom. I had failed to acknowledge its natural intelligence hidden in the depth of my genetic blueprint. I had failed to see the impact of my lifestyle choices. My ego had led me to be in a state of disharmony. Quite simply, I had pushed myself too far. I was stressed, tired, depleted, dysfunctional and depressed.

I thought I knew what to do. I was a health professional and leader in my industry and community. People looked to me for advice and support. Yet, in this moment I felt incongruent and lost. How could I help others if I couldn't even help myself? All my dreams and passions came crashing to an abrupt halt.

This was crisis point.

As I woke up on this dreary winter's morning in my home town of Fremantle, Perth, I was already an hour late for work. I had slept through six consecutive wake-up reminder alarms, but I didn't even try to get up. I couldn't. I had no choice but to surrender to my body and soul's need to rest. I was physically, mentally, emotionally and biologically stuck. Exhausted. Depleted. I had hit rock bottom and was helpless to change it.

I felt as though nothing mattered anymore. How could I move forward if I didn't have my health and a sense of wellbeing to move forward with? I was forced to realize the true value of my health; which was linked to every dream, aspiration, business, relationship and lifestyle I had envisioned. Without my health, nothing else was possible. Dreams were useless in the graveyard. I imagined all the dreams that were never lived and all the innovations never shared.

As I imagined being restricted from everything I loved doing, my heart sank. I was scared. A strong man on the outside, but a scared fearful child on the inside. I didn't get how precious this gift of health was, until I was on the brink of losing it.

Through my work, I had access to modern technology, scans and an impressive network of experts with whom I worked, but no one could help me in this moment. It was up to me, something had to change. I had to change.

As I lay there, I remember asking myself three questions:

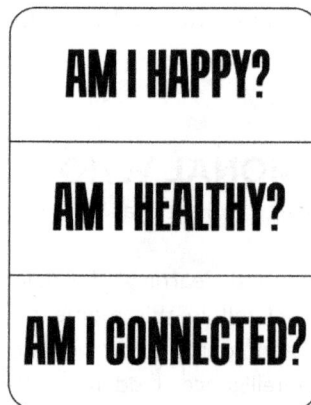

AM I HAPPY?

AM I HEALTHY?

AM I CONNECTED?

THE DOWNWARD SPIRAL

*"The first revolution is when you change your mind and
beliefs about how you look at things, and see there might
be another way to look at it that you have not been shown."*
— Gil Scott Heron —

Before answering, I took a breath and sunk deeply into these questions. My brain desperately tried to take charge and formulate clever answers, but the truth was too confronting for any mental gymnastics.

I answered a somber NO to all three questions.

I was a witness to my own situation. In my mind's eye, I could see the dark circles under my eyes, the muscle loss, the poor posture, the loss of energy and severe brain fog, the lack of mental clarity. All those signals and symptoms from my body were suddenly evident. Those aches, those pains, that digestive reflux, those intolerances to foods I once loved. All signs! But I was looking away.

It was as if I had simply existed in a state of dullness over the past 12-months, or perhaps more. Everything was finally clear in this moment. *I had chosen all of this*.

But how had I ended up here? Was I a passenger to my own human experience, erroneously thinking that I was in the driver's seat? Or had I consciously driven down this path, making my own choices every step of the way?

Something big had to change. But how was I meant to communicate this to my boss, to my long list of patients booked in to see me that day, my partner, my family and my friends? What about all the demands I had to meet, and my endless to-do list?

I felt like I had failed all of them. I felt like I was falling further behind. But, who was I racing against?

A deep sense of shame and guilt encompassed me as I lay there, unable to help myself, let alone anyone else. I replied to the 10 missed calls from my manager and said that I was sick and unable to come in. She replied with a worried but empathetic voice and said that she would move all of my patients across and clear my schedule for as long as I needed to recover. It was as if she had been waiting months for this moment, watching me ready to crash and burn, without saying anything.

My mom warned me that I had been "burning the wick at both ends for nearly five years."

In that moment, I finally received that message, albeit five years too late.

How could I have been so goal-orientated and narcissistic, yet oddly combined with an equal blend of selfless empathy, prioritizing other people's needs before my own? I knew that my heart wasn't selfish, but I had lacked in prioritizing my own self-care. My desire to serve others was driven from an unconscious desire to find my own self-worth and obtain self-value in helping others, at the expense of myself.

I knew what to say and do, but had no time, and had not prioritized myself into my own schedule. I was not walking my talk. I had never felt so incongruent. Whilst being at the peak of my career, I was at the bottom of my life. A bizarre paradox that shocked me to the core.

This had been a long time coming. I had been blinded by cultural and societal expectations of who I should be in the world and how I should serve. I had been working 100 hours per week in the healthcare system. It all of a sudden seemed odd that the healthcare system was set-up in a way where the leaders, healers, coaches and experts were forced to live as part of the very statistics they were inspired to change.

I had to step back and see the bigger picture.

THE CRISIS, THE CATALYST AND THE COMEBACK

I reflected on what had led me to this point. Growing up in one of the most isolated cities in the world, I had a warped view of reality. Was I always a candidate for a burnout? Or was this an environmental factor? Surely there was a better way.

I remembered my dad, a 27-year-old man who had met my 44-year-old mother. An amazing painter with his whole life ahead of him, who not long after my birth succumbed to mental health challenges that led him to seek mind-altering substances as a way of numbing the pain created in his mind.

I remember walking through the streets of my hometown in Fremantle with my two best friends, and seeing a homeless guy rolled up in the corner of a shopfront with a bottle of beer next to him. We started laughing and joking at the situation, until I realized that it was my dad.

I remembered my mother. A strong, powerful and independent woman with an unlimited work ethic. She had sacrificed so much for my brother and me and always showed up with a sense of unconditional love and an unwavering belief in anything we put our minds to. For most of my upbringing, we lived pay check to pay check. She had invested in our home and I soon learned that her being born just after the Great Depression meant she had a strong belief to not owe anyone anything. She showed me the transformative power of unconditional love and served from an empty cup, going without, so we had every opportunity in life. She was relentless in ensuring we owned our home and had our basic human needs met, even if it meant that she sacrificed her own.

I remembered the day we were debt-free as a family. My mother came home with three round-the-world tickets, saying, "You know what boys, life is for living!" She'd gone back into debt, inspired to show us the world she had seen as a young air-hostess traveling to all the corners of the globe. She said that we weren't meant to simply pay bills and die.

I watched as my brother had to make a hard decision: come on the world trip with us, or take the apprenticeship that paid less than $5 an hour so that he could secure a future for himself and his family. He chose his future career over this experience. I remember feeling as if this was a turning point in both of our lives. I imagined what would have happened if he had gone and I had stayed.

As I ventured on my first trip outside of the city I was born, I felt things changing inside me as mom and I boarded our first plane from Perth to Bali. The first thing I remember on this trip was meeting a man called Wayan. I learned he was living and supporting his family on $150 a month; the same amount I had in my pocket for spending money. I was confused, he had more happiness than anyone I had seen in my young life and yet he was so generous and giving. I felt a desire to give him everything I had. This experience also evoked a sense of guilt within me as I questioned my own happiness and it challenged everything I thought I knew about happiness.

We traveled to Thailand and I remember seeing a young girl dying of malaria in a small hut with no access to an ambulance or healthcare. Something I had always taken for granted. My mother and I had to walk away. I remember feeling something deep in my heart, a sense of helplessness and despair in knowing that she would not last the night. Things started to change within me. I was beginning to learn profound things on this global journey.

I remember walking along the Champs-Élysées in Paris and hearing a woman's excitement over her latest "bargain"—she had just purchased a pair of shoes for €1000. My young mind reflected deeply after hearing that the malaria medication for the young girl in Thailand would have only cost ~6 cents if she had the means to access it. I felt my worldview shift rapidly in that moment as I came to understand that we weren't born equal. I wondered how many lives could have been saved for the same cost of those shoes?

I remember seeing an old man in New Orleans playing a saxophone that looked older than he was. He had no hat out for money and seemed like he was just doing it out of passion, that his heart simply felt the need to share his music with the world. As he played, I watched bystanders start dancing and other musicians sat down to join in. I felt what passion really was, but resisted dancing with everyone else through fear of being judged.

I remembered all the knowledge I had accumulated studying when no one was watching. I remember feeling those chemical reactions spark and fire as my brain connected pieces of life's mysterious puzzle. This unique feeling inspired me to be the first person in my family to graduate from higher level education at university. I went on to attend university straight out of school, dissecting human bodies that had been donated to science. I saw cancerous tumors in real-time that had taken over a man's body. I knew it wasn't a normal part of aging. I saw what lay beneath each layer of our amazing human bodies. I extracted DNA, the evolutionary blueprint of life onto a stick to see it live. I worked with elite athletes and studied how the human body could perform at its highest level. This curiosity led me to further study as I grappled with my own injuries that inevitably derailed my young sporting desires. But in hindsight, this led me to explore how the body not only performed, but how it could repair.

I worked in hospitals with patients who were in intensive care (ICU), teetering on the border of life and death. I remember a doctor describing it as "angels gates"—a place many people never left.

I remember seeing a Buddhist monk have his life support switched off after being a victim of an unexpected assault on his morning run for the $20 he had left in his wallet.

I remember working in the children's ward with kids who had cancer, trying to morally understand how they had been dealt this card in life. I watched them laugh and make the best of their situation as their parents cried in the background, too afraid to show their child the reality of the situation.

I remember working in the respiratory ward, walking a middle-aged woman 10-meters down the hallway before her oxygen saturation dropped to a level where she could go no further. Coming to terms with her lifestyle choices and smoking from an era that promoted.

I remember working with a father who had a heart attack on the way to work, even though he looked fit on the outside. I watched as his three young children lay by his bed all day, waiting for their hero to wake up from life-saving surgery. It made me appreciate the wonders of modern medicine but I felt that we could have prevented it from happening at all.

I remember working in the neurological ward helping a young man walk again after he had sustained a head injury in a car accident he had caused. Only to find out that the person he had collided with had not survived the crash. I questioned why he had survived but the innocent mother had not.

I watched a lady get her leg amputated because her foot became gangrenous from a metabolic issue associated with Type 2 diabetes. Her lifestyle choices were deplorable, and I wondered what circumstances or emotions had led her to making those choices. It seemed like she was destined to remain ingrained in the system, supported and funded by tax-paying individuals who had made different life choices. I questioned whether she was at fault, or whether the wider community and health system had not really helped her. I wondered what past traumas she had experienced, or whether her poor lifestyle choices were conscious or a result of deeper troubles.

All of this became a personal driving force. It lit a fire within my soul to be part of the solution, part of the change.

TO KNOW AND NOT DO, IS TO NOT YET KNOW

The Japanese have a proverb that says, "Knowledge without wisdom is a load of books on the back of an ass."

Like most, I came out of 18 years of study gaining knowledge, minus the wisdom of experience. A sobering reality that made me feel like the Japanese proverb. I came fresh from college with a desire to change the world, feeling like I knew it all and was ready to show the world. I worked and worked, determined to do my part in changing the world.

It didn't seem right that there was a large proportion of the world that was not living in a state of good health and wellbeing. I was not yet sure of the extent, but I just knew it wasn't right. I had to try and fix it.

When I woke up at 26—unhappy, unhealthy and disconnected, I realized that I had become a statistic of the very system I was inspired to pivot and change. As I reflected on this moment, still laying in bed, the words of leaders and giants who had come before me echoed in my mind.

W. Edwards Deming suggested that "a bad system will beat a good person every time." I knew in my heart that I was a good person and this social and cultural environment and "system" had definitely beaten me. For now.

Albert Einstein shared, "We cannot solve our problems with the same level of thinking that created them." I knew that all of this health knowledge I had accumulated did not translate into living and serving from a place of good health and wellbeing.

I felt like I had spent years banging my head against a wall, learning and being forced to apply "health" concepts that didn't add up in the real world. But I had trusted the system. I felt like my $100,000 in student loans had been a total waste of time if this "knowledge" was the ultimate and final outcome. I felt cheated by the education system, by society and by the social constructs that had molded me to think this way. Trading time for money and working at the expense of my own health and wellbeing.

As I stepped in deeper reflection, I remembered the words of Buckminster Fuller, "You can never change things by fighting the existing reality. To change something, build a new model that makes the existing model obsolete."

It became clear; I was both the problem and solution. I had to step outside the system in order to heal and make a real difference. I dreamed of co-creating a system that empowered people in their own self-care. A model that would one day make the existing model obsolete. I was sick of fighting within an inefficient system that had the best intentions but was flawed in its very foundation of passive care, disconnected from the essence of humanity and disconnected from nature, our true source of healing and regeneration.

SelfCare and self-governed communities seemed to be an appropriate way forward. If we all simply looked after ourselves, each other and our communities, we'd thrive. My gut feeling was that we could slowly create a global change. We could change the current system and ignite a more human-centric approach founded in nature and in our innate connectedness as tribes and communities.

In essence, I wanted to remind people that they are their best SelfCare doctor. Not a doctor in the technical sense of an administering health professional, but a Dr in the sense of administering healthy daily rituals and lifestyle choices.

In hindsight, I can now see that my past and present experiences were necessary in order to come to this realization. As I reflect, it all adds up. Choices add up! Author and entrepreneur James Clear shares that if you can get 1 percent better each day for one year, you'll end up thirty-seven times better by the time you're done. Compound your health! In the same way you dream of compounding your wealth. Health is wealth.

Seeing my dad homeless on the streets did leave me with a choice, walk on by and ignore his very existence or stop to acknowledge him as the man who brought me into this world. After all, I was a 1 in 4 trillion chance of being born and he made that miracle possible.

I stopped and went over to my dad, kneeling down as I pressed on his shoulder. He woke up in a daze, smiling as he saw his son in front of him. I later found out that I am the one reason he is still alive today. That one simple caring gesture inspired him to keep going that day when he had no reason or want to exist.

He wasn't a deadbeat, he was my dad. An amazing painter and creative soul. He suffered mental health issues not long after I was born in 1987, which lead to addictive escapism. Society would call him an alcoholic and homeless. But to me, he always has and always will be, my father.

His journey taught me a valuable lesson in empathy, compassion and how resilient the human body can be to self-harm. He is still alive, even after succumbing to a head injury in his 40s. Without access to our amazing healthcare system and the allied health professional team he would not be here. I am grateful for everyone that is part of the integrated support system that means that my dad still lives on today.

Did you know that over a billion people do not have access to healthcare? This means that children are losing their parents globally. But that doesn't need to be the case.

My father's recovery from a severe brain injury also taught me how amazing neuroplasticity is. A year after his injury he could not even throw a ball, today he still paints and lives relatively independently. Something miraculous happened as well. After his head injury, he lost his long-term memory. He no longer remembers the demons that once ruled his mind and led him to seek mind-altering substances to silence them.

His paintings used to be of natural environments with solitary characters who were intimately connected with the land. It was almost as if he found peace within his paintings. After his injury, his paintings became more colorful and vibrant as if his mind was seeing the world differently. He even started to sign his name at bottom of his paintings, something that a man who lacked self-love, self-worth and value could never once do.

He helped me realize the true damage of suppressed emotions. I grew up without a father because of them. Even at the bottom of a bottle, he didn't find what he was emotionally searching for. It helped me understand that at the deepest level, we all need emotional connection. Emotions are unique and contextually relevant to the events and experiences of our life. They weave our memories and envelope our feelings of unity or aloneness.

My mother taught me my most valuable lessons. The way she spoke of my father in such a positive way, when she had every reason not to. She showed me a level of compassion and empathy that would change the way I see and treat people forever. She showed what could be done by serving from an empty cup (in the material sense) but an overflowing cup in her sense of unconditional love for her children and the world around her. She inspires me every day to serve from overflow. I always wondered what she would have been capable of, if she was ever able to receive the love she gave so freely and willingly.

THE ARRIVAL AND RETURN TO HARMONY

As I lay there, that fateful day in bed. I became inspired to create a different future and reality for myself and others. I wanted desperately to one day sit in the depths of happiness, with a sense of inner peace, connected to myself, my partner, my friends, my family, my community and the world. A healthy and unrestricted human being.

The good news is: I made it. I am happy, healthy and connected beyond my wildest dreams. Yet it could never have happened if I had stayed dwelling in a system that didn't have the deeper resources or understanding to spark my self-healing capabilities.

Now, I want everyone to wake up feeling happy, healthy and connected in a sustainable and unified world. We were never meant to survive alone, we are here to learn how we can thrive together. And yes, it wasn't just an overnight epiphany—I had to make a giant leap and make new and consistent choices to come back from the brink of ill-health. I had to move from a broken system in order to fix myself. I had to move from Healthcare to SelfCare. It was up to me. Self-acceptance and ownership was just the beginning.

This is the inner revolution many people are now taking. It doesn't mean that they're dismissing traditional medicine, it simply means that they are making self-care choices toward wellbeing and happiness.

Many people are disappointed that they don't get better, that all solutions aren't found inside our current healthcare system. Though as a health practitioner, I'm not suggesting you walk away from any healthcare providers, I am simply suggesting you begin to make empowered choices in your own life. A choice to not solely rely on others to fix you but begin to look at fixing yourself. Move from being over-reliant on HEALTHCARE and start to realize that SELFCARE holds many answers you may have never investigated (or been advised to look at).

This is the inner revolution. This is the new step forward.

Seek mentors that remind you that you don't need to be fixed. Mentors who show you where to look, without telling you what to see. Mentors who help you focus on the solution and work together with other mentors in their fields of expertise, being truly human-centric in their approach.

SELFCARE is the foundation, the 80–95% within our control. HEALTHCARE is the intervention, for the 5–20% outside our control.

CALL TO COURAGE (C2C):

WHAT is one painful event that taught you a valuable life lesson?

....

....

....

....

....

....

....

....

....

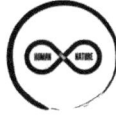

CHAPTER 2

YOU HAVE NEVER NEEDED TO BE FIXED

You have never needed to be fixed. Seek to be nourished. Spend time in places and with people where you leave feeling more full than when you arrived. The keys have always been in your hands. Choose your environments and proximity wisely. They will dictate your wellbeing more than any other factors.

Have you ever seen a little fragile flower pushing its way through the cracks in the pavement of a busy concrete city? Who cannot help but marvel at its tenacity in trying to adapt and find a way to bloom

Is our environment stronger than our willpower? Or is our willpower stronger than the environment? Are our choices dictated by the environments that we grew up in and/or even live in now?

Imagine you had all of the will power in the entire world, but the environment you dwell in was never designed to help you thrive in abundance, to reach your full potential. What would happen?

THE FLOWER THAT DIDN'T BLOOM

Perhaps this story of the gardener and the flower will shed some light on this point.

Many of us are trying (willpower) to cultivate and activate our own health and wellbeing so that we flourish and bloom from within, in our own unique way. Humans, like flowers, are designed in the same way; to flourish and bloom. However, not all do. Mystic and philosopher Mokokoma Mokhonoana shares that "we are capable of believing ourselves out of or into disease."[1] So, what do you believe?

But why? If we are all designed and have the potential to express our ultimate human potential, then why don't we? Think about this for a second; if a flower you planted doesn't flourish, bloom or grow, what would you do?

Imagine you were the gardener, tending to a group of flowers. 19 in 20 were struggling to survive and only 1 was really thriving.

How would you help the majority? Would you try and fix the flower? Or would you look at things a little bit differently?

Rather than honing in on the one flower, you could take a step back. You then see the flower in the context of its environment. Not knowing the answer, you look laterally to other gardeners and other flowers who seem to have found the ease and flow of growth.

A seemingly complex problem all of a sudden becomes simple. Almost as if the answers were hidden in plain sight all along, sitting just beyond the tunnel vision perspective of focusing on fixing the flower. But the fact remains: the flower has always been designed to bloom.

What if rather than focusing on the problem (the flowers inability to grow), we shifted our mindset and expanded our consciousness to consider the flower within the context of its environment? This way we would have to trust in the flowers innate evolutionary design.

In the 21 century we have forgotten something seemingly obvious; something the best gardeners know all too well. We are designed to bloom innately.

YOU ARE DESIGNED TO BLOSSOM AND BLOOM

What if the solution was that simple?

That you do not need to be fixed with silver bullet solutions. That you do not need to be more or do more.

That you simply need to live in abundant and enabling environments.

That your amazing human body holds all of your human potential inside of you. That you have 99.9% of the same genetic blueprint of anyone quoted in this book—Aristotle, Plato, Albert Einstein, and Maya Angelou; or anyone that you admire and look up to. That your evolutionary blueprint is ready and waiting for the rich consistent stimulus of environments that nourish and support you. Then you can do what you have been designed to do—be the ultimate expression of yourself. You can be this expression in any environment. But wouldn't it be nice to co-create environments that enable us to thrive, rather than ones that challenge us to survive?

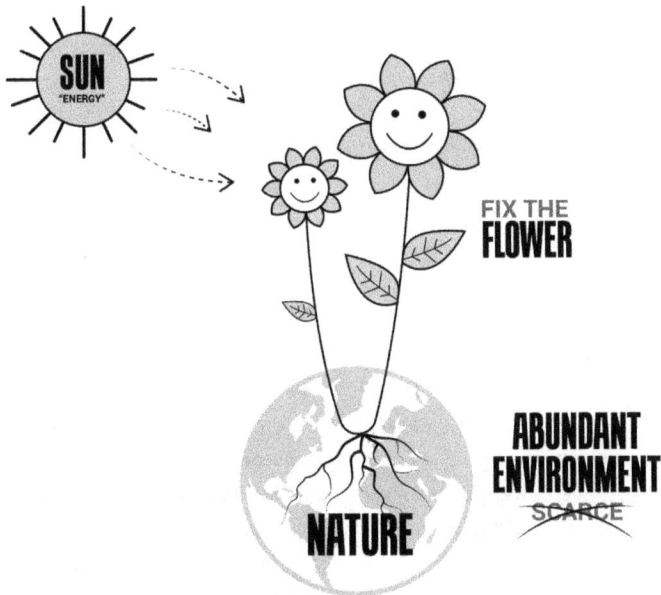

*"When a flower doesn't bloom, you fix the environment
in which it grows, not the flower."*
— **Alexander Den Heijer** —

SEEK NOURISHING ENVIRONMENTS

We have been side-tracked by industrial and now technological revolutions in the last 200 years, seeking progress at the expense of the environments we have to live in. We are fish-forcing ourselves to live in polluted, depleted fish ponds; adapting to environments that were never designed to promote human health and wellbeing. What's worse is that we have designed health and wellness systems to "fix" the flower, passively supporting it to adapt to environments that it was never designed to thrive in.

As an example, everything in our human biology is made to move. Yet here we are, designing work environments where we sit behind computers for hours on end; one-third of our day if you want to get into specifics. Then we begin to wonder why we have developed stiffness and soreness in every joint in our body.

Trying to move forward, we seek out a solution in a health and wellness system that directs us to physical practitioners who mobilize, click, clunk and stretch our backs into place and simply remind us to move at least 30 minutes a day. Yes, remind us to move for less than 5% of your day. But because we as a society are busy being busy and don't have time, (because we have to work, we have to make money to survive, to maintain food, water and shelter) we dismiss this advice. Then we're back to square one tomorrow, falling back into the same old habits and rituals that don't serve us, wondering why the pain and stiffness slowly returns. We continuously repeat the process, ending up with the same result. We're essentially running in circles. Does this sound familiar?

Until one day it clicks for you...
I was not designed to sit all day
I was not designed to live in stress
I do not need to live beyond my means
I do not need to sit in traffic for 3 hours each day in order to be abundant.

You start to question who designed all of these environments and systems. You start to realize that you are the driver and no longer the passenger in this human experience. Sure, you can learn to adapt to any environment like a fish can adapt to survive in a dirty, polluted fish pond or a flower adapts to bloom in the city. Or, you can choose differently. You can seek environments that nourish you to grow and support you for the longevity of the journey allowing your cup to stay full.

Like the flower, many of us cannot determine where our seed is planted or where it grows, in the same way we can't choose our parents. However, humans CAN choose the environments in which they live in. It is not something new either. Human beings have always been nomadic, moving between environments, seeking abundance, whilst allowing for the natural cycle of the seasons. Moving with natural cycle of birth, growth, maintenance and destruction has been in our blood for centuries. What if you knew that it is actually the one behavior that allowed the oldest still living human civilization to survive over tens of thousands of years?

Perhaps a flower is not designed to bloom in a pot plant, inside a house, or as part of a concrete jungle deprived of light. What if all it needed to bloom and thrive was to be moved outside with clean air, sunshine, clean water, and nourishing soil. Then it could finally do what it was born to do. Flourish and bloom.

Remember: Humans, unlike the flower, CAN choose.

The hardest truth we may have to come to understand is that we might not be able to heal in the environment that made us sick. However, it doesn't mean that we can't change that. If we are truly are the most intelligent species, then we wouldn't destroy our natural life support system. We would nurture it, so it can nourish all of us.

Can you remember ONE place where you found ease, flow, happiness and abundance? A place where you simply felt good?

....

....

....

....

....

....

....

ENVIRONMENTS ENABLE OR DISABLE WILLPOWER

You may have heard the term, "environment is stronger than willpower." For the most part it is true. As we grow we become a product of the geographical and cultural environments that we grow up in. We become a product of the family and social environments that we spend the most time with. As we continue to learn and grow through the experiences, we become a product of our work environments and even the 5 people we spend the most time with.

It can leave you wondering if your beliefs, thoughts and actions are really yours, or whether they have been programmed, nurtured and molded by the environments and people you spent the most with as you grew.

Cast your mind back to the blank canvas of your younger mind and reflect on some simple questions. What did you actually want to do and be before entering the "working world"? What made you happy before you were sold into a lifestyle that didn't perhaps feel quite right? What were you passionate about before you were told that it wasn't relevant?

To shine the light on the power of the environment on your behaviors and lifestyle choices, I will share some insights from the "Rat Park" experiment as it explores addiction.[2] Now addiction is relative. You might not be addicted to mind-altering substances, tobacco, sugar or other vices. But you may be addicted to a lifestyle that doesn't make you happy, addicted to work, and even addicted to technology and the dopamine hits you get from social media. It's a simple experiment that you could do at home (but I wouldn't recommend it for reasons that will soon become apparent).

If you get a rat and you put it in a cage and you give it two water bottles: one bottle of clean water and the other water bottle laced with morphine. If you do that, the rat will almost always prefer the drugged water and almost always kill itself quite quickly. So there you go, right? That's how we think addiction works.

We have been taught that there are chemical hooks. This means that if you took "the chemical hook" for a period of time, your body would become dependent on them and you would biologically need them and become an addict, right? If you smoked one cigarette, you wouldn't be able to stop. If you took recreational drugs you wouldn't be able to control them. If you ate a lot of sugar or drank alcohol, you would get diabetes and become a sugar-addict or an alcoholic. Many of us may have had an accident, ended up in a hospital and taken opioids, but the vast majority aren't addicted to the synthetic chemicals that numb our pain. But what if the pain was necessary, something to be felt and embraced; not something to be suppressed and numbed? Perhaps this modern approach to suppressing pain, rather than embracing its signal in our life is the real issue.

What if everything we have learnt about addiction from a chemical and biological standpoint is wrong. What if the effect and addiction of choice was simply just a response to stress, boredom, suppressed emotions and environments that never really served us? Would it mean that rather than looking at the chemicals and behavioral addictions, we looked at what role the environment played. This is where the Rat Park experiment gets interesting.

In the 1970s Professor Bruce Alexander looked at this experiment and he noticed something interesting. He noticed that the rats were being put in an empty cage. The rats had nothing to do, except use drugs. Imagine living like a rat in a cage, isolated, disconnected, stressed and bored. I'm sure you would seek mind-altering substances to warp your reality too. Consider how caged animals in a zoo become depressed and the whales and dolphins in the sea parks who have been known to try and take their own lives.

Professor Bruce Alexander suggested something a bit different. He built a cage that he called "rat park," which is basically a heaven for rats: loads of space, cheese and activities. Rat park includes an array of tunnels, exercise wheels, and most importantly—loads of friends, and they can even have lots of sex. Now the kicker is that the rats were given drugged water for 57 days in a row and then released into rat park. In rat park they still have access to both the water bottles, the normal water and the drugged water. Considering the first experiment. What do you think happened next?

In rat park, something interesting happened. They didn't use the drugged water. None of the rats used it compulsively. None of them ever overdosed. They preferred to get on with life in rat park.

What this shows is that the rats went from almost a hundred percent strike-rate of overdosing when isolated and caged, to zero percent overdosing when they lived in a happy, connected and nourishing environment.

Coming out of the 2020–21 "pandemic" makes you consider whether isolation, disconnection and removing people from their activities was the right response for good health?

"Lack of support is one of the number one things my patients complain about. I've seen, firsthand, how social isolation can manifest into illness. Studies show that isolation can set off a cellular chain reaction that increases inflammation and suppresses the body's immune response to disease,"[3] said changemaker Radha Agrawal

In his TED talk, journalist Johann Hari asked: "What if addiction is an adaptation to your current environment?"[4] He shared that a professor called Peter Cohen in the Netherlands said that maybe we shouldn't even call it an addiction. Maybe we should call it bonding.[5]

Human being things have a natural and innate need to bond. And when we're happy and healthy we'll bond and connect. But it's harder to do that when you're traumatized or isolated or beaten down by life, often you will bond with something else, something that will inevitably give you a sense of relief. Now that might be painkillers, gambling or pornography. That might be cocaine or cannabis, but you will bond and connect with something because that's human nature. Perhaps we need to create nourishing environments and stop focusing on the vice itself so that people don't need to escape their current reality.

CALL TO COURAGE

Simply do your best. Good health is not about perfection. I'm not perfect either. There have been many moments in my life where I could have gone one of two ways. I think perfection is an illusion. A construct that we can never truly fulfill. Like any true blue Aussie, I enjoy a beer with friends and have pushed the boundaries of my own human experience as I navigated my 20s and 30s. However, I always found that connection with self and others, nourishing environments, fresh experiences, empowering mentors and a mom who gave me unconditional love enabled me to be here today, sharing this message with you.

The question is: would you be willing to step outside of your comfort zone and experience new places, new work environments, new friendships, new connections and discover what really enables you to tune into the harmony and flow of an abundant life?

When you disconnect from what you think you "should do" and tune into what makes you feel at ease, at peace, happy and connected, everything can change in an instant. As I mentioned before, all it takes is 10 seconds of courage to overcome any irrational fear and make a small pivot or a giant leap into a new experience. Would you lean into that courageous conversation? Would you buy a one way ticket to "that place" that keeps showing up in your mind and dreams? If you do, send us a message and let us know how you feel when you get there! We'd love to hear from you.

CALL TO COURAGE (C2C):

What are 3 FEARS that hold you back in life? E.g., fear of being judged, missing out, the unknown, being seen, sharks.

1. ....

2. ....

3. ....

What are 3 HABITS, patterns of behaviors or addictions that negatively impact your life and take you further away from who you truly are? E.g., smoking, people pleasing, saying yes or no too much, betraying yourself or your values?

1. ....

2. ....

3. ....

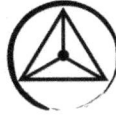

CHAPTER 3

IGNITE YOUR HUMAN POTENTIAL

"In oneself lies the whole world and if you know how to seek and learn,
the door is there and the key is in your hand. Nobody on earth can
give you either the key or the door to open, except yourself."
— *Jiddu Krishnamurti* —

In my attempts to regain my health and my life, I discovered that the foundation of healing was based on what I was feeding my body and how it was absorbed. I realized that my immediate environment was not serving me well. I quit my "dream job" and started living my dream life. I started moving more, surfing, and doing things I loved. I made time to invest into myself, and regained self-love and self-worth while rediscovering my life's purpose. Pretty heavy, I know. I was living to work and now I was working to live.

I surrounded myself with positive, open-minded, purpose-driven people. I changed my mind, my environment and my health. As a result, everything I started to do felt good. Really good. Who knew that it was all once choice away?

Real health began to invade my entire being and I couldn't believe the difference. It transformed me from inside and out.

Fast-forward to today. I am now in my early 30s, living in Bali, Indonesia and working as a health practitioner with an integrated tool belt. My mantra to my clients is: "If you don't get better under my guidance, you don't pay." I have always felt that if I was willing to receive someone's hard-earned money, then it's my duty to ensure they get better. This can mean treating them, or at times, referring them to other allied health professionals. Whatever option is best for them. Sometimes not treating them at all. Whatever is best for them.

Although it took some time to integrate everything I had learned, both intellectually and experientially. It all led to this. To build a community of people empowered in their own self-care, with a heart-spaced desire to help others along the way. This spark is the SelfCare revolution. To create curiosity and empowered learning in the 12 Medicines and to help others ignite their own human potential and optimize their own unique experiences free from restriction.

FOCUS ON WHAT YOU CAN CONTROL—WHICH IS MORE THAN YOU THINK

I remember when I watched that Buddhist monk fight for his life in the intensive care unit after being "king hit" on his morning run as someone stole his wallet. Each morning before I arrived at the hospital, close to 100 people lined the wards in unified support for someone who had impacted his community. The same day, I saw a lady addicted to heroin, suffer from multiple organ failure— return to life, despite the fact she had no desire to live. There was not one person waiting in the halls to be there for her.

It made me appreciate the allied health team who saw that both lives were equally valuable, even though they both lay there on life support with thousands of tax paying dollars being spent daily to ensure they were given every opportunity to live or pass on through the "angels gates."

After 30 days on life support, the Buddhist monk died. 100 people cried in despair. The lady with no desire to live, walked out of the hospital with no one waiting to pick her up.

It made me realize that life was unpredictable, in a constant state of change and that tomorrow was not granted for anyone.

Though we aren't guaranteed a long life and an aura of unpredictability is always present—there are many factors we can control. Many changes we can make. Just like Jiddu Krishnamurti said, "Enlightenment is an accident, but some activities make you accident-prone." Living for a long time may be unpredictable, but these SelfCare solutions make you prone to longevity and good health.

That's my job—to help you make choices that make you health prone. To help you control what you can (which is a lot!)

Over time, I realized that to heal we need to:
- heal ourselves with the support of amazing people
- heal the natural environments that we live in
- heal our communities and all whom live in it.

We need to encourage healers—not only the ones working in hospitals or health clinics, but the biodynamic farmers that are producing food without chemicals and collateral damage to the natural world, the person that stops and takes time out of their busy life to help someone in need whilst others watch or walk on by. Creating ripple effects through inspired action.

This is a book of choices, but it's also a book of connection. After working as a practitioner in the modern healthcare system for a decade and after being a patient and spending thousands of dollars trying to buy my health back, I came to see how many people were answering my three questions (Am I happy? Am I healthy? Am I connected?) with the same loud ringing NO that I once did.

This journey empowered me to step out of the current systems of healthcare and look at the bigger view of health and happiness. Over time, I curated the 12 Medicines that you will read in this book. These 12 Medicines stem from years of research (both modern science and ancient wisdom), observation, insights from leading mentors in their field, and personal experience. This SelfCare matrix and simple fillyourcup method is designed to help you move from burnout and emptiness to bubbling with an overflow of joy and good health as a "well-being."

CHOOSE YOUR OWN LIFE ADVENTURE

"What do we mean by saying that existence precedes essence?
We mean that humans first of all exist, we encounter ourselves,
surge up in the world—and define ourselves afterwards."
— Jean-Paul Sartre, Existentialism is a Humanism —

We can begin with a simple choice. Choose to change something. Anything. As has been said many times, the definition of insanity is doing the same thing over and over again and expecting a different result. If you keep on ending up with the same results, then choose to do something differently today. Even in this moment, right now.

Yes, it's that simple.

Choose to think different thoughts, choose to eat different foods, choose to move different, choose a different environment to be in, choose different people to spend your time with. If all else fails, cast a new positive future vision for yourself and the ideal life you would love to live. Then choose to get uncomfortable stepping into that dream with unapologetic action. Now, that boldness may even result in you selling everything you own and buying a one-way ticket to somewhere that captured your heart a long time ago. Or it may mean creating new experiences that surpass your old ways of living. It may be as simple as starting to walk every day.

Give yourself permission to choose different. This doesn't mean what "appears" to be the "right path." It's not about pleasing others, it's about following your own life's calling. Everyone's direction is unique.

Some sit in yoga pants, drinking a green smoothie, talking about how they just went vegan to save the planet. Some may sit at the pub, drinking a beer, smoking a cigarette and laughing with friends, secretly planning a way to create more financial freedom for their family.

Your way to create a better, happier and healthier life is uniquely yours. You may not know all the answers, but you don't need to. You just need to be willing to take one step in the right direction. As Lao Tzu so wisely said, "A journey of a thousand miles begins with a single step."

It's about choosing every step you take.

Steve Jobs left this message before he passed away.

"When you grow up you tend to get told the world is the way it is and your life is just to live your life inside the world. Try not to bash into the walls too much. Try to have a nice family, have fun, save a little money. That's a very limited life.

Life can be much broader once you discover one simple fact: Everything around you that you call life was made up by people that were no smarter than you and you can change it, you can influence it, you can build your own things that other people can use. Once you learn that, you'll never be the same again."[1]

Take the keys. Take ownership of it all. Ask for support and offer support to others along the way. We are all simply doing our best, within the context of our own upbringing and lives.

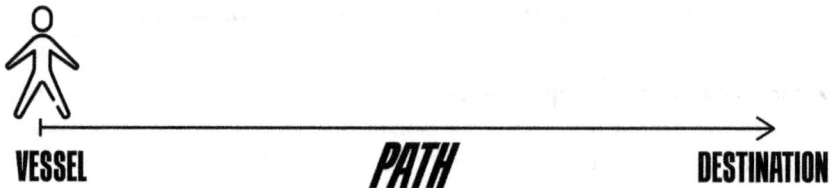

VESSEL   *PATH*   **DESTINATION**

WHO YOU ARE TOMORROW IS YOUR CHOICE

I'm going to tell you this one magical piece of information. Who you are tomorrow is your choice. Scientific studies into epigenetics show us that who you are and who you become is largely in your own hands and decided through your lifestyle choices.[2] What you eat, where you live, who you spend time with, the amount you sleep[3] or exercise.[4] All of these lifestyle factors ignite chemical reactions in our genes which "switch" those genes on or off over time. In cases such as cancer or Alzheimer's, various genes are switched away from the natural state of health.[5]

So, it does matter what you say yes to, and what you say no to. What you lean toward or what you lean away from. We are not a victim to our genes. We can determine how our evolutionary blueprint expresses itself.

We have however, created environments that are not allowing people to truly bloom and flourish.

19 out of 20 people are living in a restricted, dysfunctional or disease-ridden human body. Which means only 1 in 20 people are living in a state of good health and wellbeing, towards longevity.[6]

That's only 5 people out of 100.

"THE HEALTHY ONE"

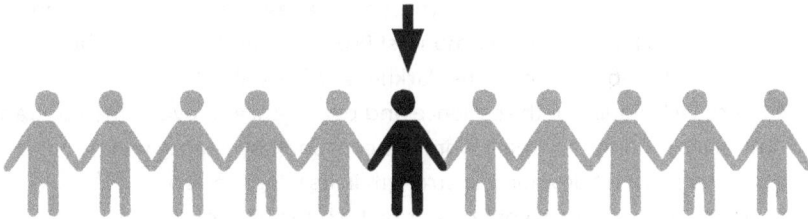

Perhaps it is time to pivot, even if only slightly. Course-correct towards a world that is sustainable, ecological, and a win for all, not just some.

After I healed myself all those years ago, I encountered so many people that needed help. I could see many of those "19 out of 20" people looking for a way to feel normal again. Dreaming of what it would be like to be unrestricted in their human potential. All deeply desiring to have a positive impact on the world but finding themselves stuck and desperately trying to fix their own internal and immediate world.

My drive shot up like a high-voltage surge. I wanted to find real and lasting solutions for everyone. I wanted to find a solution for my mom, who worked to the point of exhaustion. I wanted to find a solution for the mothers, nurturers, and carers who are so passionate about putting oxygen masks on everyone else that they forgot to put one on themselves. I wanted to find a solution for my dad and people that battled addictions and mental health issues. I wanted to help my friends who felt they were lacking in true wellbeing. I wanted to find a solution for the stranger I met in passing.

Now, I want to find a solution for you and the people you care about. So, I did.

It all begins with one moment of truth. Take time to ask yourself:

Am I happy?
Am I healthy?
Am I connected with myself and the world around me?

This is the entry-point to your own SelfCare Revolution.

It's time to take back your control.

You have greatness within you. In the essence of Wilma Rudolph, "Never underestimate the power of dreams and the influence of the human spirit. We are all the same in this notion. The potential for greatness lives within each of us."

Your greatness lays dormant until you ignite the spark in what you believe, how you think, and your embodied daily actions.

Greatness is like a bamboo shoot. It may take years to nurture and nourish, before it has an opportunity to break through the resistance of the soil and grow 10-foot tall and bullet-proof in just months! Proudly, standing tall for the world to see. No longer a bamboo shoot in the darkness of the soil.

Greatness will require both resilience and persistence to overcome resistance. Like a butterfly, no one can free it from the cocoon. If by chance you help it break free, the butterfly won't develop the strength in its wings to survive.

Life has its own wisdom. If you try to free the butterfly, you kill it. If you try force a seed to sprout, you destroy it. We all need to have the courage to break free from our own cocoon, our own darkness. We require resistance. Welcome it, so that you have the ability to stand tall like the bamboo shoot, or fly like the butterfly. Shining in the glorious way that nature intended all along.

CALL TO COURAGE

What is ONE point of resistance in your life right now? Is it health, money, love, connection, time, lifestyle?

....

I have learned that whatever I resist, persists.

What if rather than resisting it, you welcomed it as an opportunity to grow and transform? Keeping this in mind, what would you do differently next time?

....

....

....

....

....

....

....

"In the long run we shape our lives and we shape ourselves.
The process never ends until we die. And the choices
we make are ultimately our own responsibility."
— Eleanor Roosevelt —

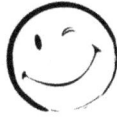

CHAPTER 4

ARE YOU HAPPY?

"Happiness is when what you think, what you say,
and what you do are in harmony."
— *Mahatma Gandhi* —

Those three questions were a sobering epiphany for me. A moment of truth. A long hard look at what happiness, health and connection truly meant for me rather than what it had been pushed and marketed as by society.

ARE YOU TRULY HAPPY?

John Lennon was attributed with this quote, "When I was 5 years old, my mother always told me that happiness was the key to life. When I went to school, they asked me what I wanted to be when I grew up. I wrote down 'happy.' They told me I didn't understand the assignment, and I told them they didn't understand life."

Although no one knows if he actually said it or not, it's a damn good quote. It sums up society's strange and somewhat excessive pursuit of status whilst devaluing the reason we pursue anything at all. Usually, most people just want to be happy.

Everyone wants to be happy, right? But what is happiness? What is *your* definition of happiness? Countless books have been written on this subject, but are we happier for it?

Positive psychology defines a happy person as someone who experiences frequent positive emotions such as joy, interest, and pride. And in doing so also experiences infrequent negative emotions, such as sadness, anxiety and anger.[1]

Pretty straightforward really. Happy people feel more good than bad, more often. Nevertheless, happiness is a subjective feeling and each person defines and measures happiness differently. What makes you happy may make another miserable. The best place to start defining happiness is by defining what it is for you and what it's not.

Many people believe that happiness is being wild at a party, or having a new thrilling experience, or being in the throes of passion and sex. Some prefer a more milder example and believe that happiness is dining out at an elegant restaurant or lying in bed for hours binging on Netflix. Now don't get me wrong, these are all amazing experiences that are meant to be enjoyed, but they're not actual happiness.

These experiences are the definition of pleasure. Sweet pleasure. But here's the problem with pleasure—it doesn't last. It happens in moments. And then these moments must continue to keep that experience feeling pleasurable. When we enjoy the pleasurable experiences all the time, our brains adapt and turn pleasure into routine. Now, there's nothing wrong with having a whole lot of pleasure...but when our brains get these pleasure "hits" continually, over time it takes even more "hits" to make us feel good again. Like a pleasure addict. It never quite reaches the level of true lasting happiness.

Have you ever seen extremely wealthy and comfortable people begin to complain all the time if their soup is too hot, or too cold, or the bowl is too big or small? They are so ingrained in pleasure, they try and ensure nothing interferes with their pleasurable moments. It's not happiness because pleasure never lasts. It relies on moments being filled with sweet unadulterated pleasure.

So this may lead you to think, okay then Rory—what does last?

BLISS, JOY AND MEANING

Have you ever experienced the beauty and joy of absolute bliss? The suspended moments in life where everything feels just right, perfect. When you're present and perfectly content with where you are right in that moment. It might be driving to an amazing location listening to your favorite song after a great day or week. It might be the way you feel in particular environments or surrounded by certain people. It might even be one of those moments where time stops as you step back, content, peaceful and grateful with everything surrounding you.

If you're blissful, you're happy and at peace. There is an inner peace distilled into the present moment. It's here that you can be happy for no particular reason, *just being*.

Can you think of a moment like this in your life?

You can never have too many blissful moments.

Many of us spend our whole lives seeking these moments of complete inner peace and true presence, combined with an overwhelming feeling of joy. Legendary psychologist Mihaly Csikszentmihalyi, and expert on flow and happiness describes the flow state as "a state in which people are so involved in an activity that nothing else seems to matter; the experience is so enjoyable that people will continue to do it even at great cost, for the sheer sake of doing it."[2]

WE NEED TO FEEL PAIN TO ENJOY HAPPINESS

Have you ever experienced a painful event in your life? Perhaps it was a traumatic life event or even something small that evoked a feeling of grief, shame, sadness and even prolonged emptiness? I want to normalize this emotion as part of the human experience.

Pain is not weakness leaving the body, nor is it something that needs to be numbed with mind-altering substances or avoided with busy work schedules. It is something that needs to be embraced, felt and learned from. I feel that this is an extremely important point considering that suicide is a leading cause of death for males under the age of 35, 1 and the burden of mental health issues are rising exponentially without a direct cause.

SAVE uses the most recent data available from the Centers for Disease Control and the World Health Organization. Here are some somber statistics they share:[3]

- Nearly 800,000 people die by suicide in the world each year, which is roughly one death every 40 seconds.
- Suicide is the second leading cause of death in the world for those aged 15–24 years.
- Depression is the leading cause of disability worldwide.

I wanted to share that, yes; chase happiness and seek experiences that evoke a feeling of bliss. But please learn to embrace pain, heal ancestral and past traumas. Learn from these experiences, make peace, let go, surrender and build resilience for the next step in your journey. Like me, you can even use this pain to find your purpose.

"The most beautiful people I've known are those who have known trials, have known struggles, have known loss, and have found their way out of the depths."
— **Elisabeth Kübler-Ross** —

SURVIVE FIRST, THEN THRIVE

Famed American psychologist Abraham Maslow was best known for creating a hierarchy of needs that outlines the human quest for happiness. He suggests that once our basic human needs for survival are met (when we're out of the stress-fight-or-flight mode) we then have the breathing space to be fully present and live at a more self-actualizing level.

He suggests that there are seven parts make up this hierarchy of human needs: air, water, food, shelter, safety, sleep and clothing (in some cases). Depending on the situation, the importance of these basic human needs may be lower or higher (except for air, water, and food which you obviously always need). He suggests that we have a natural human tendency to strive toward health, growth and excellence. However, we need to work together to ensure that each of our survival needs are met before we can thrive together. Take note on which of the 7 basic human needs are being met in your life.

ME MASTERY

4

SELF-FULFILLMENT NEEDS

SELF-ACTUALIZATION
Achieving one's full potential including creative activities

PSYCHOLOGICAL NEEDS

ESTEEM NEEDS
Prestige and feeling of accomplishment

BELONGINGNESS AND LOVE NEEDS
Intimate relationships, friends

BASIC NEEDS

SAFETY NEEDS
Security, safety

PHYSIOLOGICAL NEEDS
Food, water, warmth, rest

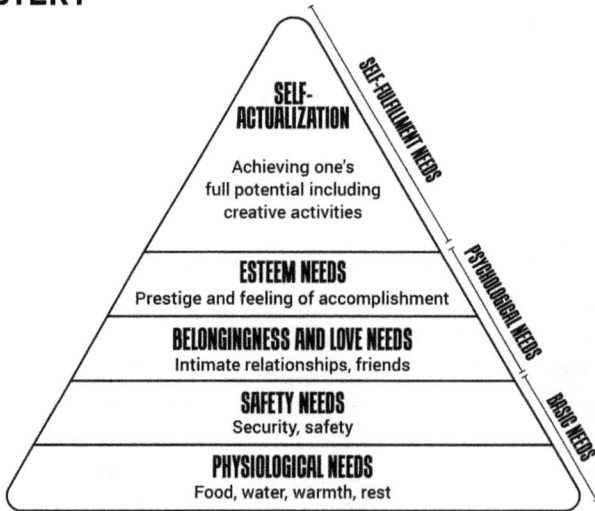

" Human life will never be understood unless its highest aspirations are taken into account. Growth, self-actualization, the striving toward health, the quest for identity and autonomy, the yearning for excellence (and other ways of phrasing the striving "upward") must by now be accepted beyond question as a widespread and must by now be accepted beyond question as widespread and perhaps universal human tendency..."

MARSLOW, 1954

HAPPINESS IN HARDSHIP

But can we find happiness in tragedy, darkness and chaos?

Imagine you were born into one of the most war torn countries in the world. In the 21st century, Syria, Iraq, Afghanistan, Mexico, Somalia, Nigeria, Sudan, South Sudan, Libya and Pakistan comprise the top 10 war torn countries in our modern society.

How would you meet your basic human needs for survival, let alone find happiness and moments of bliss when chaos is going on around you?

Famous psychologist and Holocaust survivor of WWII Viktor Frankl wrote in his bestselling book, *Man's Search for Meaning*—"When we are no longer able to change a situation, we are challenged to change ourselves."[5] He describes happiness and meaning as two very different things. He also says that finding personal meaning within his horrible experience of being a prisoner of war during the Nazi regime, gave him the will to live through it.

He suggests that in the absence of meaning, people fill their deeper void with hedonistic pleasures, power, materialism, hatred, boredom, or neurotic obsessions and compulsions. He says, "It is the very pursuit of happiness that thwarts happiness."[6]

Many modern day researchers agree with Frankl's views and some even caution against pursuing happiness as the "ultimate cure." In the *Journal of Positive Psychology*, researchers discovered that happiness and meaning did overlap but had very separate signatures.[7] They interviewed nearly 400 people over a month long study (aged 18 to 78) and asked whether they thought their lives were meaningful and/or happy. They found some interesting differences.

Satisfying one's needs and wants increased happiness but was largely irrelevant to meaningfulness. Happiness was largely present oriented, whereas meaningfulness involves integrating past, present, and future.

For example, thinking about future and past was associated with high meaningfulness but low happiness. Happiness was linked to being a taker rather than a giver, whereas meaningfulness went with being a giver rather than a taker.

Higher levels of worry, stress, and anxiety were linked to higher meaningfulness but lower happiness. Concerns with personal identity and expressing the self-contributed to meaning but not happiness.[8]

Interestingly, being a "taker" was linked with happiness whilst being a "giver" was linked with meaning. The authors state very boldly that "Happiness without meaning characterizes a relatively shallow, self-absorbed or even selfish life, in which things go well, needs and desire are easily satisfied, and difficult or taxing entanglements are avoided."[9]

Over millennia, many insightful souls from Mahatma Gandhi, John Lennon, Kenneth Benjamin and many others have explored the concept of happiness in an attempt to summarize the shared wisdom of this feeling we all know. We need to first acknowledge that it not a rational thought. Which means that science is limited in measuring this feeling in the context of our individuals lives. It also means that what evokes this feeling for you is unique, and may be different to me and others.

9 FACTORS FOR BLISS AND HAPPINESS

Here are 9 factors that influence how we feel on a daily basis and our ability to remain present enough to feel happiness.

1. Health and wellbeing—Feeling good inside is a great start
2. Connection—Having two people to confide in and a supportive community
3. Environment—Living in nourishing environments where you can meet your basic human needs, will remove stress in your life and create space to be happy.
4. Adaptability—We can find happiness in hardship. It's how you react to life's natural chaos and cycles. Do you dance in the rain or complain about it?
5. Optimism—It's not about being overly positive. Remember people who have felt pain, embrace it and choose to see the good in life. Stay curious and adventurous!
6. Purpose—Finding you purpose with the wisdom to make it meaningful
7. Engagement—Being an active part of a community or tribe is essential
8. Pleasure—Never feel guilty about beautiful experiences such as fun, sex, love, and eating delicious food. Explore what life has to offer!
9. Success—In whatever version you define it. Feedback from yourself and others that what you do has value, can help. This is less meaningful, but still important

These categories above include the range of human needs in a general way and naturally overlap. Just as meaning and happiness can overlap in real-life. These universal needs will inevitably make you fertile to attract epic episodes of bliss.

To keep attuned to these blissful experiences:
- Immerse yourself in environments with good people where moments are more common. Be mindful of where you're experiencing these moments,

who you're with and what you're doing when feelings of complete presence emerge within.

- Once you've caught onto how you can bring these moments into reality, don't stop tuning into them. Follow how you feel; forget the details.
- Happiness is a feeling, not a rational thought. Slow down, breath, be present and remind yourself what it feels like. It can be found at any second, even right now.
- Always remember that we are feeling beings that think. Feel more and avoid suppressing or distracting yourself from these normal human emotions.
- Pursue things that mean something to you. Cease to think that pleasure is happiness. A meaningful, happy life can be created!

SURVIVE TO THRIVE
Share 3 basic human needs that you still need to fulfill in your life!

1. ....

2. ....

3. ....

Meet your basic needs in order to create breathing space for life's abundance ☺

TAKE HAPPY ACTION TODAY
Share 3 things that make you happy!

1. ....

2. ....

3. ....

Do more of that ☺

EMBRACE PAIN AND LEARN FROM IT

Share three things that give your life meaning and promote blissful moments!

1. _____

2. _____

3. _____

Keep embracing the full human experience ☺

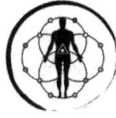

CHAPTER 5

ARE YOU HEALTHY?

"When health is absent, wisdom cannot reveal itself, art cannot manifest, strength cannot fight, wealth becomes useless, and intelligence cannot be applied."
— *Herophilus* —

HOW HEALTHY ARE YOU REALLY?

I just did a quick internet search for "health" and received a whopping 9,120,000,000 results. If you do a more refined search for the definition of health, the definition of health will be along the lines of, "the state of being free from illness or injury" or "free from disease."

But I believe that health is more than just the absence of disease and dysfunction.

Perhaps the smartest way to maintain good health is to preserve it through a nourishing, healthy lifestyle rather than waiting until the wheels fall off through degradation and illness. Measuring the absence of disease and dysfunction might just be the start but it's certainly not the answer to good health.

The World Health Organization (WHO) once claimed that health is "a state of complete physical, mental and social well-being, not merely the absence of disease or infirmity."[1] 40 years after their initial definition WHO further clarified health. They said: *"To reach a state of complete physical, mental and social well-being, an individual or group must be able to identify and to realize aspirations, to satisfy needs, and to change or cope with the environment. Health is, herefore, seen as a resource for everyday life, not the objective of living. Health is a positive concept emphasizing social and personal resources, as well as physical capacities. Therefore, health promotion is not just the responsibility of the health sector, but goes beyond healthy life-styles to well-being."[2]*

They have equally been praised and condemned for their holistic point of reference. But what makes us really healthy is a deep sense of physical, mental and emotional wellbeing.

The McKinley Health Center at the University of Illinois IL defines wellness as: *"A state of optimal well-being that is oriented toward maximizing an individual's potential. This is a life-long process of moving towards enhancing your physical, intellectual, emotional, social, spiritual, and environmental well-being."[3]*

Wellness includes an active participation in health, as an individual and within the lifestyle of each community. Maintaining wellness and optimal health is a lifelong, daily commitment to self-care rituals. This doesn't mean a quick fix, or a 28-day challenge. We're talking about a lifestyle here, a way of living and being.

Does this mean that we choose to live in a state of restriction, dysfunction or disease based on our daily rituals? Inevitably, it is our choice what we do each day, or what we don't do.

It seems so simple yet so many of us stay stuck in the same rituals we've had in place for years. If we stop and think about it for just one moment, does this mean we can choose our health and wellbeing by adopting different daily rituals and lifestyles?

What about science? For the science nerds like me, if you wanted to take it to a whole new level, then maybe this definition is more your style:

"A healthy adult is a complex biological system capable of highly elaborate functions such as the ability to move, communicate and sense the environment—all at the same time.
These functions are tightly regulated by genetic and epigenetic networks through multiple feedback loops that precisely coordinate the expression of thousands of genes at the right time, in the right place and in the right level [1].
Together, these networks maintain homeostasis and thus sustain 'life' of a biological system."[4]

Okay, that may have made some of you space out a little. I know not everyone is a health geek but align with whichever definition resonated most with you and LIVE your definition.

BUT HOW DO YOU KNOW IF YOU'RE TRULY HEALTHY?

When I ask people whether they feel like they are in a state of good health and wellbeing, every answer is very subjective. If people can do everything they enjoy doing without restriction, most will say that they are healthy. Even if all other vital signs and waistlines say otherwise. On the flipside a seemingly healthy person might say they are not in a good state of health and wellbeing if their knee is sore, which restricts them from partaking fully in activities that make up their life.

So how do we measure health and wellbeing? Is it possible?
Is it:
1. The length of life that matters?
2. The quality of the life lived?
3. The number of experiences outside of our comfort zone?
4. The vital signs (e.g., pulse rate, temperature, respiration rate, and blood pressure) that indicate the state of our essential body functions?
5. The years lived free of disease, dysfunction or restriction?
6. The legacy we live and leave for others?

There is a massive detachment in how we define our own health and wellbeing. In Australia, over 85% of the population subjectively reported themselves as being in a good state of health and wellbeing.[5] Yet only 5% are. Even in Australia, the land Down Under, where bronzed active, healthy Aussies live, the statistics show the gap between reporting good health and living good health.

The Dalai Lama, when asked what surprised him most about humanity, answered: "Man! Because he sacrifices his health in order to make money. Then he sacrifices money to recuperate his health. And then he is so anxious about the future that he does not enjoy the present; the result being that he does not live in the present or the future; he lives as if he is never going to die, and then dies having never really lived."

There is a massive disconnect between living in a state of good health and our subjective views on what being healthy is. We need a new normal. We need to raise our standards and change our rituals accordingly. We need to consciously create environments that empower these rituals with ease and flow.

Now, let's be honest, 95% of the world's population don't wake up each day and decide that they will make poor health choices. It happens as we complacently "agree" to our definition of health without questioning what is really means for us individually and collectively.

So how do we do this?

If we were to measure health on a bigger scale, like wellbeing and lifestyle, joy, happiness and connection, wouldn't this seem a healthier alternative? We need to take the scale of health and move it up for all of us!

4 ZONES OF HEALTH AND WELLBEING

Here's something you need to know. Think of 100 people you know or love.

- Less than 1 in every 100 people live beyond 100 years, let alone over 80 years!
- 4 in every 100 people (4%) are living in a state of good health and wellbeing towards longevity.
- 45 in every 100 people are living in the limbo arena of the "orange zone" bouncing between restriction, dysfunction, disease and good health and harmony. Living with 1 or more ailments or health challenges.
- 50 in every 100 (50%) people are living with one or more chronic or preventable diseases.

It's not pretty but it's pretty important. Imagine if we could flip these hard statistics. Where 1 in 2 people were living in good health and wellbeing towards longevity?

BLUE ZONE	LONGEVITY	1%	Less than 1% of people reach their 100th birthday, let alone live over the age of 80
GREEN ZONE	GOOD HEALTH & WELL BEING	4%	Less than 4% of people are living in good health, 1 in 20 people worldwide had no health problems from 2013-2020
ORANGE ZONE	MODERATE HEALTH	45%	45% (9 in 20) people are living with 1 or more than 1 health ailment, restricton or dysfunction
RED ZONE	SURVIVAL	50%	50% (1 in 2) are living with 1 or more chronic,preventable and lifestyle -related non-communicable diseases
	RESTRICTED	7 IN 10	Over one-third of the globla population has more than 5 ailments and 1 in every 2 people are living with a non-communicable and preventable disease
DEAD ZONE	DEAD	1 IN 148	Roughly 54 million people die each year. non-communicable diseases now make up 7 of the world's top 10 causes of death. The other 3 in 10 are due to communicable diseases,maternal deaths and injuries

6

EMBRACE DEATH TO FULLY LIVE

This may be an uncomfortable conversation, but it is one that is necessary to have. Many cultures embrace death as a part of life, whereas others are taught to fear it in the hope of finding "anti-aging elixirs," the "fountain of youth" and ways of resisting the inevitable. Change is necessary part of life and life is circular, not linear.

Consider how many minds have been referenced in this book, names that no longer live in their physical form. One could argue that they still live today. It has been said that you die twice, once when you take your last breath and secondly, the last time your name is said. I hope that by embracing death as a part of life, it will inspire people to truly live, taking advantage of 1,220,000 (~140 years) potential hours we all have access to, spending each breath and minute as if it were the most valuable gift in the world. The unfortunate truth is that many of us limit our human experience to ~613,000 hours (72 years) through the lifestyle we choose to live. What if we changed that? Perhaps the graveyard would no longer be the richest place on the planet; full of all the dreams ideas and innovations that never were.

The Tibetan Book of the Dead shares some insightful perspectives so that we can embrace death as a part of life. Padmasambhava says: "It is undeniably the case that in our society we do not easily accept that death is a natural part of life, which results in a perpetual sense of insecurity and fear" and asks "are you oblivious to the sufferings of birth, old age, sickness and death? There is no guarantee that you will survive, even past this very day!"[7]

If we can all understand death in the social, cultural and geographical context of the 21st century, we can enable and empower each other to make decisions today, that our future self will be proud of. We can learn to embrace death, so that we can be inspired to live fully in this present moment, knowing that tomorrow is not guaranteed for anyone.

When we look at life and death from a broader perspective the Dalai Lama shares that "dying is just like changing our clothes! When this body becomes old and useless, we die and take on a new body, which is fresh, healthy and full of energy! This need not be so bad!"[8]

Whatever perspective you have about life and death. It is important to consider that we have been given a gift. By understanding what impacts our rate of aging, degeneration and the factors restricting and shortening our length of life, we can create lifestyles and environments that allow us to best live.

THE DEAD ZONE (MORTALITY, 50+ MILLION)

To reverse engineer disease and dysfunction, it is important to understand how to live a life free of restriction so that we can live fully. It's not all bad news either. According to the World Bank, based on 2014 data for every 1,000 people in the world, an average of 7.748 people will die each year and 19.349 will be born.[9] That's a ratio of about 2.5 births for every death. There is more life than death!

In 2019, the top 10 causes of death accounted for 55% of the 55.4 million deaths worldwide.[10]

1. Cardiovascular (ischaemic heart disease, stroke)
2. Respiratory (chronic obstructive pulmonary disease, lower respiratory infections)
3. Neonatal conditions—(birth asphyxia and birth trauma, neonatal sepsis and infections, and preterm birth complications).[11]

If we understand how we die, perhaps we can build a more sustainable and regenerative ecosystem to support each individual over their lifespan. Some people see this population growth as a challenge for humanity. I see it as an opportunity to adapt and evolve the way we live in harmony with the natural world and its resources. As an example, we don't have a food shortage issue where 1 billion people need to go to bed hungry tonight, 40% is wasted by inefficient systems of distribution and degenerative agriculture. If we have regenerative systems and efficient distribution of resources. We can all survive and thrive together.

So, what is disease? I'm sure you can do a quick web search and see many gruesome photos of people living in a state of dis-ease. Like defining health, our medical dictionaries find it hard to clearly articulate a satisfactory definition of disease. For example, what's the difference between a cold, tuberculosis or chronic respiratory diseases and cancers? If good health is about living in harmony and homeostasis, then perhaps people living with a "disease" are simply living in a very large grayscale of disharmony. From temporary restrictions to longstanding dysfunctions and even states of disease. Where the longer you live out of harmony internally and externally with your choices, the increased likelihood that your internal cellular systems will adapt to think this "state" is the new normal. We see this in both chronic pain and chronic inflammatory states.

To understand when something becomes potentially chronic and longstanding, you must first understand that nearly everything in your body will heal within six months. This means that if something (a pain, a restriction, an injury) persists beyond six months, then your body will start to epigenetically change its cellular pathways to support this new state. Further to this, you will start to think differently and behave differently, which may even cause the disease state to persist and accelerate. It can become a slippery slope!

So how do we get out of it?

First, let's take stock on where we are as a global population. If we understand how we got here, then we can learn the lesson required to create local and global change so we can learn how to fully embrace living.

Senior Research Fellow Jackie Scully from the University of Basel Switzerland says that, "What counts as a disease also changes over historical time, partly as a result of increasing expectations of health, partly due to changes in diagnostic ability, but mostly for a mixture of social and economic reasons."[12]

Lower income countries have much higher rates of communicable and neonatal diseases, whereas wealthier countries rank very high in non-communicable diseases like cardiovascular disease, cancer, musculoskeletal disorders, mental disorders and substance abuse.

Experts break down the burden of disease into three main categories: 1. non-communicable diseases (NCDs); 2. communicable, maternal, neonatal and nutritional diseases, and 3. injuries. According to our World in Data reports, on global scale:

1. More than 60 percent of the burden of disease results from non-communicable diseases (lifestyle-related).
2. 28 percent result from communicable, maternal, neonatal and nutritional diseases
3. And just over 10 percent from injuries.[13]

Communicable diseases are the diseases that are caused by infectious agents and can be transmitted from an infected person to other people, animals, or other sources in the environment. HIV, hepatitis A, B and C, measles, salmonella, measles, and blood-borne illnesses. Most common forms of spread include fecal-oral, food, sexual intercourse, insect bites like malaria. People living in a low-income country are far more likely to die of a communicable disease than a noncommunicable disease. Despite the global decline, six of the top 10 causes of death in low-income countries are communicable diseases. Communicable diseases are strongly linked to geography of birth right, access to adequate healthcare and the health of the natural environments that children grow up in.

Non-communicable diseases such as stroke, heart disease, diabetes, chronic respiratory disease, and cancer account for over 70% of all deaths, of which nearly half are in people younger than 60 years.[14] They are diseases that are NOT transferred from an infected person to another via any means and are mostly caused by factors like improper lifestyle choices combined with social, cultural and environmental factors.

It should become clear why we are focusing on helping solve the 60–70% of affluent lifestyle related diseases in middle to high income countries, so that together we can free up the wasted resources to influence the 30% of birth-related and communicable diseases found in less developed parts of our planet.

However, note the key word is that most of these dis-ease states are "preventable," which means there is hope to move away from this zone with the right lifestyle changes and universal health strategies. Wouldn't it be amazing to see a world where every child has the possibility of good health and wellbeing irrespective of which country or postcode they were born into?

THE 50% – RED ZONE ("DIS-EASE AND DIS-ABILITY")

Do you find it interesting that non-communicable diseases now make up 7 of the world's top 10 causes of death? According to WHO's 2019 Global Health estimates non-communicable diseases (NCDs) kill 41 million of the 54 million people each year, equivalent to 71% of all deaths globally. Each year, 15 million people die from a NCD between the ages of 30 and 69 years and over 85% of these "premature" deaths occur in low- and middle-income countries.[15]

These are essentially diseases of choice and lifestyle. It would take a courageous person to admit that they chose this state of being without blame and victimization.

Would you be willing to make five small changes in your daily lifestyle choices in order to increase both the length and quality of your life, so that you could spend more quality time with the people that you love? If you did, you would cut your risk of developing a chronic preventable disease by 78%. You could reduce our risk of dying young by 52%.

Non-communicable diseases are lifestyle related diseases of affluence and choice (the 70%)

To move out of the red zone on a PERSONAL level you would need to;

1. Learn how to sustain a healthy weight through better daily lifestyle choices
2. Address inactivity and make movement a meaningful part of your life
3. Address poor food choices and learn how to nourish yourself
4. Avoid, stop, swap or quit smoking all together
5. Limit or at least moderate alcohol consumption

If we addressed these five factors, the ambitious target of Sustainable Development Goal (SDG), to reduce by a third of premature non-communicable disease (NCD) mortality by 2030 would become very achievable.

Communicable diseases are linked to birth right, not personal choices (the 20–30%)

When it comes to communicable and infectious diseases, the good news is that there has been a significant reduction in the global burden from communicable diseases in recent decades, falling from over 1.1 billion in 1990 to below 670,000 in 2016 (around a 40 percent reduction).[16]

To help more people move out of the red zone will require a team effort. To solve the remaining challenge for communicable disease we need to address these 5 factors:[17]

1. Prevention and early intervention
2. Community education
3. Promoting healthy immune systems
4. Reproductive and maternal health care
5. Creating enabling healthy environments for all children, addressing basic human needs, like clean water as a starting point!

It's important to note that non-communicable "lifestyle related" conditions account for nearly two-thirds of deaths worldwide but communicable diseases are also preventable! Which means that for most of us we can create change in our own lives.

What if to help the developing world and the 30% of maternal and communicable diseases, all we had to do was to be empowered in our own health and wellbeing in order to free up trillions of dollars to build the environments and infrastructure others need in order to thrive?

To help more global citizens move out of the red zone requires us to focus on the five factors I listed above. As an example, diarrhea kills 2,195 children every day—more than AIDS, malaria, and measles combined.[18] Diarrheal diseases account for 1 in 9 child deaths worldwide, making diarrhea the second leading cause of death among children under the age of 5.[19] The solution is simple, give every child access to clean water.

> *"I water you, you water me; We grow together."*
> *— Jay Shetty —*

It's up to you to choose your own standards and levels of healthy moderation. But this is a simple start to prolong the potential for life; start by minimizing or at least moderating self-harm.

Keeping this in mind, if you currently live with a cardiovascular disease, have had a stroke, heart attack, diabetes, cancer or have chronic respiratory disease, or if you currently fighting a communicable disease; then you are currently living in the red zone. The good news, is that you don't have to stay here. Remember that 80% of non-communicable diseases are lifestyle related and are preventable. Even type 2 diabetes is reversible. Also, communicable diseases like HIV are no longer a death sentence with the right lifestyle changes. Our human vessel is capable of health and harmony. If every child had access to healthcare and clean water then we would take a giant leap in our human history. The choice is yours on a personal level and ours on a community level, as to whether we stay here, or move out of the red zone together.

MOVING FROM RED ZONE TO ORANGE ZONE

- Move out of red zone by addressing lifestyle and environmental factors keeping you there.
- Move to the orange zone by addressing factors reducing your length and quality of life.
- On a personal level; minimize self-harm. Stop, swap, quit and make major lifestyle changes toward the orange and greens zone. Find a mentor and a community to support you!
- On a community level: people in orange, green and blue zones can create enabling environments to support each other on an individual level. And on a global level we can share resources to ensure that each child access to healthcare, education, clean water and a healthy environment to grow in.

Like Dr Mark Hyman shares: "The power of community to create health is far greater than any physician, clinic, or hospital. You need to build yourself a support system to succeed long term. And while this may sound easy to some, many of my patients and community members have said that they don't have a community that is encouraging them to achieve their health goals."[20]

THE 45% – ORANGE ZONE (DYS-FUNCTION, RESTRICTION)

In the red zone, a focus on mortality (what kills us) does not take into account that the burden of disease not only kills people but also causes deep suffering to people who live with them. People are living longer on average, but they are doing so with more disability and restriction.

"Notions of health are highly context-dependent, as human diseases only exist in relation to people, and people live in varied cultural contexts. Studies in medical anthropology and sociology have shown that whether people believe themselves to be ill varies with class, gender, ethnic group and less obvious factors such as proximity to support from family members,"[21] says researcher of Biosciences Jackie Scully.

Most people in the orange zone think they are living in a state of good health and wellbeing. Even if their waist line, energy and biomedical measures say otherwise. They often accept that it is normal to be overweight, have mildly high blood pressure, be tired, live depleted of nutrients and live a sedentary lifestyles. Mostly, because they have never really felt what good health feels like. As an example of my own story, I only grasped the deep value of my health once I lost it and got it back.

To measure the impact of living in the orange zone we will use DALYS and YLD.

DALYs = Disability Adjusted Life Years

YLDs = Years Lived with Disability

The World Health Organization defines them as, "The sum of years of potential life lost due to premature mortality and the years of productive life lost due to disability."[22]

DALYs are a standardized metric that allows us to measure the loss of health and burdens of disease across countries and over time. One DALY is considered equal to losing one year of good health through premature death, disease or disability. In contrast, YLD (Years Lived with Disability) measures the time spent in less than optimal health.

One DALY represents one lost year of healthy life.

One YLD represents one year living with disease, disability of restriction.

In the past 23 years, the leading causes of health loss have hardly changed. These 5 factors resulted in the largest overall health loss worldwide and are measured in terms of YLD (Years Lived with Disability).

"95 percent of the world's population has health problems—
with over a third having more than 5 ailments!"
— THE LANCET[23] —

1. Lower back pain
2. Depression
3. Iron-deficiency anemia
4. Neck pain
5. Age-related hearing loss[24]

The challenge is that lower back pain and neck pain are more than just physical issues. Leading experts like Max Zusman, Professor Peter O'Sullivan, David Butler and Lorimer Mosely share that pain is an output of the brain, influenced by cognitive (thoughts), behavioral (actions), environmental (financial stress etc.) and metabolic factors (chronic inflammation etc.). In the same way you can't tell a depressed person to "just be happy and think better thoughts." We need to treat each person in the context of their environment and their life. What works for one person, may not work for another. This is the challenge of moving out of the orange zone. Finding what works for you in the context of your unique life and circumstance.

To understand what keeps you out of the green zone. Know that the chronic disease burden in developed countries largely results from a short list of 10 risk factors. If you can address these, you can move out of this zone.

1. Tobacco use and poor air quality (respiratory challenges)
2. Poor nutrition intake, less natural food, more "frankenfoods" (digestive and metabolic challenges)
3. Physical inactivity and sedentary lifestyles (strongly associated with obesity and mental health)
4. Excessive alcohol consumption (kidney and metabolic challenges)
5. Uncontrolled high blood pressure (cardiovascular challenges like strokes)
6. Hyperglycemia (blocked arteries and cardiovascular challenges)
7. Blood glucose levels (metabolic challenges like Type II diabetes)
8. Chronic stress (endocrine system)
9. Isolation and disconnection and substance abuse (unknown mental health burden)
10. Degradation and pollution of natural life support systems leading to accumulation of "chemical toxins" inside us.

In terms of attributable deaths, the leading metabolic risk factor globally is elevated blood pressure (to which 19% of global deaths are attributed), followed by overweight and obesity and raised blood glucose.[25]

All of these of these factors can be effectively addressed. A good start would be to see your local allied and functional medicine professional to get a baseline measure for these factors. Then make a plan to improve these "signals and symptoms" over the next 12 months with corrective lifestyle changes.

MOVING FROM ORANGE ZONE TO GREEN ZONE

Stay out of the orange zone by addressing daily lifestyle choices, seeking community support and changing environmental factors that kept you there.

Learn about the green zone and adjust your lifestyle habits to start moving towards the green zone over the next 12 months.

Find a mentor and a like-minded community to help you go somewhere you have never been before. Proximity has the power to break old thought patterns, habits and behaviors.

HEALTH AND WELLBEING DASHBOARD

Imagine you had some wearable technology that gave you feedback on the current status of your human body. Like the dashboard in a car. If your blood pressure goes up, it starts to flash orange or yellow. If your weight starts creeping up with a busy and stressful lifestyle, it flashes yellow or red. If you are dehydrated or lacking sleep, it lets you know. Biofeedback can be ignored, or you can make a decision to change something.

High risk metabolic risk factors contribute to four key metabolic changes:
1. Raised blood pressure
    » A normal blood pressure level is less than 120/80 mmHg
2. Overweight/obesity
    » Body composition is a better measure than BMI. DXA is gold standard.[26]
3. Hyperglycemia (high blood glucose levels). Generally it doesn't cause symptoms until glucose values are significantly elevated.
    » Usually above 180 to 200 milligrams per deciliter (mg/dL), or 10 to 11.1 millimoles per liter (mmol/L).[27]
4. Hyperlipidemia (high levels of fat in the blood).
    » HDL: Men: more than 40 mg/dl Women: more than 50 mg/dl
    » LDL: Otherwise healthy people: less than 100 mg/dl. People with heart disease or diabetes or poorly controlled risk factors: less than 70 mg/dl.[28]

High risk, but modifiable behavioral risk factors (things you can change):
Modifiable behaviors, such as tobacco use, physical inactivity, unhealthy diet and the harmful use of alcohol, all increase the risk of NCDs. The World Health Organization reveals the following:
1. Tobacco accounts for over 7.2 million deaths every year (including from the effects of exposure to second-hand smoke), and is projected to increase markedly over the coming years.
2. 24.1 million annual deaths have been attributed to excess fake food consumption, synthetic sugar and refined salt/sodium intake.
3. More than half of the 3.3 million annual deaths attributable to alcohol use are from NCDs, including cancer.
4. 1.6 million deaths annually can be attributed to insufficient physical activity.[29]

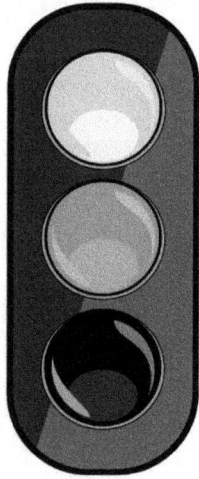

LOW RISK

GOOD WORK! Metabolic and lifestyle behaviours are in good standing. Keep going.

MODERATE RISK

BE MINDFUL! Metabolic signals are in disharmony. Make some lifestyle changes.

HIGH RISK

WARNING! If you don't change your lifestyle habits soon you may develop a "dis-ease". Up to you!

THE 4% – GREEN ZONE (GOOD HEALTH AND HARMONY)

Asking people, "How is your health?" may be a simple question, but the answers seem to be a good predictor of people's future health care use. According to the OECD Better Life Index about 69% of the adult population say their health is "good" or "very good."[30] They reveal that in Canada and New Zealand, 88% of adults report being in good health; while in Japan and Korea less than 40% of people rate their health as "good" or "very good."[31]

According to a major new analysis from the Global Burden of Disease Study (GBD) 2013, published in *The Lancet*.

- Just 1 in 20 people worldwide (4·3%) had no health problems in 2013.
- A third of the world's population (2·3 billion individuals) experience more than five ailments, which means that over 95% of the world's population has one or more health challenges.[32]

So where is the disconnect? Have we accepted "good health" as a state of living with one or more ailments? Especially when the research shows the proportion of lost years of healthy life (disability-adjusted life years; DALYS) are due to these ailments and illnesses, and death from these ailments rose by 21 percent.[33] That's 3 in every 10 people accepting that it is normal to have both their length and quality of life restricted.

WE NEED TO AGREE ON A NEW DEFINITION OF "GOOD HEALTH"

We can agree on what good health isn't. Like the World Health Organization's says we can all agree "that 'good health' is not merely the absence of disease or infirmity." However it is a good start to live free of restriction and health ailments.

What if good health was simply living in a state of complete physical, mental, emotional and social well-being, supported by healthy natural environments and enabling social environments that empower each individual to make better daily lifestyle choices? What is good health meant complete harmony within our bodies integrated systems, combined with harmony and nourishment from our external environments.

Create your own standards. How would you define living in good health in your own words? Create your own definition.

....

....

....

....

....

....

....

....

....

....

MOVING FROM THE GREEN ZONE TO THE BLUE ZONE

- Stay out of red zone by addressing lifestyle and environmental factor keeping you there.
- Stay out of orange zone by addressing factors reducing your length and quality of life.
- Learn to stay in the green zone by mastering the 12 Medicines of SelfCare shared in the next sections.
- Learn and model the behaviors and lifestyles of centurions and longevity hotpots. It may require changing your environment and community, or

applying their principles to the community and environment that you live in.

- Remember the story of the flower that didn't bloom in the way that nature intended.

THE 1% – BLUE ZONE (LIVING TO LONGEVITY)

Have you ever considered living beyond your 80th birthday? Or even celebrating 100 revolutions around the sun? Well, it is available to more people than you would think. Life expectancies have been on a rise in the past century according to Statista.[34]

The elusive dream of living beyond 80–100 years begins by managing your lifestyle habits and behaviors today. A thought, that seems too hard for many of us to deal with right now. Especially considering that many of us are still learning how to survive, let alone thrive, without disability, disease or dysfunction.

According to the World Bank less than 3% of the global population lives beyond 80 years of age.

- 2.298% of women in 2019 and beyond are living beyond the age 80
- 1.419% of men in 2019 and beyond are living beyond the age of 80 [35]

However, the United Nations expect the number of centenarians to rise to approximately 573,000 worldwide. With a global population of 7,794,798,739 in 2021. Which is just 0.0073% of the global population reaching their 100th birthday! You may find this contradictory considering their increasing burden of disease. But, according to World Atlas the U.S. has the highest number of centenarians in the world, with 97,000 living in the country. Followed closely by Japan (79,000) and China (48,921).[36]

ON A NATIONAL LEVEL

- Japan have the highest rate of centenarians: 6 for every 10,000 people or approximately 0.06 percent.
- The U.S have approximately 1 person in every 6,000 reach their 100th birthday. Which is 0.0167% of their total population.
- France, Spain and Italy, average around 0.03 percent of centenarians—the highest in Europe.
- Uruguay, Hong Kong and Puerto Rico share some of the highest levels of centenarians with rates between 0.06 and 0.045 percent.[37]

ON A COMMUNITY LEVEL

Communities from every geographical context have become famous due to the high number of centenarians within their community borders. Here are 10 communities that have found the fountain of youth and longevity. We will discuss their not so secret-secrets in coming chapters. Here are 10 longevity communities to be aware of:

1. The Chinese village of Bama
2. Okinawa in Japan
3. The Vilcabamba valley in Ecuador
4. Icaria of Greece
5. The Hunza valley in Pakistan
6. Seventh Day Adventists in Loma Linda, California
7. Abkhazia in the Caucasus mountains
8. Costa Rica's isolated Nicoyan Peninsula
9. Modern-day cities like Hong Kong
10. The island of Maui in Hawaii

LIVING IN THE BLUE ZONE TOWARDS LONGEVITY

1. Master staying out of the red zone (self-harm)
2. Master staying out of the orange zone (healthy moderation)
3. Master the green zone (good health and harmony)
4. Find environments, communities and lifestyles that enable you to live towards longevity.

Note that many of the Blue Zone communities are islands, peninsulas and valleys. There is a strong correlation between the health of the natural environment and your longevity. Combine this with a community that supports you over your lifespan and you might just be 90% of the way there.

To live towards longevity remember these 5 core principles:

1. Nature is our primary life support system. Consider how your health would improve simply by moving from a polluted fish bowl to an abundant natural environment with easy access to clean air, water, sunshine and uncompromising food sources.
2. When a flower doesn't bloom, you don't need to fix the flower. Find an environment that helps it thrive in the way that nature intended.
3. Environment is more important than willpower. Imagine moving to a longevity hotspot and community. Do you feel that it would be easier to maintain good lifestyle habits?
4. Proximity is power. Having an empowering community and close social relationships that support you over the lifespan is the longevity elixir.

5. The last one is you. Most of us start here. Remember that 80–95% of who you are, who you become and your lifestyle choices are within your hands. Choose and act wisely!

IT'S OKAY TO PING-PONG BETWEEN ZONES

In all honesty and transparency, I have bounced like a ping-pong ball between the red/orange and green zone. Learning, unlearning and redefining my standards and daily rituals. And all of that is okay.

Health and wellbeing is a lifelong process, and with that comes trial and error. An imperfectly perfect process of maintaining ourselves so that we can optimize our human experience and activate even a small piece of our human potential.

YOU NEED TO MEASURE WHAT MATTERS

What matters most to you? How you live or how long you live for?

A successful 52-year-old Western businessman went to his allied health doctor who practiced both western and eastern medicine. He was concerned that he was getting older and was wondering how long he would live for.

The businessman asked the doctor if he would live beyond the age of 80. The doctor noticed from observation and in his file that the man was not overweight and never had been. He had a good body composition with excellent muscle tone and low body fat. Which suggested that he was active on a regular basis and consumed food from good sources.

His fasting blood sugars were in normal limits, his blood pressure was within normal limits (120/80). He had no previous major injuries or ailments. His physical body was unrestricted and his energy and mental clarity was great. He had visited the previous doctor regularly each year for cancer screening and other preventative checks.

The doctor looked up from his file and smiled.

"First of all let's look at your lifestyle choices," he said. "Do you smoke or regularly inhale any chemicals?"

"No," he replied.

"Do you drink or consume any beverages that may do harm?"

"Occasionally I have a beer or red wine."

"Do you take any synthetic drugs, both prescribed and recreational?"

"Not really" he replied. "Occasionally I use aspirin If I have a headache."

"Do you work too much or have a highly stressful lifestyle?"

"No, I have a simple life and live within my means."

"Do you have trouble sleeping?"

"No, I am well rested every night. At least 8 hours."

"Do you ever eat any processed, rich or naughty foods?"

"Not really, I am vegan and occasionally eat some raw chocolate."

"Do you find yourself sitting down all day, lacking variable movement in your day?"

"No, each morning I go for a bike ride and make sure I am not sitting for more than 50% of my day."

"Do you find yourself having a lot of negative, low vibration or dark thoughts each day?"

"No, I rarely, if ever find myself in those states of mind."

"Do you sleep with many promiscuous women?"

"No, I am happily married for 20 years with 2 children."

"Do you partake in adventurous or risk taking sports like snowboarding, surfing, skydiving?"

"No, I have never tried."

"Okay, well here is my prediction" said the doctor. "Providing that nothing unexpected happens. The good news is that YES you will live to over 80 years and beyond with these lifestyle habits."

The doctor laughed with a cheeky smirk and said "the bad news is, what's the point of living if you never get to experience all that life has to offer?"

WHAT DOES LIVING MEAN TO YOU?

If you are healthy in that you appear to be unrestricted in your physical, mental and emotional body, that's great and ideal, but more importantly...

Are you happy?

Are you connected to yourself and living your ultimate truth?

Are you connected to your family and the people you care about most?

Are you connected to the natural world around you and stars above?

Are you living your ideal day every day? Or are you limiting your potential?

Is it length or the quality of life that matters?

Is it being like the oldest female on record, French born, Jeanne Louise Calment who lived to 122 years and 164 days. Or the oldest person living female Kane Tanaka (Japan, b. 2 January 1903) aged 117 years and 41 days, from Fukuoka, Japan, (as verified on 12 February 2020).[38] Or the oldest living male, Robert Weighton (UK, b. 29 March 1908), who is 112 years and 1 day old, (as verified in Alton, Hampshire, UK, on 30 March 2020.)[39]

Or is it Martin Luther King Jnr who lived to 39 years, or Amy Winehouse, Kurt Cobain or even Jim Morrison who didn't make it much beyond their 27th birthdays?

WHAT MEASURING STICK MATTERS?

Is it the quality of the life lived, even if short, but full of experience? Is it the length of life lived, even if it was short on experiences outside our comfort zone? Is it based on who had a bigger impact? Or is it based on whose names still live on today? Or it is just based on the opportunity to live and find happiness?

Perhaps dying with no regrets is a measuring stick we can all relate too?

Perhaps the unique nature of living our own life, embracing all our choices in their imperfect perfection is what we most need to own and love. As long as it doesn't negatively influence the people or world around us.

Perhaps Bob Marley sums it up best when he said "Who are you to judge the life I live? I know I'm not perfect—and I don't live to be—but before you start pointing fingers...make sure your hands are clean!"

CALL TO COURAGE

How do you define good health? What is normal for you? Describe in your own words.

....

....

....

....

What matters most to you? To live fast and die young or to live to longevity? Or to live a life full of experience?

....

....

....

....

What type of old person do you want to be?

....

....

....

....

SELF ASSESS – 4 ZONES SELF ASSESSMENT

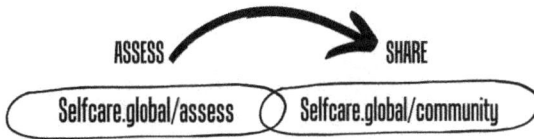

ASSESS → SHARE

Selfcare.global/assess ◯ Selfcare.global/community

Which zone are you living in today?

....

4 ZONES	100 PEOPLE
BLUE ZONE	50
GREEN ZONE	45
ORANGE ZONE	4
RED ZONE	1

FUTURE 2030+

Which zone are you moving to next?

....

What are 3 health ailments, challenges, restrictions or lifestyle related diseases that you would like to solve or at least manage? (lower blood pressure, improve cholesterol, low back or neck pain, type II diabetes etc.)

....

....

....

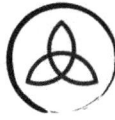

CHAPTER 6

ARE YOU CONNECTED?

"United we stand, divided we fall."
— Aesop —

CONNECTION & UNITY

The sequoia redwood trees in California are among the tallest trees in the world, they are also among the oldest. They can grow beyond 300 feet and some are as ancient as 2000 years old. Despite their soaring heights and weight, they endure gale force winds, earthquakes, fires, floods and storms. Most people assume they are so strong because of their deep rooted system. But this is not the case. In fact, their roots are rather shallow and only delve into the earth around six feet, they also only extend about one hundred feet from their trunk.

So, what makes these colossal giants so strong? The answer is each other. They reach their roots out for each other underneath the dirt and intertwine together. They depend on each other for support and nutrients and literally hold each other up against any impending storms.

They are among the oldest and tallest organisms on earth because of their ability to thrive together. I believe humans are the same.

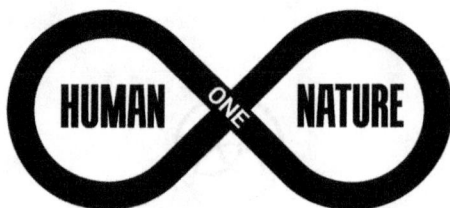

Connection matters. Connection helps us thrive.

4 WAYS TO CONNECT FROM THE INSIDE OUT

Is it a connection with self, a human connection, a social connection, a connection to the natural world around you, or a connection to the universe and the stars above?

Most definitions of connection will refer to it as being "a relationship in which a person, thing, or idea is linked or associated with something else." However, I feel this might be missing something. We need to find unity in our diversity, connected as one with ourselves, each other and the natural world around us.

Perhaps "interconnectedness" is a better term? The state of being connected to all things in the universe.

1. INTERCONNECTEDNESS

The concept of interconnectedness is powerful. If we are truly "one" and all things are interconnected, then this one thought has the power to break down the greatest illusion in this world: the illusion of separation. If you take a look at simple 101 biology or the basics of quantum physics, we have never been separate. It's only our mind and collective consciousness that has perpetuated this illusion for centuries. Let's change that in this generation and be reminded of what the ancients inherently knew in their wisdom.

2. UNIVERSAL CONNECTION

Look up at the stars, then focus back to yourself. You are connected to the stars. Let's look at our basic elemental composition as humans for a second. You might already know this, or heard it in passing somewhere—*humans and the universal stardust share 95% of the same elemental composition.*[1]

We also share the same composition as Earth. So when you hear people throwing around the concept that we are made from stardust or you are born of this earth, they are simply referring to the fact that the stars and you are made from the same elemental building blocks, just in a different configuration. In the same way no two stars are the same, no two humans are the same either.

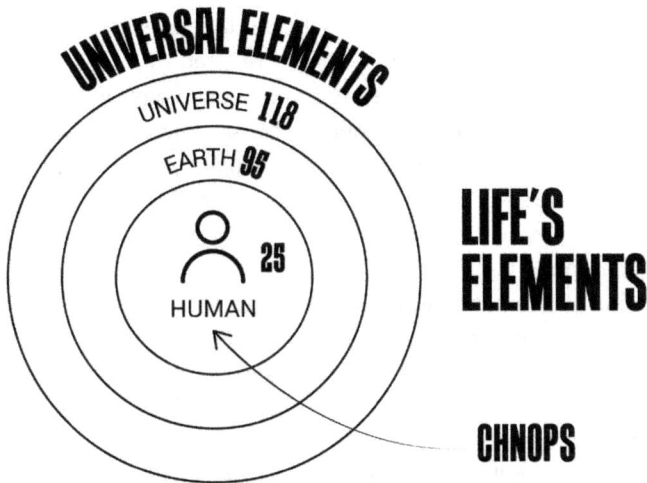

UNIVERSAL ELEMENTS

UNIVERSE *118*

EARTH *95*

25

HUMAN

LIFE'S ELEMENTS

CHNOPS

3. EARTHLY CONNECTION

To understand this through a different lens, let's focus on the famous astronaut Piers Sellar's perspective of Earth from space. While he was sitting in the international space station, looking down at the earth and watching the great Amazon river pass between his feet, he noticed one peculiar thing: there were no visible borders between countries like there are in our geography textbooks in school. In this moment he realized that the concept of separation and borders was simply a mental construct created by humans. It suggested to him that the human mind creates separation in a universe that is intricately interconnected.

Piers started to wonder who owned these countries with borders. This illusion of separation must then be closely followed by the illusion of ownership.

Honestly, who owns the earth? Who actually owns the land we live on? Who owns these countries or the resources that are readily available? Does the United States of America own the moon because they were the first to put a flag on it?

An ancient Indian Proverb speaks of overcoming the illusion of ownership.

"Treat the earth well: it was not given to you by your parents, it was loaned to you by your children. We do not inherit the earth from our Ancestors, we borrow it from our Children."

At the end of the day the oldest living human culture sums it up quite well.

> *"We are all visitors to this time, this place. We are just*
> *passing through. Our purpose here is to observe, to*
> *learn, to grow, to love...and then we return home."*
> — **Australian Aboriginal proverb** —

To reinforce this further, let's look at ancient Buddhist philosophy.

Buddhism is based on the universal view that everything is interconnected. When Buddha became enlightened, he realized this deep united oneness as the true nature of all beings. He didn't just know it intellectually, is was self-realized to be evident. He could see that everything and everyone was one intrinsic Source. Therefore, dualism didn't exist at the highest level, but attempting to sever our innate inter connectivity was the cause of much suffering and even death. Buddha's philosophy was based on *all as nature* and nothing separate.

To appeal to the rational scientific minds, let's turn to Dr. David Bohm, a renown quantum physicist who co-discovered that "everything interpenetrates everything." He noticed that while our human nature may seek to categorize and subdivide, the deeper level of reality is that all things in the universe are infinitely interconnected and all of nature is ultimately a seamless web. He concluded that "Ultimately, the entire universe...has to be understood as a single undivided whole."[2]

More recent philosophies have been established to explore our interconnectedness with the world we inhabit. Gaia is the name of the ancient Greek goddess of the Earth, and this name was recently used to refer to the hypothesis formed by James Lovelock and Lynn Margulis. Lovelock and Margulis suggest that the whole biosphere may be alive in that Earth's life forms are themselves responsible for regulating the conditions that make life on the planet possible.[3]

This basically means that humans are a living microbiome, as part of a bigger living earth biome. As humans we can influence the health of the earth in the same way that bacteria in and on our body can influence the health of our human system.

4. HUMAN LEVEL CONNECTION

If we now bring this down to a human-centric or a personal level, all you need to do is simply look around you. Our genetics break down the illusion of separation between us and other living beings by showing that you and I and any other human on this planet share 99.5% of the same genetic makeup, which means that the 0.5% that separates us by size, height, gender, and race is very minor. We also share much of the same DNA and elemental composition with all other living beings.

All in all, from quantum science to ancient philosophies, everything points towards collapsing boundaries between yourself, others, the world we inhabit and the universe we are part of. Now it is fundamental that our communication becomes embodiment and communion.

We need to treat others as we ourselves would like to be treated—where empathy, intimacy and harmony exist. It is through this illusion of separation—this assumption that boundaries are absolute—that we create disharmony in ourselves, in our relationships, and ultimately our lives. The notion that we can be separate from others or the world creates conflict, so let's simply let go of this thought and replace it with interconnectedness.

So from this moment onwards, please understand that when we talk about connection in this book, it is a connection between humans and nature, and the energetic universal or spiritual source. On a human level it is an internal connection with "self" and a connection with others. How we connect with ourselves, others, nature and the universal source of all energy is totally individual. So is what we name it. Some call this connection "God," some call it "Gaia" some call it nothing at all. Either way let's all agree that we are all speaking about the same universal "source" and energy.

I hope one day we can all look down at the earth from space like Piers Sellars, seeing the Amazon River travel between your feet, seeing no borders, and no separation; just humans and this biome which is Earth.

Everything is connected to everything. We truly are one interconnected seamless web. Unified.

It all starts by going first.

CALL TO COURAGE

"Trust your intuition and be guided by love."
— **Charles Eisenstein** —

Use your energy to serve from overflow, become a global citizen and have an impact. Not all heroes wear capes and most of us are just regular people who simply want to help solve challenges for our local community. Some may even want to help solve major global challenges. A mantra we can all share is "Act and Sustain Local," so that together, we can help solve global problems. If we all did just that, the ripple effects of change would surge like a wave around the globe. Show empathy, love and compassion when you can. Make relationships a big part of your life. Don't neglect your family and friends.

1. Personally: How can you prioritize connection with yourself in your 168 hour week?
2. Locally: What are your neighbors names?
3. Naturally: How do you connect with Earth's life support system each day?

4. Universally: How often do you look up and star gaze and ask curious questions?

5. Interconnectedness: How do you treat other people, animals and plants?

Always remember that connection is an inside-out approach, not just an outside-in approach.

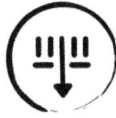

CHAPTER 7

A PERSONALIZED APPROACH

"A true teacher would never tell you what to do.
But he would give you the knowledge with which
you could decide what would be best for you to do."
— Christopher Pike —

In order to be live in a healthy environment where everyone can grow, we must be empowered and inspired to think different, remain open to new beliefs and welcome new ways of living and being. Every problem that we individually face or collectively face as humankind can be solved. "There is no food shortage," says Buckminster Fuller. "There is no energy crisis. There is a crisis of ignorance."

SelfCare is about taking ownership for the 95% of lifestyle choices within your control.

In order to take care of ourselves, it's important to know ourselves. The Ancient Greek aphorism "know thyself" are two powerful words of timeless wisdom. Although I believe wholeheartedly that we are more than a body and mind, it's still important and valid to understand what our human vessel is made of and how we can "feel it, know it and embody it" to then care for it. It's important to know how your body is built in order to optimize its functionality.

Learn to care for yourself so that others may never have to. It's the most selfless thing you can do!

HOW TO BUILD A HUMAN

Have you ever wondered what your body is made from?

Ask a group of scientists and you may get many different answers. We are complex creatures with exceptionally intelligent human bodies and minds.

Elisabeth Ratcliffe, of the Royal Society of Chemistry says the human body is made up of a "long list of ingredients" commonly referred to as CHNOPS.

"CHNOPS are considered the building blocks for life. Carbon, Hydrogen, Nitrogen, Oxygen, Phosphorus and Sulfur are the 6 key elements for life in the universe, from the stars in the sky to every cell in your body. In the human body the most abundant being oxygen (65% by mass), carbon (18%), hydrogen (10%), nitrogen (3%), calcium (1.4%) and phosphorous (1.1%)."[1]

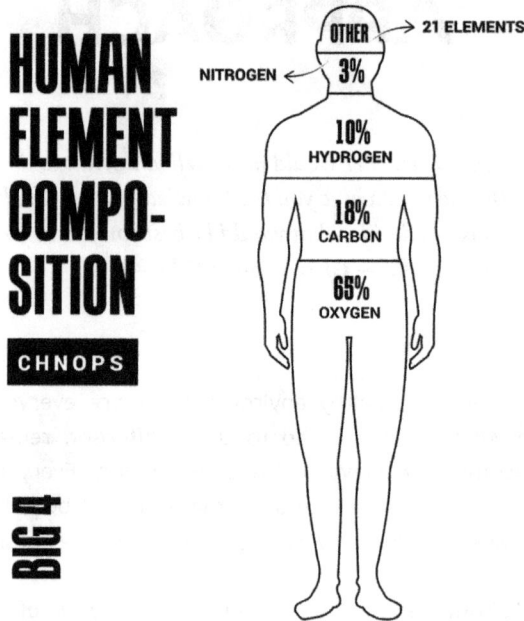

HUMAN ELEMENT COMPO-SITION

CHNOPS

BIG 4

OTHER → 21 ELEMENTS

NITROGEN ←

3%

10% HYDROGEN

18% CARBON

65% OXYGEN

Our human "ingredients" includes trillions of cells, water, bacteria all living symbiotically with one organized organism we call a body.

To go through the parts, performances and complexities of the human vessel is an entire book in itself (or perhaps a series)—but I believe that if we can each understand what our human bodies are made from, what buildings are needed to sustain, maintain, regenerate and even heal this human vessel, then it will ignite conversations about what choices and behaviors we have. Understanding this concept might even make all of those food diets obsolete!

OUR HUMAN INGREDIENTS LIST

Imagine you have been given the blueprint to build your favorite vehicle or car. You now need to source and grab all of the parts/ingredients to build this vehicle which is your human body. This is what you would need. (I hope you have a big shopping basket.)

Look to the universal building blocks available. 118 elements have been identified, of which the first 94 occur naturally on earth, with the remaining 24 being synthetic elements. We only need 25 of those universal elemental building blocks to build our human body. It is important to note that of the other 60–70 elements available on Earth, many are mildly or severely toxic to the human body. They can even disrupt normal cellular function. Examples: Mercury, cobalt, uranium, thallium, radium, beryllium and even fluoride in higher amounts. This is important to recognize so we understand what can or can't be consumed, absorbed or enter our human system.

118 available in the Universe

—

95 available on Earth

—

25 used for the Human body

So if you wanted to build a human body you would have to grab 7 octillion atoms (CHNOPS) from universal stardust, the earth and its life supporting elements; then add heaps of empty space (99.9% of atoms are "empty space")— then combine these atoms to form fundamental molecules, the biggest being the chromosome in the human body. This molecule holds our evolutionary blueprint for replication of the human form across generations as we reproduce.

From these molecules grab 23 pairs of chromosomes to create ONE human cell. Then repeat it ~37.2 trillion times to create all the cells in the human body. From here arrange the cells in groups called tissues, then teach the tissues how to work together and create one functioning organ. Then create 78 organs and teach them to work together as 12 integrated organ systems with unique, yet complementary functions. But it doesn't stop there...then switch every cell on to spark a chain of chemical reactions that bring the human vessel to life.

Now that your human vessel is alive, it needs to interact with the natural environment around it, learning to survive, adapt and thrive. To do this, all the atoms, cells, and organs need to interact and work together as ONE synergistic system.

Before you finish, don't forget to invite 370 trillion microbes and bacteria into and onto the body to help sustain it. Even open the door for 6-8 retroviruses to take root in your DNA and you're your body adapt over time.

You may even need to sprinkle in some traces of gold, dirt, and even of stardust to fill in some missing pieces. Don't worry, if we tried to sell all the elements in our body, on the current market value it would be worth less than 1USD, so your value is beyond what you are made from. It is about what you choose to make of this human experience once you are alive and engaged in the human experience.

NINE KEY PARTS REQUIRED TO BUILD A HUMAN

If we use the human blueprint and identified its universal building blocks, captured the ingredients needed to build a human and then arranged them in a way where this complex orchestra of atoms vibrated to construct a living version of the person that looks at you in the mirror each morning, then it would look a little something like this.

WHAT ARE YOU MADE OF?	
380+ Trillion	VIROME
370+ Trillion	MICROBIOME
12	ORGAN SYSTEMS
78	ORGANS
	TISSUES
372 Trillion	CELLS
	MOLECULES
7 Octilllion	ATOMS
25	HUMAN ELEMENTS
95	EARTH'S ELEMENT
118	UNIVERSAL ELEMENTS

Consider that we are all created from the "Source." We are made from the same universal elements that are found in the stars you see in the sky each night and the in the earthly soil under your feet each day. We are made of an octillion amount of atoms (mostly empty space). These form our human elements and are less than 20% of the elements available in the universe. These elements combine to form molecules.

Cells, tissues and our 12 organ systems become host to trillions of micro-organisms living in and on us, the microbiome and virome. All of this works as one to produce YOU!

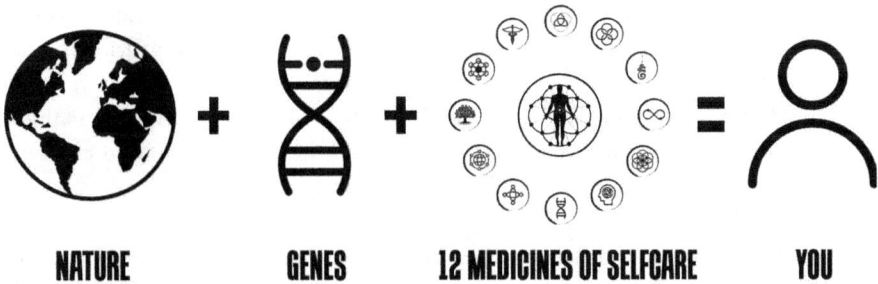

NATURE + **GENES** + **12 MEDICINES OF SELFCARE** = **YOU**

1. **ATOMS**—An adult is made up of around 7,000,000,000,000,000,000,000,000,000,000 (7 octillion) atoms.

2. **SPACE**—As Dr Jess Wade, a physicist at Imperial College London, admitted that about 99.9% of an atom was "empty space."[2] Which means that this is true for us too. We are more nothing than anything! What a thought.

3. **ELEMENTS**—Where "the crucial elements for life on Earth, often called the building blocks of life, can be abbreviated as CHNOPS: carbon, hydrogen, nitrogen, oxygen, phosphorus and sulfur." Humans and their galaxy have about 97 percent of the same kind of atoms, and the elements of life.

4. **MOLECULES**—These atoms combine to form molecules. The biggest molecule in nature resides in your body. It is a chromosome. A normal human cell has 23 pairs of chromosomes in its nucleus, each a single, very long molecule of DNA. Chromosome is the biggest, containing around 10bn atoms.

5. **CELL**—To create a human cell, each with 23 pairs of chromosomes, the biggest cell must then take up 46 x 10 billion atoms. We need to create 37.2 trillion cells to build a human body. Each cell is its own living universe.

6. **TISSUES**—Cells team up to form tissues. The body contains several different types of cells, such as blood cells, nerve cells, and muscle cells. When cells of the same type "hang together" so to speak, and perform the same function, a tissue is formed.

7. **ORGANS**—Tissues integrate and work together to form organs. An organ is a part of the body that performs a specialized physiologic function. For example, the stomach contains epithelial tissue, muscle tissue, nerve tissue, and connective tissue, and the stomach has the specific physiologic function of breaking down food. For a human, we then need to create 78 organs in differing size and physiological functions to create a human. These 78 organs then synchronize into 12 different systems of the human vessel; each with its own function to balance the human system.

8. **MICROBIOME**—Our 37.2 trillion human cells[3] regenerate at a rate of 50 million cells per second and are outnumbered 10-fold by bacteria and 100-fold by viruses. We also host single-celled organisms called archaea, as well as fungi, viruses and other microbes that attack bacteria. Together, we refer to them as the human microbiota.

9. **VIROME**—Did you know that there are 10 times as many viruses as there are microbes in a human microbiome: The human microbiome contains about 38 trillion bacteria—and about 380 trillion viruses.[4]

Viruses can be found nearly everywhere in the biosphere, giving an estimated number of 1.2×10^{30} in the open ocean, 2.6×10^{30} in soil, 3.5×10^{31} in oceanic subsurfaces, and $0.25-2.5 \times 10^{31}$ in terrestrial subsurfaces.[5] Our smartest scientists who have made it their life work also admit that we understand less than 1 percent of ALL viral diversity! Hopefully this helps reduce any fear you may have about everything living in and on us! Especially considering the recent "pandemonium" and fear created around one virus, all based on an outdated germ theory that teaches us to fear the unknown. How can anyone speak in absolutes when we understand less than 1% of it all?!

As an example; Your healthy human lungs are home to a family of 19 newfound viruses—which are present at higher levels in the lungs of critically ill people. Redondoviruses are associated with certain ailments, but whether they cause disease is unclear.[6]

Science journalist Ed Yongs says, "For most of human existence these microbes were hidden, visible only through the illnesses they caused. When they finally surfaced in biological studies, they were cast as rogues."[7]

Although we don't fully understand their role in human health. We know that it is about coexistence. These small microbiota and viruses do a lot of good too; they sculpt our organs, defend us from disease, break down our food, provide nutrients for our cells, program and educate our immune systems, prevent colonization by harmful bacteria and viruses, and even guide and influence our behavior through the gut-brain axis, bombarding our genomes with their genes and granting us incredible abilities.

The key message is that we have never been separate, and these invisible organisms do more good than harm. We couldn't survive or thrive without them. There isn't any part of the body not inhabited by microorganisms!

We must move away from the old paradigm of the "germ theory" that sees microbes as invading rogues that must be killed off at all costs, to a more balanced microbiome theory of health, understanding their bigger role from a wider lens. Our survival and longevity depends on understanding and supporting the good ones not just focusing on eliminating the bad ones. When they are in balance, health flourishes and lives transform.

LIFE & LIVING

To simplify living in good health. It is important to note that our genes are the hardware (the 5–20% of who we are that can't be replaced); environment and lifestyle are the software (the 85–95%) that is in our control through our thoughts, choices and behaviors. The good news is that we can influence how our genes express them and thus our ability to live into our human potential. This is called epigenetics. It shows that our thoughts can change our DNA. It is the change and the degree of change caused by external factors that switch genes on and off. It is now known that the environment and our lifestyle choices determine our health, wellbeing and performance more than our actual genes.

So the question remains. Are we driver of this human vessel that has been created, or does it drive us?

Deepak Chopra and Dr Rudolph Tanzi sum it up well. They said: "You are not simply the sum total of the genes you were born with. You are the user and controller of your genes, the author of your biological story. No prospect in self-care is more exciting."[8]

In addition to this, it is important to learn how to "spark" the ignition and be the driver of your own life and vessel. Did you know that living cells have different molecules than non-living things? And furthermore, these different molecules perform chemical reactions that characterize living things?

So add these four sets of molecules "the spark plugs" in to fire up the engine, so to speak.

The definition of life is something that has all four of the following characteristics:

1. Metabolism (anabolism and catabolism)—constant cycle of creation and destruction
2. Response to stimuli (internal, external)
3. Growth and adaptation
4. Reproduction

Once your life was ignited, there were numerous processes, functions and systems that fired up and work together harmoniously to keep you in balance. These processes are then maintained over your lifespan. Scientists call this homeostasis, "the tendency of an organism or a cell to regulate its internal conditions, usually by a system of feedback controls, so as to stabilize health and functioning, regardless of the outside changing conditions." Good health and wellbeing ensures empowering health and wellbeing at all ages, across all environments.

This is the human design. This is your human experience. This is life.

WHAT TYPE OF OLD PERSON DO YOU WANT TO BE?

The truth is that living in good health and aging of our biological systems occurs in relation to our lifestyle choices over our lifespan. The human body has your best interest at heart. Irrespective of how you treat yourself. It is running three core systems to ensure that you can survive and thrive.

1. Maintenance and regeneration
2. Repair
3. Defense

Maintaining good health and wellbeing. Your body is constantly replacing old cells with new ones at the rate of millions per second. By the time you finish reading this sentence, 50-million cells will have died and been replaced by others. Some are lost through use, some reach the end of their lifespan, and others self-destruct. The life cycle of every cell is carefully controlled, so you always have just the right number of each type of cell.

Mostly, everything regenerates. Essentially if every cell in your body, all 37.2 trillion of them, will regenerate in a sliding scale of ~10 years at a rate of ~50 million per second, then every 10–20 years you will be a completely new human (relatively speaking—kind of a cool thought either way!) Maybe the damage we did to ourselves in our youth or in the live-to-work phase of our life can be reversed over time.

Out of the cells that are continually replacing themselves, fat cells take the longest and are replaced at the rate of about 10% per year in adults. So you could say that on average, human beings replace all their fat cells about every ten years. Everything else is a bit quicker. Colon cells have it rough: they die off after about four days. Sperm cells have a life span of only about three days, skin cells live about two or three weeks. Red blood cells live for about four months. White blood cells live on average more than a year.

CELL TIME	TURNOVER TIME
SMALL INTESTINES EPITHELIUM	2-4 Days
STOMACH	2-9 Days
BLOOD NEUTROPHILS	1-5 Days
WHITE BLOOD CELLS EOSINOPHILS	2-5 Days
GASTROINTESTINAL COLON CRYPT CELLS	3-4 Days
CERVIX	6 Days
LUNGS ALVEOLI	8 Days
TONGUE TASTE BUDS (RAT)	10 Days
PLATELETS	10 Days
BONE OSTEOCLASTS	2 Weeks
INTESTINE PANETH CELLS	20 Days
SKIN EPIDERMIS CELLS	10-30 Days
PANCREASE BETA CELLS (RATS)	20-50 Days
BLOOD B CELLS (MOUSE)	4-7 Weeks
TRACHEA	1-2 Months
HEMATOPOIETIC STEM CELLS	2 Months
SPERM (MALE GAMATES)	2 Months
BONE OSTEOBLASTS	3 Months
RED BLOOD CELLS	4 Months
LIVER HEPATOCYTE CELLS	0.5-1 Year
FAT CELLS	8 Years
CARDIOMYCYTES	0.5-10% Per Year
CENTRAL NERVOUS SYSTEM	Lifetime
SKELETON	10% Per Year
LENS CELLS	Life Time
ODCYTES (FEMALE GAMATES)	Life Time

MOSTLY EVERYTHING REGENERATES

We really need to take care and look after four special organs.

1. Our central nervous system, brain and spinal cord, including all 100 billion neurons
2. Our heart
3. Our eyes
4. Our teeth

The reason is that while brain cells typically last an entire lifetime, neurons in the cerebral cortex, for example, are not replaced when they die. Heart cells "cardiomyocyte" are replaced at a reducing rate as we age. At age 25, about 1% of cells are replaced every year. The cells in our eyes do not replace themselves and we only get one set of teeth!

Imagine what would happen if your heart stopped pumping, your eyes stopped seeing or your brain or even your limbs stopped working. That is the true value of these organs. Look at your loved ones today and be grateful for sight. Take a deep breath as you wake up tomorrow morning and be grateful that your heart kept pumping while you slept. Look down at your finger and move it, stand up to walk, think and communicate to others. Now be grateful for your brain and your spinal cord. In every moment we could complain about life, but in every moment, we could also look down at our fingers and move it, walk, think, talk, see and communicate with the world. Being grateful that every breath, every movement, every moment shared with a loved one, everything we see, is a gift.

The good news is that this amazing human body can still adapt to function, survive and even thrive after injury. We are starting to see that some areas in the brain might regenerate to its original function, but neuroplasticity and neurogenesis is showing us how powerful the human vessel is for rearranging things if necessary so that it can still function and utilize different pathways to achieve the same end goal. It opens up a whole new area of human design and even suggests that we are using less than 1% of our true human potential.

The heart and eyes can even adapt. Modern science is showing us that they may even be replaced with organ donation! Another crazy thought.

When it comes to defense. Your human body is fighting and invisible war every second of every day.

The immune system protects us from the constant onslaught of viruses, bacteria and other types of pathogens we encounter throughout life. It also remembers past infections so it can fight them off more easily the next time we encounter them. In its simplicity the immune system can be thought of as having two divisions: the general or non-specific immune system, and the adaptive or specific immune system. All multicellular animals have dedicated cells or tissues to deal with the threat of infection. Some of these responses happen immediately to quickly protect the immunity of the host and quickly limit the infection or 'invasion'. Other times, the response is slower but more specific to combat the infection or immune 'invader'. These protective responses are referred to as the immune system. The good news, is that your innate wisdom and design has your back to repair, regenerate and thrive from any starting point. Even after disease, dysfunction and injury.

Now that you understand the complex overlay of all these amazing systems. Let's explore the 12 organs systems and 78 organs that enable you to live, function and perform each day.

"Since the dawn of time, organisms have been subject to evolutionary pressure from the environment. The ability to respond to environmental threats or stressors such as predation or natural disaster enhanced survival and therefore reproductive capacity, and physiological responses that supported such responses could be selected for. In mammals, these responses include changes that increase the delivery of oxygen and glucose to the heart and the large skeletal muscles. The result is physiological support for adaptive behaviors such as 'fight or flight'."[9]
— *Suzanne C. Segerstrom and Gregory E. Miller* —

12 SYNERGISTIC ORGAN SYSTEMS WORKING AS ONE

Yes, you are the orchestration of 12 synergistic organ systems working as one! When one system is out of harmony, you need to treat the whole, not just the individual parts or systems. These 12 systems are:

An organ is a part of the body that performs a specialized physiologic function. For example, the stomach contains epithelial tissue, muscle tissue, nerve tissue, and connective tissue, and has the specific physiologic function of breaking down food. To create a human we need 78 organs in differing size and physiological functions. These 78 organs then require to synchronize into 12 different systems of the human body; each with its own function to balance the human system.

1. **Digestive system**—Salivary glands, esophagus, stomach, liver, gallbladder, pancreas, small intestine, and large intestine. Processes foods and absorbs nutrients, minerals, vitamins, and water.

2. **Reproductive system**—Fallopian tubes, uterus, vagina, ovaries, mammary glands, testes, vas deferens, seminal vesicles, prostate, and penis. Produces sex cells and sex hormones; ultimately produces offspring

3. **Respiratory system**—Mouth, nose, pharynx, larynx, trachea, bronchi, lungs, and diaphragm. Delivers air to sites where gas exchange can occur between the blood and cells (around body) or blood and air (lungs).

4. **Endocrine system**—Pituitary gland, pineal gland, thyroid, parathyroid gland, adrenal glands, testes, and ovaries.) Provides communication within the body via hormones. Directs long-term change over other organ systems to maintain homeostasis.

5. **Skeletal system**—Bones, cartilage, and ligaments. Supports and protects soft tissues of the body. Provides movement at joints, produces blood cells, and stores minerals

6. **Nervous system**—Brain, spinal cord, nerves, and sensory organs (eyes, ears, tongue, skin, and nose). Collects, transfers, and processes information. Directs short-term change over other organ systems in order to maintain homeostasis.
7. **Lymphatic system**—Lymph, lymph nodes, and lymph vessels. Defends against infection and disease. Transfers lymph between tissues and the blood stream.
8. **Urinary system**—Kidneys, ureters, urinary bladder, and urethra. Removes excess water, salts, and waste products from the blood and body. Controls pH.
9. **Musculoskeletal system**—Tendons, skeletal, cardiac, and smooth muscles. Provides movement, support, and heat production.
10. **Cardiovascular system**—Heart, blood, and blood vessels. Transports oxygen, nutrients, and other substances to the cells, and transports wastes, carbon dioxide, and other substances away from the cells; also helps stabilize body temperature and pH.
11. **Integumentary system**—Skin, hair, and nails. Provides protection from both injury and fluid loss and provides physical defense against infection by microorganisms. Controls temperature.
12. **Immune system**—Leukocytes, tonsils, adenoids, thymus, and spleen. Defends against pathogens and other diseases.[10]

"The whole is greater than the sum of its parts."
— Aristotle —

Internally, our survival as an organism depends on the balanced integrated activity of all the 12 organ systems, often coordinated by the endocrine and nervous systems. However, as we will discuss later, there are external factors that can influence the natural harmony of all these systems. When one system is out of balance, the internal harmony of our entire biological starts to dysfunction and may even lead to dis-ease. Your mind is like Mozart conducting an amazing band of 78 organs. If one organ "instrument" is out of tune (balance) then the entire orchestration functions "sounds" different.

So let's apply all of the above principles and frameworks into helping you grow a healthy human vessel by asking ourselves TWO key questions.

1. Where do we find the 25 elemental human building blocks needed to build, grow and sustain our human vessel over our lifespan? From plants, animals, soil, water and everything else in between.
2. Where does this energy begin?

There are THREE primary sources of energy.

1. **Universal energy and the sun:** Light energy; photons & waves are the source of life's energy on earth. Especially plants.
2. **Earth's energy, air, water and soil:** The source of 95 earthly elements, over 5000 inorganic minerals, the oxygen we breathe, the water we drink and the nutrients we consume in various forms (plants, animals, insects, fish etc.)
3. **Human energy:** Energy is delivered to the body through the air we breathe, the foods we eat and liquids we drink. We literally absorb energy from the sun, air and the soil. We are like a plant, just with more complex emotions! Our body then breaks down these fuels into smaller components and absorbs them. ATP is the principal molecule for storing and transferring energy in our cells. It is often referred to as the energy currency of the cell and can be compared to storing money in a bank.

SOURCING THE 25 HUMAN BUILDING BLOCKS

Let's first remember that:

- 65+% of our body composition is water
- 65+% of our elemental composition is oxygen
- 95+% of the element al building blocks we need to source from our environment comes from 6 key elements CHNOPS (Macro-nutrients)
- The remaining 5% comes from the rest (micro-nutrients in our air, soil and water).

So it becomes obvious that the quality of the water we consume, the quality of the air we breathe, and where we source the six key elements common to all living beings is vital to our health and wellbeing.

We are essentially Carbon-based life forms brought to life by oxygen and water. The sun's energy and the elements from earth simply permit the complex chemical reactions that permit us to function, live, grow and adapt. All of this links back to what we call a "healthy adult human." As you can see it is a complex biological system of systems, capable of highly elaborate functions, whose integrated networks maintain homeostasis of the human vessel in the context of any environment.

What this all means, is that despite all of this foundational work I have broken down into "parts" we must go beyond treating the human being as parts. We need to empower each individual to find harmony within from their cells to the integrated orchestration of their organs, to how they live and dance with the external reality.

The future of medicine is energetic and WHOLE-listic, not just biological and a pathoanatomical parts manual. It's an interesting perspective in discerning "who sustains who?" A stark reminder that we are simply part of the whole of one complex and interconnected web of life.

So the question is: how do we use this information to function optimally each day. How can we perform and remain resilient as the natural world changes around us?

Some communities have found the elixir to life. Indigenous cultures have lived within tribes for 100,000 plus years.

I hope that our modern civilisation can do the same, adapt, pivot and course-correct together to overcome the challenges of today and ensure a future of tomorrow.

So, let me ask you this question. Considering we are spiritual beings having a human experience, are we simply borrowing this land from future generations? If so, what type of life will you live and what type of world will you be leaving to your children and their children? Or are we too late into this crisis? Can we return to be custodians rather than owners?

The Chinese word "crisis" consists of two separate Chinese characters. One represents *danger* and the other represents a *critical moment*. When a crisis comes, it's important to remember that it's a time to make a decision. Change emerges from growth. You can allow ground-zero to be both an ending and a beginning. Perhaps 2020 was the end of one chapter and the beginning of a new chapter in human history together, both personally and collectively?

CALL TO COURAGE

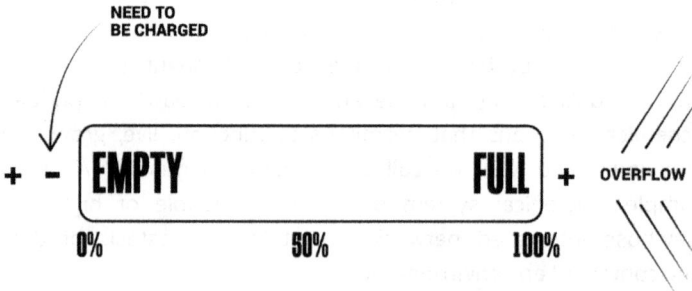

1. When you wake up each day, how full is your energetic human battery? (0–100%)

2. How many times does you human battery hit empty over the day? (perhaps you need a nap etc.)

....

3. How much energy is left in your human battery when you finish each day? (0–100%)

....

4. When you sleep each night, does you battery full recharge to 100%?

....

5. Share one way that you could improve your human energy

....

....

....

....

SELFCARE'S 7 ENERGY DOCTORS

CONNECTION Inside out, Outside in
REST Sleep, Fast, Wind Down
MOVE Energy creates energy
FOOD Saturate & Eliminate
WATER Hydrate
AIR Oxygenate
UNIVERSAL SOURCE Sun, Waves, Frequencies & Light

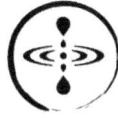

CHAPTER 8

ANCIENT WISDOM FOR A MODERN WORLD

"There is zero, and there is eternity, and there is mortality, but there is no ultimate."
— *Stephen King* —

YOUR CREATION AND CREATION

Did you know that the chance of you being born is closer to zero than anything you can conceive?

You won the lottery the day you took your first breath. It was a 1 in 4–5 trillion chance that you in all your beauty, imperfectly perfect, with all that unique genius here on spaceship earth.

Let alone the fact that your parents (also walking miracles) connected passionately igniting a chain of chemical reactions that created your life, 9 months later! What an amazing opportunity each of us has to live and be alive! Yes it is an opportunity to live, it is not guaranteed that you will choose to truly live it.

As a unique human being on a big blue planet in an expansive universe, it's natural that at some time or another you may have pondered some curious questions and marveled at the answers. For example:

- How old is the Universe? Predicted to be 13.8 billion years.[1]
- How old is Earth? 4.543 billion years.[2]
- How long has life been on Earth? 4 billion years.[3]
- When did we see the first complex life forms? 400 million years (insects).[4]
- How old is the oldest living human civilization? 100,000 + years.[5]
- How long does the average human live? 72 years.[6]

How long will you or I live? We don't know. The human potential is estimated around 142 years, yet we only live half of that as a species. Perhaps it is not about how long we live, but the richness of the life we live. Being grateful for every moment granted to us.

How long will the Earth keep living for? Predicted to be 7.79 billion years.[7]

I will pre-frame here that science is our best guess and as mentioned above, time is a concept that humans created. However, here is what our smartest minds have come up regarding these estimations.

A BRIEF HUMAN HISTORY

Galen Strawson from *The Guardian* wrote a review of *Sapiens: A Brief History of Humankind* by Yuval Noah Harari, giving a powerful overview of humankinds' history.[8] It starts by sharing that human beings (members of the genus Homo) have existed for about 2.4m years whereas Homo-sapiens (our own species from great apes to modern human) has only existed for 150,000 years. Roughly, 6% of that time period. In other words, the history of Homo-sapiens plays only a small part in the history of humankind. Mind-boggling when you think about it.

The first half of our existence is steady but then...the radical transformation is quite remarkable. We evolved in new and evolutionary ways.

1. **Cognitive revolution/transformation**—About 70,000 years ago, our species started to behave in new and interesting ways, and our radical ingenuity spread quickly across the planet.
2. **Agricultural revolution/transformation**—About 11,000 years ago we entered the agricultural revolution, from a hunting and gathering species to a farming species.
3. **Scientific revolution/transformation**—Science is still a newborn in many ways, its origins tracing back to about 500 years ago. The science revolution triggered the industrial revolution about 250 years ago, which triggered the information revolution about 50 years ago, which triggered the biotechnological revolution. That's a cascade of revolutions.

4. **Bio-technological revolution/transformation**—The biotechnological revolution signals the rapid emergence of biotech, including cyborgs, AI and a new type of immersion between technology and human.

With rapid evolution and growth comes problems and pitfalls as well as advancement and education. However, in our modernization we must not forget or dismiss the ancient wisdom that has been here on Earth for thousands of years.

If we continue to grow and revolutionize the way we live so rapidly, without supporting and nourishing what permits us to be here, then we unconsciously create revolutions that harm future generations. As an example, the industrial revolution came at the cost of the natural world, resulting in the 6th mass extinction, and the technological revolution came at the expense of our waistlines, and our mental and emotional health, as we normalized sedentary behaviors.

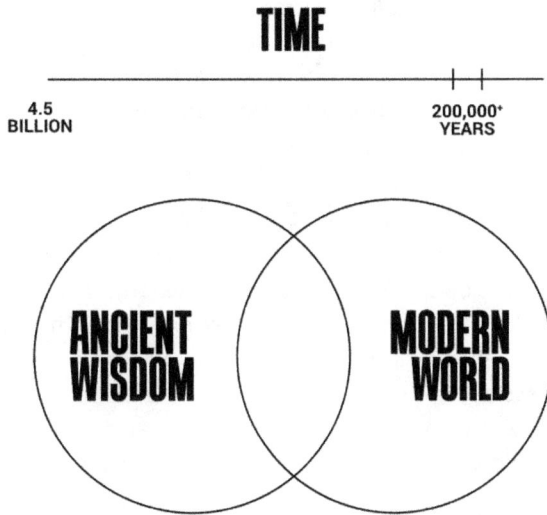

TIME

4.5
BILLION

200,000+
YEARS

ANCIENT
WISDOM

MODERN
WORLD

When you think of the oldest modern culture, we might cast our mind back 5 or 10 generations. Perhaps even consider the Chinese, Indian, Roman or Babylonian empires. However this is only a very small piece of human history. Indigenous Australians and other indigenous cultures have been surviving for over 100,000 years.[9] Just imagine what simplicity and wisdom they hold in their stories and culture.

Cast your mind back tens of thousands of years and imagine our ancient ancestors surviving through floods, ice ages, heat waves, scarcity, disease, famine and anything else you can possibly imagine. This is the most adaptive and resilient human form of humans. Their epic journeys gave them great wisdom.

Just taking a handful of ancient wisdom from our oldest culture, Indigenous Australians and you'll notice how relevant is still is today. Why? Because they learned how to live in harmony with nature, with Mother Earth and each other. Their stories of survival and wisdom was carried through story, art and ceremony generation after generation.

> *"Our spirituality is a oneness and an interconnectedness*
> *with all that lives and breathes, even with all*
> *that does not live and breathe."*
> — ***Mudrooroo***[10] —

> *"So I take this word 'reconciliation' and I use it to reconcile*
> *people back to Mother Earth, so they can walk*
> *this land together and heal as one. Because she is*
> *the one that gives birth to everything we see*
> *around us. Everything we need to survive."*
> — ***Max Dulumunmun***[11] —

A BRIEF HISTORY OF MEDICINE

Could we take lessons from all of the current and ancient civilizations so that we can connect the dots forward to create healthy, happy and connected humans who all believe in unity and a sustainable existence? This would show up in the world is as a human-centric and spiritually aware energetic approach to health, harmony, happiness and unity.

What if we could model the best pieces of each ancient culture and apply it to our modern world and lifestyles? Let's explore thousands of years of cultures and approaches.

> *"The land is my mother. Like a human mother, the land*
> *gives us protection, enjoyment and provides our needs—*
> *economic, social and religious. We have a human relationship*
> *with the land: Mother, daughter, son. When the land is taken*
> *from us or destroyed, we feel hurt because we belong to the*
> *land and we are part of it."*
> — ***Rev Dr Djiniyini Gondarra*** —
> ***Senior Yolngu Elder and retired Uniting Church***
> ***Minister from Galiwinku on Elcho Island***[12]

INDIGENOUS AUSTRALIANS REMINDS US OF PRIMARY HEALTH SYSTEMS

The oldest living human civilisation understands what it takes to thrive and survive. They remind us to support, nourish and be intimately connected with our primary life support system.

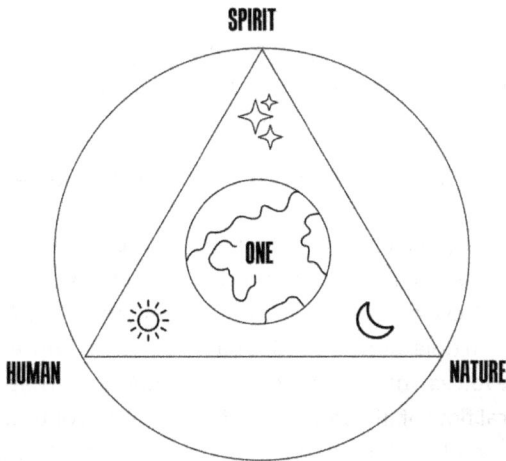

BABYLONIANS HELPED US DISPEL MAGIC FROM REAL MEDICINE

If we look backwards we can see where modern scientific medicine found its place over 4000 years ago. We had to figure out whether these ancient methods actually had any effect or impact on this human beings long-term health and wellbeing. This reflection and investigation allows us to discern between ancient myth, the magic and sorcery used in those time and the interventions that were most effective. We can be science-based in discerning magic from medicine, but still focus on the outcome for the individual.

Researcher of the mind-body connection, Dr Joe Dispenza sums up the 4000+ years of magic medicine by sharing that most of the magic starts between our ears. He stated that "If you begin the inward journey and start to change your inner world of thoughts and feelings, it should create an improved state of well-being. If you keep repeating the process in meditation (in your mind), then in time, epigenetic (gene expression) changes should begin to alter your outer presentation—and you become your own placebo."[13]

Biology researcher Dr Bruce Lipton added to this by showing how our "beliefs can change our cellular biology." In other words, thoughts literally become things internally and externally.

INDIA TAUGHT US TO TREAT THE WHOLE PERSON

India and Ayurveda gave us the science of life, connecting the mind-body health systems, seeing the whole person in the context of their life and their environment. The approach was, and is, more than a system for treating illness, it integrates a science of life (Ayur = life, Veda = science or knowledge).

The two main guiding principles of Ayurveda are:

(1) the mind and the body are inextricably connected, and

(2) nothing has more power to heal and transform the body than the mind.

Freedom from illness depends upon expanding our own awareness, bringing it into balance, and then extending that balance to the body.

CHINA TAUGHT US WELCOME CHANGE AS A NATURAL PART OF LIFE

China taught us the philosophy of change, think of the I-Ching and the Tao philosophy. What if we simply accepted that everything and everyone moves through the eternal cycle of birth, growth, decay and death? That everything has a beginning a middle and an end. That everything and everyone changes, transforms and evolves into another state of being. Perhaps we could stop resisting the natural flow of life and let go of the need to control. We could remain in a state of being and flexibility, allowing room for growth, change, adaptation and natural transitory cycles.

BUDDHISM GAVE US A SOLUTION TO END HUMAN SUFFERING

The story of Buddhism gave us insight into the nature of suffering. Siddhartha Gautama, a young prince of the Shakhya clan in India, was raised in comfort and royalty, shielded from the realities, temptations and cruelties of the world. Upon seeing outside the palace walls he was confronted with a dose of reality: suffering, disease, death, sadness and desperation. He became enthralled with human suffering, and the question that burned in his consciousness— "How may suffering be ended?" Siddhartha Gautama entered many spiritual practices and rituals and yet remained inflicted with the dichotomies of life and in search for their cure.

To cut Gautama's epic spiritual quest grossly short, one day, Gautama saw a tree and decided to sit under it until he worked out the answers to life. Some ancient traditions say he achieved "enlightenment" overnight, others say three nights, others say seven weeks. The time frame isn't the point, because what he gave us insight into remains enduring. He gave humanity the Four Noble Truths which forms the foundation for Buddhism.

His first teaching of the Four Noble Truths follows this pattern:

1. The First Noble Truth—"life is dukkha." Dukkha is variously translated as suffering, pain, impermanence.
2. The Second Noble Truth—the pain of life is caused by "tanha"—our cravings, our attachments, our selfish grasping after pleasure and avoiding pain.
3. The Third Noble Truth—a complete release from attachment and dukkha is possible, a liberation from pain and rebirth.
4. The Fourth Noble Truth—how to attain liberation; it describes the Noble Eightfold Path leading to Nirvana and the cessation of suffering.

Another main teaching of Buddhist metaphysics is known as the Three Marks of Existence. They are *anicca*—impermanence: all things are transitory, nothing lasts. *Anatta*—the no-self or no-soul: human beings, and all of existence is without a soul or self. And *dhukka* is suffering.

The over-arching idea is that self is an illusion, one which causes immeasurable suffering.

JAPAN INSPIRED US TO FIND OUR REASON FOR BEING
Japan gave us their philosophy of *Ikigai* (生き甲斐, pronounced ee-kee-guy) which translates to "our reason for being." Ikigai can also mean the "thing that you live for" or "the reason you get up in the morning," or your "purpose," or even your "usefulness to others." What if we lived our Ikigai and simply gave it forward to the world? Wouldn't that transform the planet and its people entirely?

AFRICA—A CULTURE OF WE NOT ME
In Sierra Leonne, Africa, the Ubuntu culture of "We not me," grew. What if we could learn from the war, greed, corruption, loss of culture and deep connection in Sierra Leone. Seeing that disconnection does not promote longevity. What if we lived by their cultural values of Ubuntu, "We not me" and allowed it to bleed into other cultures.

BHUTAN TAUGHT US TO MEASURE HAPPINESS OVER PRODUCTIVITY
Bhutan taught us to measure Gross Domestic Happiness. What can we learn from a country that assesses all of its government policies based on how much they contribute to the happiness of its people? Seeing that focusing on happiness results in a flow on effect, a ripple effect into all the areas of society that are measured in gross domestic product, or a countries GDP.

FRANCE GAVE US PERMISSION ENJOY HEALTHY MODERATION

France gave us permission to enjoy healthy moderation. What if we learnt from the French that life isn't so serious, and that we can have our cake and eat it too, with humor, elegance, grace and style? The French show us that it's all about moderation, not excess. It is more about good things being enjoyed and shared. It's quality, not quantity.

A LESSON FROM TIME ITSELF

Understanding that we may only get 600,000–1,000,000 hours in our lifetime (if we are lucky) may help us reflect on where we spend our time and what we truly value, beyond what we say we do (money, success etc). As an example, if you say that you value quality time with your family above all else, but you spend 80 hours at work each week, then perhaps you value work more than your family? Harsh truth, I know. However, it may also help you appreciate the time that others spend and invest in you. If a friend sits with you on the couch or phone for two hours, then they are spending their most valuable resource with you.

SELF-MASTERY

All of these cultures and communities lead us to consider the unique balance of self-care, self-harm and self-expansion. Are you promoting more self-harm than care? Take note of your own balance right now.

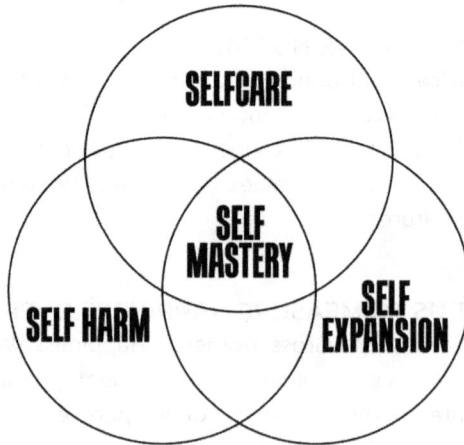

As we "modernized" on a global scale, ancient wisdom was often left in the past like an ancient relic. We must however take the time to saturate ourselves in ancient wisdom and try to integrate it into our modern world without manipulating it to suit ourselves. As history went on, humans created mental constructs and often compartmentalized and separated things. One concept we created was Time. Regardless of what our calendar or clock now says, one thing has always remained the same: the fact we have a certain amount of time on this Earth. Yes, no one gets out alive. Time is ultimately our most valuable and scarce resource.

In 2019, the average human lives 72 years, which is exactly half of our predicted human potential (142 years). 8 This is equivalent to 630,720 hours.

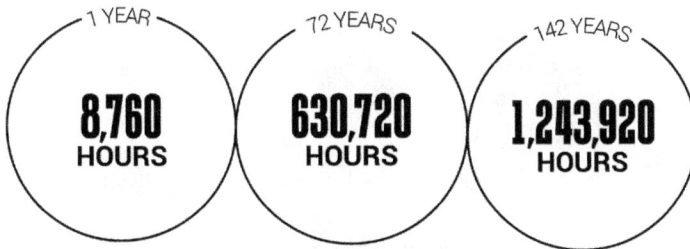

So, why waste a minute living a life that does not serve you? Why live a life that will leave you with regrets? Time is a relative concept. Something that we can slow down in the presence of experiencing or sharing a blissful moment. It is something that we can speed up, living busy life that is never truly lived and appreciated.

HOW WE SPEND OUR TIME IS WHAT REALLY MATTERS...

WE ALL HAVE 168 HOURS IN A WEEK.

ABUNDANCE Passion projects Conscious enterprise Social Impact & Giving	SELFCARE & LIFESTYLE 12 medicines & daily rituals Fun and Living
BASIC HUMAN NEEDS What's your monthly number to cover your basic human needs Food & Water, Shelter, Basic Living costs	SLEEP Average 6-8 hours a night

What remains constant is that we all have 168 hours each week. How we spend that time will ultimately determine our health, wellbeing, abundance and even our freedom to be and do. If you want time to stop; kiss, hug or eye gaze with someone. Travel in time: read or dream. Escape time: listen to music, dance, move. Feel time: write, stop, feel. Release time: breathe.

QUADRANT 1—REST AND SLEEP

Although we spend one-third of our lives sleeping, this rest and restorative time is the greatest player in how healthy and successful the other two-thirds of our lives are. Sleep is important, but make sure you don't sleepwalk through life too. Sleep deeply, wake up, be present and live fully.

> *"I was asleep at the wheel before cancer shook me awake."*
> — *Kris Carr* —

Sleep Recommendations[14]
- Newborns: 14–17 hours
- Young children: 11–15hours

- Teens need at least 8 hours—and on average 9¼ hours—a night of uninterrupted sleep to leave their bodies and minds rejuvenated for the next day
- Adult's: 7–9 hours, no less than 6 and no more than 11 hours!

QUADRANT 2—LIFESTYLE & SELFCARE

Casting a vision for your ideal day and lifestyle is a beautiful starting point. If we define success on our own terms. Rather than other versions of success dedicated by societal and cultural norms, then we can use this quadrant to master the 12 Medicines, master our morning rituals and live in our highest vibration each day. I feel like a lot of us forget to schedule our own self-care, fun and ideal lifestyle into our busy weeks.

QUADRANT 3—WORK TO COVER 7 BASIC HUMAN NEEDS

We each get the same number of hours in a day, yet we are not born into the same circumstances. Our attitude will determine whether we tune into the abundance or whether we tune into the scarcity. Money is energy. Happiness is dependent on many other factors that do not involve money. So live your legacy. Make a difference. Work to live your ideal day every day surrounded by the people you care about most. If you can find a way to attract cash flow to cover your 7 basic human needs (food, water, shelter, safety, rest, security, belonging) and that of your family in the least amount of time, then you can break free from the 9-5, that 40–100 hour work week and free your time for more purpose-driven projects that contribute positively to the world around you. If you can do both, then that's a bonus, because work, abundance and lifestyle become integrated into one.

QUADRANT 4—PASSION, PURPOSE, IMPACT, LEGACY AND CONTRIBUTION

The first three quadrants are about self-mastery and positively influencing your own front door step, covering your basic human needs for yourself and your family. The last quadrant is the one that our heart wants to dive into each day. As mentioned above, it is possible to integrate all 4 quadrants into a purpose-driven life that allows each of us to find harmony in our lives, whilst optimizing our human experience.

However, if you are still busy mastering the first 3 quadrants, then know that we all still have 2 hours week that we can GIVE, SHARE and CIRCULATE with purpose-driven projects in the service of others, that ultimately leaves us with a sense of fulfillment. Even in the busiest of lives. A surgeon can give 2 hours to support and educate another surgeon in a less developed country. A busy business person can share their wisdom in a weekly online conference or workshop for the benefit of future generations. A mother can support another mother in need, whilst still making time to serve her family. Ultimately these acts are the things that truly fill our cup and our hearts. No one is too busy, we just don't prioritize this quadrant into our lives. Hopefully this inspires you to give at least 2 hours a week to project in your local community that lights your soul on fire and energizes the other 3 quadrants in your life.

We can also leverage this quadrant to INVEST our time spent and money earned into abundant projects where our money "energy" **appreciates, compounds and multiplies passively or residually whilst we sleep.** Perhaps it's a business, a property or even decentralized financial systems that are positively geared in your favor. Wouldn't that be nice? Having your money work for you, rather than just working for the money. No one is too busy, we just don't prioritize this quadrant into our lives. Hopefully this inspires you remain open to the abundant strategies that others have tuned into!

CALL TO COURAGE

How we spend our time is what truly matters. Prepare today for tomorrow and schedule YOU into your 168 hour week using the TOOL below.

Selfcare.global/tools

BONUS: Print 168 HOUR SelfCare weekly method of operating (SMO) and schedule the four quadrants into your lifes.

So, what do we do that? How can we actually live a better way? Unrestricted in our health, with time freedom and abundance to share and circulate?

Let me discuss the amazing "better way" where we can all live in the Blue Zone Together. Thriving as one.

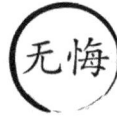

（无悔）

CHAPTER 9

WE ARE THE SOLUTION

"When replaced by WE, even illness becomes wellness."
— Unknown —

CAN WE ALL LIVE IN A BLUE ZONE COMMUNITY?

The idea of blue zones first began with Belgium demographer Michel Poulain and Italian doctor, Gianni Pes and their team of researchers who identified Sardinia as the region with the most amount of living centenarian males, publishing their original findings in the *Journal of Experimental Gerontology.*[1] What initially began as Pes and Poulain simply highlighting longevity "hot spots" with blue circles on a map of the world soon became a name synonymous with health and longevity—blue zones .

Blue Zones were further developed and described by Dan Buettner in the *National Geographic Magazine* issue "Longevity, The Secrets of Long Life."[2] Buettner also studied the areas where people live longer and healthier lives and his article drew worldwide attention. Not only do these blue zone areas have a large percentage of people living over 100, they also have less ill-health, degenerative diseases and issues common to the rest of the population. They are happy, healthy and connected citizens of the world!

Currently only 1% of the world is living in these blue zone. But I ask you...if 1% can live in these blue zone, then why can't 10% or 100%?

So, why not use the secrets of the blue zone societies and cultivate this rare longevity lifestyle into our modern world too?

THIS TO THAT IN THE FUTURE GENERATIONS

4 ZONES	100 PEOPLE
BLUE ZONE	50
GREEN ZONE	45
ORANGE ZONE	4
RED ZONE	1

FUTURE 2030+

Here is how; the five regions identified in Buettner's book *The Blue Zones: Lessons for Living Longer from the People Who've Lived the Longest*[3] are:
- Okinawa in Japan
- Sardinia in Italy
- Icaria of Greece
- Costa Rica's isolated island—Nicoyan Penisula
- Seventh Day Adventists in Loma Linda, California

However, there are more identified longevity hotspots around the world. They are not the communities you may expect either. There are the five named above, plus other places like The Vilcabamba valley in Ecuador, The Hunza valley in Pakistan, Abkhazia in the Caucasus mountains and other modern-day areas like Hong Kong or Maui.

Despite the geography, there is a community out there just like yours in the world that has managed to integrate longevity principles and ways of living and being into their daily lives. Which means you can too.

So why do some people live longer and better than anyone else on the planet. What's their secret? Do they take massive doses of supplements, did they retire wealthy or do they have special genes? The answer is none of the above.

They simply have healthy daily practices and rituals. With Dan Buettner and his team of medical researchers, anthropologists, demographers, and epidemiologists they found evidence-based common denominators of all the blue zones regions. These are the superpowers of longevity.

I have utilized these as a foundation and complement to my 12 Medicines (in chapters ahead). I see the 12 Medicines as a way to use these Blue Zones practices in modern ways that suit today's society.

THE PRACTICES OF BLUE ZONE COMMUNITIES

MOVE NATURALLY (Move)	PURPOSE (Work)	WINE AT 5PM (Food)
80/20 RULE (Mind)	MOSTLY PLANTS (Food)	REST
FAMILY FIRST (Connect)	RIGHT TRIBE (Connect)	BELONG (Spirit)

Right Tribe—The world's longest lived people have close friends (people to confide in) and strong social networks. Experts from all fields agree that isolation is the worst thing we can do to human beings.

Family First—Having close and strong family connections (with spouses, parents, grandparents, grandchildren and community) is common among centenarians. But family is more than just blood too. We are all 99.5% genetically the same anyway!

Modern families are seen to be nuclear and separate from each other. Whereas indigenous and ancient cultures saw family as kinship; where community, teachers, neighbors and mentors were family too. I love the Maoris of New Zealand term "whanau" which can be anything from an intergenerational lineage of family to a group of like-minded people that come together for a common purpose. It is a multi-layered, flexible and dynamic version of "family" that ensures physical, mental, emotional and even spiritual health and wellbeing of all people. The concept is extremely powerful, especially if you are born into families that are less than nourishing, have had parents pass away or a fall out with blood related "family." Connect with your family first, look after your front door step and serve your proximity before trying to change the world.

Belonging—Centenarians have shown that being part of a faith-based community can adds 4 to 14 years to life expectancy. This does not specify whether religious or spiritual. It refers to a sense of belonging and support that inspires hope, even in the darkest of times.

Eat more plants—Plants and beans are at the forefront of most centenarian diets. Eating more plants; vegetables, fruit, and whole grains, while animal based food is eaten in small amounts.

Keep moving—Moving naturally throughout the day—walking, gardening, doing housework, surfing—is a core part of living towards longevity. No one likes to sit down all day behind a computer. We all know that, our backs, hips and body feels that! Motion is lotion!

Slow Down—Move less, rest and digest. Stress is part of life, but centenarians have stress-relieving rituals built into their daily routines. Adventists pray, Ikarians take afternoon naps, and Sardinians do a happy hour, socially connecting and sharing a wine at 5pm.

Work in Purpose—The Okinawans call it Ikigai and the Nicoyans call it "plan de vida"—it means your purpose in life, the reason you wake up in the morning. According to research, having a sense of purpose can add seven years to your overall life expectancy.

Enjoy Healthy Moderation—80/20 Rule. The world's oldest living people have been found to stop eating when their stomachs are around 80% full. They tend to also eat their smallest meal in the early evening. Moderation is all about enjoying life without being ridiculously extreme. Enjoy life, drive off the beaten track, jump in that puddle, take a risk and enjoy that desert. After all, life is for living.

HEALTHY MODERATION

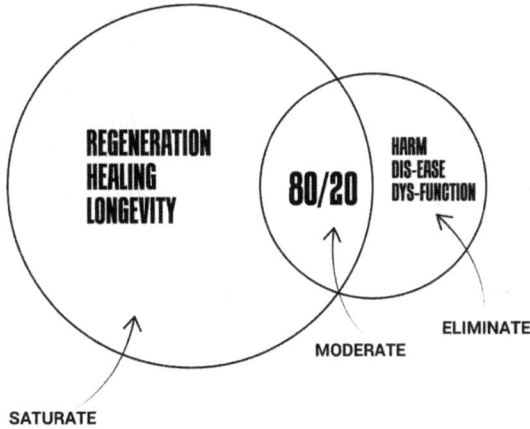

REGENERATION HEALING LONGEVITY **80/20** **HARM DIS-EASE DYS-FUNCTION**

ELIMINATE

MODERATE

SATURATE

Wine at 5—Did you know that moderate but regular consumption of wine (with friends and/or food) is part of some centenarian lifestyle. Perhaps it is less about the fermented grapes and more about the social connection and natural food. None the less, it is a practice that has stood the test of time.

The key point is that self-care is not about perfection. It's about finding what works for you in the context of your life. Which means that these Blue Zone principles and the SelfCare matrix of 12 Medicines, simply becomes a framework to help you make better lifestyle choices each day. Create your own standards for living and take radical responsibility without guilt, self-judgment or comparison. Ultimately your life = your choice!

7 COMMON ELEMENTS FOR SUPERCENTENARRIANS

Curious adventurers like Master Del Pe and others have noticed that centenarians and supercentenarians groups were found in specific geographical environments with overall good Feng Shui or geomancy that tuned into the natural flow of the world. Imagine tuning into the sun's energy each morning and evening, the fresh flow and circulation of clean air, the flow of water and growing food in living soil with an abundance of nutrients needed for daily function.

Beyond geography, these longevity hotspots have eight simple correlations.
1. They lived with an abundance of fresh food from natural sources, grown in nourishing environments free of chemicals and toxic pollution.

2. They had fresh air and natural spring water with a higher alkalinity.
3. Having friends and family around, connection, was a key.
4. People lived with a stress free sense of lightness, laughter and fun. Simply living.
5. They lived functional lives, movement was a way of life, not a chore or exercise regime.
6. They lived with a sense of purpose, beyond the materialistic world. It kept their minds sharp and active until their final breath.
7. They had a sense of faith in the goodness of life and spiritual connection to their version of the "source" and circulation of energy in our lifetimes.

Let's explore 5 of those communities in more detail, so that you can see these principles in modern communities and apply them to the context of your own community.

OKINAWA IN JAPAN
THE PLACE WHERE WOMEN AGE GRACEFULLY

If you are a woman looking for longevity secrets then the solution is in plain sight. **Okinawa is home of the world's oldest living women!**

It is also home to beautiful blue waters and some of the most divine diving spots in the world. It has been coined the "Japanese Hawaii." Despite years of hardship after WWII, Okinawans established a lifestyle and environment to live long and healthy lives. Perhaps the collective pain felt during that time, brought people closer together and reminded them of nature's importance.

What is most noticeable is that compared to the rest of the world. Okinawans have less cancer, heart disease and dementia than others on the planet.

Perhaps their greatest secret is their stoic dedication to maintain relationships.

- **Connection:** They maintain a powerful social network called a "moai."
- **Food:** Okinawans rely on plant-based food.
- **Nature:** Okinawans have a green thumb and are intricately linked with the natural world by planting their own medicinal garden.
- **Movement:** Movement is a part of life. Not a chore or an "exercise." Movement serves a functional life purpose.
- **Work:** Okinawans also have a strong sense of purpose in life, the Japanese call it "ikigai" which means "your reason for being."

A "Moai" is a lifelong band of good friends that always support you. Maintaining strong social networks are natural to our human existence and it's what allows us to thrive. In our modern world the antidote to isolation is connection and learning to thrive together. This is the basis of the Okinawan cultural practice.

Food is also an amazing part of Japanese culture. When I visited Japan, I always left a restaurant feeling lighter and more vibrant than when I went in. Okinawans rely mainly on plant based food sources and occasionally consume animal based food like pork, on special occasions.

The Okinawans take pride in their gardening which keeps them moving with purpose and allows them to develop and innate sense of connection with the natural world. They also plant medicinal plants (the expensive ones we buy at markets or online) such as; ginger, turmeric and even mugwort. They grow their own staples and consume these plants every day. You only have to take a quick minute to research the benefits of a plant-based eating regime and saturating with medicinal plants like this to truly understand and be ready to embody these longevity practices for yourself.

Movement is not a chore either, it is a part of life. Working in their gardens, walking to visit neighbors and being an active participant in community groups gives them more than enough dosage of moving medicine. Their daily movements allow for their greater range of motion later in life, better cardiovascular health and it even helps distract the mind from daily stressors. Imagine still climbing trees in your 90s, like you did as a child!

Simplicity is mastery in this community too. Okinawans pride themselves on minimalism. There is little furniture and many Okinawans share a meal sitting on mats on the floor. It is believed that as people get older, getting up and down off the floor, plus spending time outside under the sun (Vitamin D) promotes balance, lower body strength and prevents falls later in life. The best falls prevention program might be self-evident right here.

Modern cultures are tuning into the ancient wisdom of "ikigai." Older Okinawans can easily articulate their ikagai and this sense of deep purpose allows them to feel needed and fulfilled all the way through their long lives.

Their community promotes health and wellbeing across their lifespan, rather than putting the elderly people in the community in homes. Elderly Okinawans are seen to be respected spiritual leaders in their community. They are custodians of wisdom and stories that they share with the younger generation. This gives them a greater sense of purpose later in life and spending time with the younger generations, may in fact help them stay young in spirit!

Many centenarian women in Okinawa still climb trees in their 90s, catch eels and collect produce to feed their families. This may be the simplicity of their "ikigai." These seemingly simple daily tasks give them a sense of interconnectedness as a valuable member of their thriving community, linked to their own unique passions.

How connected do you feel to your community?
Have you found your reason for being?
Why do you get out of bed in the morning?
What is your best falls prevention strategy as you get older?
What are you going to suggest for your grandparents?

SARDINIA IN ITALY

As Okinawa was home to the world's oldest living women, Sardinia is home to the world's oldest living men! Sardinians live as a culturally isolated community, on an island, as a group of villages in the Barbagia region. So what is it about Sardinia that makes it so special?

- **Connection:** For Sardinians **connection** is a powerful medicine for them too. They honor family and strongly believe that this connection is a clue to their long life.
- **Lifestyle:** Men in Sardinia gather in the street each afternoon **to laugh** with and at each other and share a glass of red wine.
- **Movement:** Movement is a lifestyle where Sardinians walk for five miles a day or more.
- **Nature:** Sardinians have a great connection with the **natural** world that supports them.
- **Food:** They still hunt, fish and harvest the food they eat. They laugh and drink wine together
- **Genes:** Good genes are good; 8 in 10 Sardinians are directly linked to original Sardinians.

Sardinians longevity secret may again be found in the simplicity of connection being the ultimate medicine; by putting family first, celebrating elders and laughing with friends, Sardinian men ensure that they have a supportive social network over their lifespan.

The beauty about Sardinia's strong family values is that it helps assure that every member of the family is cared for. Modern research has shown us over and over again that people who live in strong, healthy families suffer lower rates of depression, suicide, and stress. It is important to know that we all have a family that loves us—they just might not be related by blood. You could meet someone tomorrow who has better intentions for you than someone you have known your entire life! Build your social support network with this in mind.

Like the Okinawans, grandparents in Sardinia provide love, wisdom, support, childcare and financial help, to their grandchildren and childrens' lives. They aim to continue family traditions and help raise healthy, well-adjusted family members. Imagine how much money people could save on childcare and the unconditional love that could be utilized to nourish the future generations if we all applied this with our grandparents, godparents or even community.

Living a connected and light-hearted lifestyle is powerful. Laughter reduces stress, which can lower one's risk of cardiovascular disease. Contrary to modern beliefs on alcohol, they also drink red wine at 5pm! They toast— "Kent'annos" which means "Health and life for 100 years." Maybe you don't have to make excuses for that glass of red wine with dinner after all? Just enjoy healthy moderation without drinking the whole bottle (or two!). The connection alone helps reduce stress from the day.

Movement is also a lifestyle for Sardinians. Imagine walking for at least 5 miles a day without it being a chore. Imagine the cardiovascular and mobility benefits. The Sardinians believe in staying active and working their entire life. Sardinian men commonly share that "We walk and work our entire life, even when we don't feel great."

Most Sardinians still hunt, fish and grow their own food. They eat a mostly plant-based foods alongside their classic Italian cuisine including whole-grain bread, beans, garden vegetables, fruits, cheese and homemade oil. Their pecorino cheese is made from grass-fed sheep and is high in omega-3 fatty acids. Meat is largely reserved for Sundays and special occasions.

How well connected are you to your "family" (blood or non-blood related)?
How often do you laugh and live lightly?
How connected are you to the natural world?
Is movement a lifestyle or a chore?
Do you live in the realms of healthy moderation?

IKARIA IN GREECE

Ikaria is known as the island of long life for all! No gender bias! 1 in 3 make it to their 90s!

Icaria is an isolated entrenched with beauty, culture and family tradition. On a health scale, Ikarians are almost entirely free of dementia and other chronic diseases. They live an active outdoor lifestyle and like the Sardinians maintain an abundance of social connections. Their strong social networks foster connections that last their lifetime. They prioritize family and close friends, which has been shown to benefit overall health and longevity.

- **Environment:** Some of the longest living Ikarians were those living in the high lands coming from poorer socio-economic backgrounds.
- **Movement:** Their movement came naturally into their lifestyle; walking to see a neighbor, gardening, general work, consciously engineer environments and lifestyles that promote more movement, without it being a chore or "exercise."
- **Food:** Ikarians follow a largely Mediterranean regime when it came to eating. Lots of fruits, vegetables, whole grains, beans, potatoes and of course olive oil. Herbal teas were commonly consumed rather than coffee.
- **Rest:** A mid-afternoon nap is a common practice for Ikarians, some scientific literature has suggested that people who nap more regularly have better health.

There is common belief that those from lower socio-economic backgrounds are less healthy than those living in the "developed world." However, this is not so. One could even argue that the modern lifestyles may have increased our length of life, but reduced the quality of life lived. Especially considering that 1 in 2 people are living with a chronic preventable disease that restricts them as they get older.

Some of the longest living Ikarians were those living in the high lands coming from poorer socio-economic backgrounds. As such, movement naturally integrates into their lifestyle; walking to see a neighbor, gardening, general work, consciously engineering environments and lifestyles that promote more movement. Again, without it being a chore or "exercise."

Ikarians follow a largely Mediterranean diet including lots of fruits, vegetables, whole grains, beans, potatoes and olive oil. Herbs like wild rosemary, sage and oregano were used regularly. All of these plants have a high antioxidant punch and help keep the body's cardiovascular system in good condition. Ikarians also consume animal based food such as goat's milk rather than cow's milk. Taking it one step further, they even enjoy periodic intermittent fasting or "caloric restriction" as part of their religious calendar. Imagine adding intermittent fasting and a plant based regime as a foundation to your week.

Resting, digesting and relaxing is important too. We all know that rest day can be more important than another "working day." Whether in the gym or at work. Ikarians enjoy a mid-afternoon nap. Some scientific literature has suggested that people who nap more regularly can reduce their chances of dying from heart disease by 35%! However, upon reflection. If you have time to nap in the afternoon, you are probably living a pretty stress-free lifestyle.

When was the last time you used public transport or walked to see a friend?
Do you schedule a rest day into your week, or enjoy an afternoon siesta?

Are you currently enjoying a mostly plant based eating regime, allowing for some animal based food?

NICOYAN PENISULA IN COSTA RICA

Nicoya is an 80-mile peninsula just south of the Nicaraguan border. This community is home to some of the happiest people in the world and a thriving natural environment!

Nicoya Peninsula biodiversity is large and they have a common goal to preserve nature for future generations. They are even close to running completely off renewable energy. They understand that healthy environments nourish and provide longevity for its people.

They have **common daily practices** and rituals that promote their individual and collective longevity.

- **Work:** Nicoyan enjoy physical work of all their lives. They are always involved in daily chores and regularly take in the sunshine, which helps their bodies produce vitamin D for strong bones and healthy body function.
- **Connection:** Nicoyan centenarians tend to live with their families, and children or grandchildren provide support and a sense of purpose and belonging. They maintain their social networks and get frequent visits from neighbors.
- **Work & Lifestyle:** Successful centenarians have a strong sense of purpose. They feel needed and want to contribute to a greater good. They call it a "plan de vida" or reason to live, which propels a positive outlook among elders and helps keep them active.
- **Food:** They eat a mostly plant-based diet including plentiful supplies of squash, corn, and beans. They eat fortified maize and beans and utilize the indigenous Chorotega roots.
- **Lifestyle:** A simple life allows them to also live a relatively stress-free life.

Like the Okinawans, Ikarians and Sardinians. Nicoyan centenarians tend to live with their families, and children or grandchildren provide support and a sense of purpose and belonging. This is a circular economy of wisdom sharing and support!

Rather than restricting diets, Nicoyans look to saturate their body each day with clean air, fresh water and nutrient dense food from their thriving natural environment. Their water has the country's highest calcium and mineral content. Healthy environment, healthy spring water and healthy people! It makes sense when we consider that we are over 70% water internally!

Perhaps the biggest takeaway from this beautiful culture is that by living a simple life, it allows them to also live a relatively stress-free life.

Sustaining healthy natural environments, food from mostly plant based sources, working with a sense of purpose "plan de vida," maintaining social networks for support over their lifespan, spending more time outside and simple daily practices are the secrets to longevity for Nicoyan people.

Do you too live a simple life?
Do you have a positive outlook and bias for our future together?
Do you work to live, enjoying the movement in between?
Do you support your natural environment, understanding that it is your life support system too?

LOMA LINDA IN CALIFORNIA

Can you imagine a modern day community without the burden of chronic preventable disease? Well there is one—Loma Linda in California, USA. The place where a group of Seventh Day Adventists have been found to have the nation's lowest rates of heart disease, diabetes and very low rates of obesity!

They live 10 years longer than the average. But why? Here are the components that make up their style of living:

- **Spirit:** All Adventists have faith; Believing in "god directs, god protects." This safety net removes unwanted stress. The belief that a higher power has your best interest at heart is powerful, especially in times of hardship.
- **Food:** Adventists sustain a healthy lifestyle by eating more plants, eating meat sparingly, if at all.
- **Movement:** They keep active and take pride in their daily chores. They believe that many hands make light work for the collective community. Adventists get regular, moderate exercise as part of their lifestyle.
- **Connection:** Adventists spend a lot of time with like-minded friends. They enjoy sharing each other's values and supporting each other's habits.
- **Work:** Many find a sense of purpose, and stave off depression by focusing on helping others.
- **Lifestyle:** Adventists are reminded to "Remember the Sabbath day and keep it holy." The 7th day of the week is a SelfCare Sunday!

As a result they have lower blood pressure, lower blood cholesterol , and less cardiovascular disease. Plus a healthy waist line compared to the rest of America. This community is a great example for any modern day community where chronic preventable disease are usually all too common.

Adventists spend a lot of time with like-minded friends. They find well-being by sharing each other's values and supporting each other's habits & take pride in giving something forward. Like many faiths & belief systems, Adventists encourage and provide opportunities for its members to give forward and volunteer their time or resources towards meaningful causes in their life.

Who knew that giving could make us feel so good! Might be worth trying this week.

When it comes to food, they tend to eat an early, light dinner and believe that they should "Eat breakfast like a king, lunch like a prince and dinner like a pauper." In support of a biblical diet of grains, fruits, nuts, and vegetables. The Adventists encourage a "well-balanced diet" including nuts, fruits, and legumes, low in sugar, salt, and refined grains. Natural with low human interference as "God" intended it to be.

SelfCare Sunday is a common phrase spoken these days. It originates from Adventists who are reminded to "Remember the Sabbath day and keep it holy."

All in all, Adventists have a strong faith. They maintain an optimistic viewpoint by having a deep sense of faith that the source "God," directs and protects. Their mental constructs, cultural beliefs and deep sense of faith help them walk into the unknown with a good heart, trusting in universal laws and a powerful safety net in hard times. Perhaps inspiring faith and hope is a powerful tool for longevity too?

Do you have a deep sense of faith?
Do you take a SelfCare Sunday? (or other day)
Do you eat low human interference natural food and drink plenty of water?
Do you seek to serve and help others each week?
Are you an active encourager and supporter of your friends and family, without judgment?

Isn't it amazing to consider that in every corner of the globe there is a community that has found the elixir to living a long and happy life, free of restriction and disease. These communities shine the light on how we can nurture healthy, happy and connected human beings. Reflect on the 9 core principles shared and TICK which ones you have mastered in your own life.

☐ RIGHT TRIBE—Who are one healthy tribe/group that you connect with daily? (friends, lifestyle, gym, social)
☐ FAMILY—Who do you consider family? Are you putting family first? Family can be more than just blood too.
☐ BELONGING—Do you feel a sense of belonging and community?
☐ EAT MOSTLY PLANTS—Does your diet include plant-based foods? Clean air and natural spring water?
☐ KEEP MOVING—What do you love to do that keeps you active in your lifestyle?
☐ REST, SLOW DOWN—How do you slow down, rest, digest, recover each day? (meditate, nap, fasting etc.)
☐ WORK WITH PURPOSE—Why do you get out of bed each morning?

☐ HEALTHY MODERATION—Are you living in moderation and using the 80/20 Rule?

☐ WINE AT FIVE—Are you taking social time to de-stress and enjoy yourself?

The summary and graphic below shows which of the 12 Medicines are the common core for individuals and their collective wellbeing. Do you see a pattern?

CORE MEDICINES FOR BLUE ZONES

SARDINIA, ITALY

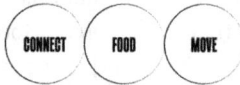

CONNECT · FOOD · MOVE

IKARIA, GREECE

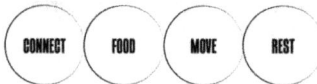

CONNECT · FOOD · MOVE · REST

LOMA LINDA, USA

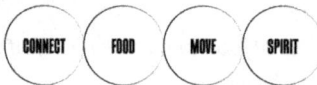

CONNECT · FOOD · MOVE · SPIRIT

NICOYA, COSTA RICA

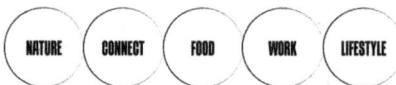

NATURE · CONNECT · FOOD · WORK · LIFESTYLE

OKINAWA, JAPAN

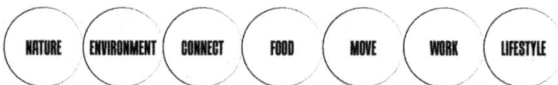

NATURE · ENVIRONMENT · CONNECT · FOOD · MOVE · WORK · LIFESTYLE

CALL TO EMBODIMENT

Write down 3 Blue Zone practices that you would like to embody in your life!

....

....

Which Blue Zone Community would you like to emulate in your community?

....

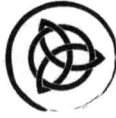

CHAPTER 10

CO-LIVING IN THE BLUE ZONE

It takes a community to raise a child. It takes a community to heal the sick, and it takes a unified community with a common goal to thrive together as one towards longevity

LIVING AS BLUE ZONE COMMUNITIES

Blue zone communities are the modern collective "we"—not just the individual "me." They use the foundation of a community-wide approach to collective and therefore individual wellbeing.

Imagine a community where all citizens, schools, employers, restaurants, grocery stores, and community leaders have come together to optimize residents longevity and well-being. Wow!

Well this is happening more than ever before.

In 2009, Dan Buettner partnered with Healthways to start the Blue Zones Project. They set to actively integrates the 9 longevity principles to whole communities. As an example, in 2010, the Beach Cities Health District in Southern California applied Blue Zones principles to three California communities: Redondo Beach, Hermosa Beach, and Manhattan Beach. Success was measured using the Gallup Healthways Well-being Index (WBI) and other economic indicators.[1]

These three beach cities in Southern California continue to show dramatic improvements since launching with Blue Zones Project in 2010. Their website reports:

- **50% drop in childhood obesity rates at Redondo Beach K-5 schools.**
- **15% drop in adult obesity and overweight rates.**
- **17% drop in smoking.** A significant unhealthy indicator in the Beach Cities was significant daily stress, higher than the national average.[2]

Significant daily stress has dropped 10 percent since 2010.

In 2011, the Blue Zones Project joined together with Wellmark Blue Cross and Blue Shield to deliver the Blue Zones Project across the State of Iowa. In 2013 Projects began in Fort Worth, Texas and the State of Hawaii. In 2014, work began in Naples, Florida, South Bend, Indiana and Klamath Falls, Oregon.

Blue zone communities understand that the health of the individuals within any community will dependent on the health of the natural environment and the ease and flow for health based behaviors within that environment.

Let's shift the perspective and co-create nourishing environments for all of us to thrive in! Blue zones are places of "We, not me."

> *"If you look at the cultures around the world where*
> *people are living the longest it's never because*
> *individuals are trying to do it."*
> **— Dan Buettner —**

BE THE NEXT BLUE ZONE COMMUNITY

Who is going to initiate the Blue zone initiative in your community? Perhaps your community could be the next Blue Zone? Join the Blue Zone project (bluezonesproject.com) with your community leaders and see if you can become the next blue zone.

Residents from Central Maui are designing a Blue Zone community with the purpose to create a community that is great to live and work in and also one that promotes the happiness and longevity of its residents. And many others are following that same direction.

For example, as of 2016, men in Hong Kong are living, on average, up to 81.3 years and women even longer at 87.3 years. Dr. Timothy Kwok, professor of geriatric medicine at the Chinese University of Hong Kong said, "Over the last few decades, Hong Kong has caught up in a big way."[3]

According to Kwok's research, "Hong Kong ranks first for enabling environments."[4] He believes that this may explain their increasing longevity. The environmental factors include things such as:

1. Easy access to everything
2. Streets are safe
3. Easy access to public transport and public amenities
4. Footbridges and walking routes remove the temptation to use a car
5. Affordable taxis and public transportation
6. Public spaces promote connection and outdoor activities like tai chi, qi jong, calisthenics and other movement based sports like soccer. Many people enjoy a meal together after exercise too!
7. Good hospitals
8. Access to good food and healthy produce.

Hong Kong is a Confucian culture, with an Asian philosophy of respect for one's parents, elders and ancestors. Older people are genuinely respected, and younger members of the family put an emphasis on ensuring the well-being of older members of the family.

However, Hong Kong is not perfect. As mentioned previously, living a long life does not necessarily mean that you live a quality life. Professor Kwok also noticed that the quick rate of overpopulation led to many second and third generation family members living without social support and financial security. Suicide rates are highest above the age of 65[5] which differs to the western world which shows the highest suicide rate is between 25–35 year old males.[6]

Hopefully now we have enough solutions, practices and rituals that you can embed into your daily routine or local environment.

Do you have access to health care?
Does your environment "actively enable" your healthy lifestyle?
Do your elderly citizens have respect?
Do you look after and care for each other?

It is time to live in nourishing environments, even if surrounded by concrete skyscrapers. We need to treat and empower each person within the context of their own environment to transition to blue zone living.

TRANSITIONING TO BLUE ZONES TOGETHER

So, how do we inspire community leaders to listen and be attracted to these solutions around the world? The messages that shine the light on some simple truths and provides the answers we are all looking for. Yet, for some reason, knowing and realizing isn't enough to take action and create a change for the benefit of all humankind.

Why is that? If we all know and we all hope for a brighter future, why are we not changing our thoughts, actions, habits and behaviors collectively to create a change that our future children need; that we need?

Compassion in World Farming worked together with Catsnake Film highlighted the answer to this universal problem that reveals my point.

They enlisted the help of Kate a real-life actress pretending to work as a marketing consultant to major food companies. The video was made similar to a TedTalk and was called *The Secrets of Food Marketing*.[7] The audience and the subject matter was real.

Kate the "marketing consultant" discusses how she is able to make any food product irresistible and needed by the consumer even if you wouldn't feed this to your child, or even your dog.

It might be a low quality burger, with a sugary drink that exceeds the daily standard for an adult let alone a child from low quality and synthetic food sources.

She shared 3 techniques that she used to make her audience emotionally buy these products.

She highlighted that the first two techniques were actually quite simple.

1. Everyone believes what they read on the label
2. If they use the words in the right way, they can convince anyone it's okay for human consumption.

The mic-drop moment came when she told the crowd that her best marketing tool was YOU, more specifically your **willful ignorance** and willingness to look the other way.

She shared this message and then walked out of the room to no applause.

What more was to be said? Despite this project being a provocative piece of video, it reveals something deeper—that it is often our willful ignorance that keeps us caught in the web of ill-health.

It reinforces why despite the glaring obvious facts, too many choose to live in red zones when they don't have to. Our willful ignorance enables us to choose things that do not serve us and allows people to market to our irrational emotions. Clever marketing knows that we will be more likely to move or buy from emotion in our busy lives, rather than the rational and often common sense knowledge we have in our minds. We search for quick fixes to help us stay busy, in lifestyles that obviously are not serving us. Perhaps we need to slow down and create time and space to step back and make better choices. As individuals, as influencers, as community leaders and as conscious enterprises we need to be responsible for the information we share and the choices we make. As Ayn Rand wrote in *The Fountainhead*, "The hardest thing to explain is the glaringly evident which everybody has decided not to see."

We must choose to overcome **ignorance with education.**

Plato famously said, "We can easily forgive a child who is afraid of the dark; the real tragedy of life is when adults are afraid of the light."

It can be explained in a million ways for us to become aware. But how do we help people see what they are willfully ignorant to? How do we collectively work towards blue zone communities? Is it by starting to change our individual behaviors?

I believe that Nelson Mandela is right when he said, "education is the one tool that will change this world." However this depends on the quality of the information being taught and shared.

> *"The purpose of education is not to validate*
> *ignorance but to overcome it."*
> **— Lawrence M. Krauss —**

The burden of chronic preventable disease can only plague humanity whilst good humans stand by and do nothing.

We need to be:

- Openly skeptic yet aware.
- Educated and download information from people walking their talk.
- Model the success and outcomes of healthy, happy, thriving communities, and integrate what they're doing into our own lives and communities.
- Act and embody the knowledge so that we can inspire people around us to do the same.
- Take ownership of our reality and provide resources to change it.
- Start to create a ripple effect to alter our existing external reality.

It starts with ourselves, but will only change collectively when we all work together from this foundation toward a future vision that serves not only ourselves but all of humanity.

So what's the solution?

WHAT IF LIFESTYLE WAS THE ULTIMATE SOLUTION?

What if lifestyle was the medicine we've been looking for. The anecdote to our universal pains and problems?

For the future, we need a different approach. Rather than trying to convince current day willfully ignorant minds to change, what if we simply focused on the future? What if we focused on children and gave them the knowledge, the tools and frameworks to consciously engineer a better future for us all?

I remember hearing a story from an indigenous elder in the north west of Australia who had been working to improve the health and wellbeing of his people. Reconciling with "stolen generations" through colonization. Interestingly, he held a different view to many others looking at the same problem.

He had made peace with the past and reconciled with the colonization that had separated his people from the land. He also acknowledged that this had happened everywhere in the world throughout time; all races, all religions, and all people. This was not just an issue for his people, but an issue for humanity as a whole.

He realized that the past had already happened, and that it cannot be changed. We needed to reconcile the future, by focusing on future generations and educating the children from past mistakes.

People have fought for their freedom in every conflict and war, which later allows for future generations to have the freedom to be and do. Even when unjust and unfair. We can learn from both pain and pleasure.

He commented by saying that to create real change, **we needed to focus on the future generations;** the children to come. He was future focused, even though I could tell he deeply cared for the current suffering and trauma of his people. He knew the solution lied in what was to come, not what had been. Educating the future children by reframing the current reality and sharing a more positive future vision for all.

Perhaps transitioning to thriving Blue zone communities means focusing on a positive future vision together? We can start now by modeling communities that already have the answers hidden in plain sight and have reconciled the past. The ones who celebrate its disruption for awakening people and humanity to a future focused collective way of living and thriving in a sustainable unity as global citizens. Humans simply being, together. Humankind.

> *"When the last tree is cut down, the last fish eaten and*
> *the last stream poisoned, you will realize that*
> *you cannot eat money."*
> *— **Cree Indian Proverb** —*

CALL TO CURIOSITY

How are you going to reflect on your own willful ignorance to keep choosing things that do not serve you or the people you care about?

Write down 5 things that you know do not serve you, but you keep choosing them.

....

....

....

....

....

Write down 5 simple solutions and realizations that are hidden in plain sight, things that do serve you and ones you are willing to action into your personal human experience. Learning to say yes to this and no to the things you mentioned above.

....

....

....

....

....

....

....

....

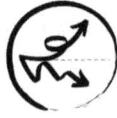

CHAPTER 11

LIVE YOUR ULTIMATE HUMAN EXPERIENCE

"And in the end it's not the years in your life
that count; it's the life in your years."
— *Abraham Lincoln* —

Mushi is a centurion in the Blue Zone village of Ogimi, Okinawa, in Japan. Nowhere else in the world will you find more centenarians per capita—almost 3x more than anywhere else recorded in the world. At the age of 103 she shares some valuable insights into how she got here. At 103, she shares that "she wants to stay healthy and live longer than anyone, for at least another 4 or 5 years." Why? Because she enjoys speaking to her grandchildren at night.

Each morning, Mushi spends time catching up with other elders in the community, drinking tea and sharing stories. Collectively Mushi and her friends share a combined age total of almost 500 years! Professors in the local community believe that this strong sense of community ensures that no one is left alone, feeling isolated or disconnected, freeing them of mental health issues like depression and other challenges.

We also know that isolation and disconnection is the worst thing we can do to a human being. Orphan babies without love and touch don't thrive.

Isolation is a killer and it's the reason why our worst criminal offenders are put in solitary confinement as punishment.

What a paradox. The antidote to the burden of preventable disease may be as simple as reducing isolation and the elixir for longevity is about creating a sense of connection and community.

100 AND BEYOND—HOW TO LIVE LIKE CENTURIONS!

Have you ever wondered why some people live to 100 and beyond whilst others don't? According to special health and longevity issue by *Time Magazine* the frontiers of longevity in replicative senescence indicate our genetic human potential could reach 142 years of age.[1] Yet, the average life expectancy of humans globally is almost half that, 72.0 years according to the World Health Organization.[2]

The paradox is self-evident. If we have the potential to live beyond 100 years, yet we only live to an average of 72 years, why do we accept that as normal? What would we have to change in order for all of us to live to 100 and beyond?

Rather than focusing on the myriad of challenges we face; let's look forward to the solution.

Yes, aging is a complex process at a cellular and genetic level. Aging leads to the deterioration of many body functions over the lifespan of an individual.[3] In an essence we can't really reverse aging per-se. The goal is just to make sure that we don't speed it up!

We can't reverse aging, just don't speed it up.

Let me explain.

Most cells cannot divide indefinitely due to a process termed cellular or **replicative senescence.**[4] It is the reason why your pet dog may have a lifespan of 10 years if they are lucky, or why a bowhead whale can live for over 200 years and how the immortal jelly fish may have figured out a way to live forever. It is also the reason why we believe that human beings have the potential to live to 142 years, yet our average lifespan is only half of that.

Does this mean that the environments we have created for ourselves and lifestyle choices we are making each day are accelerating our individual rate of aging and degeneration to the point where the average human lifespan is almost exactly half that, between 71–72 years. As mentioned previously the oldest living human beings have shown that we can live for over 120 years and blue zone communities like that of Okinawa in Japan have shown that we can build environments and communities that can become home to most centurions per capita.

7 YEAR CYCLES

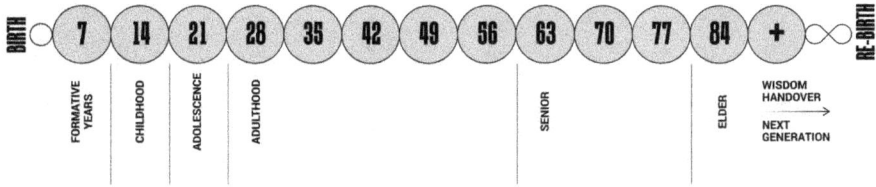

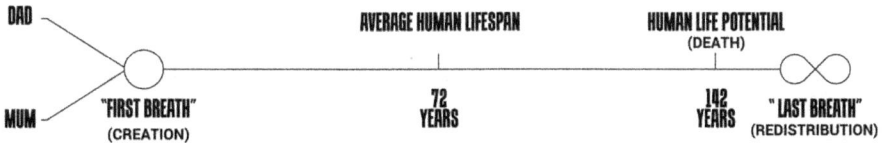

Siegfried Hekimi, PhD from The Hekimi Lab shares that it's not about finding ways to live longer but by knowing that we have an upper limit of human lifespan potential—but to slow down the process and learning how to not accelerate it.[5]

He told Radio Canada International that we are probably going to extend our human lifespan. He said, "in developed countries, we are becoming better and better at controlling our environment, resulting in less stress on the body. We control heating and cooling in our buildings, our work is generally far less arduous, we vaccinate against diseases, and we have access to better diets all year round, and better hygiene. All of this results in less wear and tear and stress on the body."[6]

> "It's humanity's greater and greater control over its
> environment and living conditions that increases
> people's average and maximal lifespan."
> — *Dr Seigfried Hekimi* —

To summarize our constant battle between our innate wisdom, the environments we live in, and our daily lifestyle choices, Dr Michael Greger shared we are battling "Inflammation, oxidation, damage and dysfunction are constantly hacking away at our telomeres (genes), at the same time our antioxidant defenses, a healthy diet and exercise, stress reduction are constantly rebuilding them."[7] We get to choose the balance of harm and care. Out innate wisdom will respond accordingly.

A SIMPLIFIED LONGEVITY EQUATION

When the rate of cellular DEGENERATION > Rate of cellular REGENERATION = *we age.*

Imagine how it feels to live a high stress lifestyle, eat processed foods, be dehydrated, depleted and perhaps even add in a hangover from a night of emotional suppression as we come to terms with the life we have chosen and the thoughts we need to numb. When you wake up the next morning... It is simple to see that the stress, the mild alcoholic toxin, and franked-food building blocks, plus dehydration puts your body in a state of accelerated cellular regeneration, and thus accelerate aging.

When the rate of REGENERATION > Rate of DEGENERATION = *we live longer.*

Imagine how it feels to wake up well rested in a hyper-oxygenated body, hydrated and ready to move. Spending time in nature, connected to high-vibing people and a passion that internally motivates you to live a lifestyle of purpose. The low stress, accompanied with internal and external nourishment are signals that the body can slow down the rate of cellular regeneration.

Pharmacist and longevity expert Farid Wassef, author of *Breaking the Age Barrier* says that "Science shows we aren't completely at the mercy of genetics."[8] That's good news! The accumulation of lifestyle choices over time means that the body's genes begin to break down once you hit forty. Leading-edge research suggests there are things you can do to reduce and slow down the aging process. Wassef shares a study that reviewed the lifestyle habits and genetic backgrounds of twins separated at birth—to sum it up quickly, genes weren't the main contributing factor of whether they were likely to develop cancer or not. In fact, their genetic DNA contributed to only 28 % of the risk. What was the other 72%?

As physician Scott Kahan, MD, says,"Genes load the gun, environment pulls the trigger."[9]

I would also add that genes load the gun, *environment and lifestyle choices* pull the trigger for how our genes express themselves over our lifespan.

Close to 95% of who we become and how we age is within our hands!

Or more so within our minds with the choices we make, leading to our actions, habits and daily rituals for self-care and longevity. Genes obviously play a role, but the rest is up to you.

I hope this leaves you feeling empowered and inspires you to take ownership of this amazing human body you have. If you wake up today as an accumulation of the choices that you made over the last 12 months, then cast a vision forward to this same time next year and start making different choices.

By minimizing harm and embodying daily rituals that slow down the aging process, we can indeed extend our lifespan within the current limits of our human potential. Perhaps one day, technology, nature and a human curiosity to live longer may lead to further advancements. But for now, this is what we know to be true, leaving chapters open for future conversations and insights.

I imagine a future where a young child picks up this book in the near future and understands what environments they need to live in, co-create and what lifestyle habits they need to embody in order to live beyond 100 years with ease. Imagine if that was our new normal. Let's choose wisely!

LIVE YOUR IDEAL LIFESTYLE FOR LONGEVITY

Scientists determine the term "lifestyle" broadly as a "typical way of life or manner of living characteristic of an individual or group."[10]

This concept includes different factors such as diet, behavior, stress, physical activity, working habits, smoking and alcohol consumption. Individual genetic background and environmental factors are intertwined to lifestyle in determining the health status of individuals.[11]

Simply speaking, these Blue zone communities have learnt to develop habits, rituals and ways of living that protect their genes, their cells and thus the longevity of their human vessel. You don't need to know all the scientific mechanisms; these blue zone centurians surely don't.

You simply need to understand the rituals and apply them to your life.

Is it really that simple? Is the most advanced secret to good health and longevity nothing more than lifestyle? No special potion or pill? No advanced bio-technology or gene splicing machinery required? Yes, that's correct.

Living this lifestyle is simple and not complex, it is not hard to understand. But, it is a choice. And sadly most people are choosing the opposite. Whether these choices are manipulated through environment, emotions, boredom or even willful ignorance is yet to be determined. But, either way, if you ever hit a point of desperation or are even inspired. Then know that you too can live towards longevity. From any starting point.

The body has an amazing ability to heal and regenerate from anywhere at any time, sometimes even spontaneously! Plus the innate wisdom of nature mixed with your genetic blueprint can be influenced to optimize your human potential and work with you to build a completely new human body within 7 years. It might seem far-fetched, but you are a regenerating self-healing miracle every day.

For those that are already living in a state of good health and wellbeing or living towards longevity, then good for you! Keep on embodying those choices and perhaps even look to inspire others in your proximity to do so too.

If you aren't living your ideal lifestyle, or you are lacking the energy and vitality you know you deserve, then it is never too late to start.

Several studies indicate that rapid improvements in health and longevity can make a "comeback" after course-correcting poor lifestyle choices. It's a testament to how resilient, adaptable and flexible our human body is to our choices. As long as the mind is willing, the body will keep going until it can go no more. When you "wake up" to the signals and symptoms that your body is giving you—those aches and pains, those food intolerances, that extra weight, those nagging thoughts or emotional triggers. Then you might be in the right place to say "enough is enough." Be inspired, before you get desperate.

CONSISTENCY IS THE CORNERSTONE

Like the Zen Buddhist saying: "Before enlightenment, chop wood, carry water. After enlightenment, chop wood, carry water." You can wait until you are sick, restricted and living in disharmonious disease. Or you can take the daily actions today that you already know help you feel good.

Long living, healthy people don't achieve wellbeing through fads, shortcuts or quick fixes. We all know this, even when those clever marketing campaigns get more savvy. You can't eat greasy fast food all week and then hope your green smoothie on Sunday will detox you. You can't begin your exercise program on Monday morning and expect a six-pack by Friday. You can't meditate for 10 minutes every day and spend the rest of your day full of stress-induced hormones and expect to remain Zen. It's unrealistic and somewhat delusional.

To live long and healthy life requires a constant, daily lifestyle of positive enrichment with human connection, nature, movement, purpose, attitude and an energetic spirit.

Your challenge is to find ways that work for you. Find ways to fit exercise into your busy week. Find ways to live a more peaceful life, even if you have to change your current habits. Find a way to fill your weekends with good friends and joyful living.

The hard truth is that no one can do it for you. Everything you need to live to over 100 years old is already here! The question is—are you willing to pivot your daily practices, habits and rituals to achieve this?

COMPOUND YOUR HEALTH BY 1% EACH DAY

If changing our lifestyle habits was easy, then we wouldn't be living in a world where 95% percent of us were living with ailments, restriction and even disease.

What if rather than focusing on getting it all together at once. You gave yourself permission to do your best and simply make better choices that you did the day before. If you did commit to simply being 1% better each day, you would start compounding your health in the same way we would all love to compound or wealth by 1% each day.

James Clear the author of *Atomic Habits* shares it simply; "Here's the punchline: If you get one percent better each day for one year, you'll end up thirty-seven times better by the time you're done. This is why small choices don't make much of a difference at the time, but add up over the long-term."[12]

It isn't as easy as it sounds either. It means that you will need to forgive yourself for past transgressions. Celebrate yourself for simply doing your best in the context of your life, your thoughts, your environment and your proximity. But now, be inspired and empowered with the knowledge and tools to make just ONE small change when you wake up tomorrow.

The power of small can have an exponential impact in your life. Will you choose a juice over a coffee tomorrow. Will you choose a surf over a cigarette. Will you choose yourself over a busy to do list. All of these small choices and actions can start to add up and build momentum. Without the need to be perfect, just a simple reminder to make better choices than you did the day before. Without judgment or comparison. One small change, just 1% daily can result in you being in a position that is 37x better than where you are today in 12 months' time

Your life. Your choice. Choose the same or choose different.

THE POWER OF SMALL HABITS
COMPOUNDED DAILY: 1% RULE

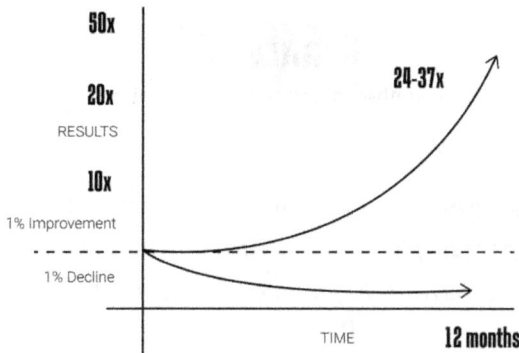

CALL TO LONGEVITY

TAKE THE IDEAL LIFESTYLE QUIZ: **selfcare.global/assess**

What is ONE SMALL change (1%) that you are going to make today?

....

....

....

What about tomorrow?

....

....

....

HOW TO MASTER YOUR MORNING IN 1 HOUR

MIND   20" Mindfullness Practice

FOOD   Hydrate, Breathe, Saturate

MOVE   30" Motion is Lotion

CONNECTION
Together is better, find your tribe

"The purpose of a doctor or any human in general should
not be to simply delay the death of the patient, but to
increase the person's quality of life."
— *Patch Adams* —

12 MEDICINES

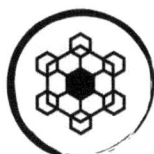

TECH

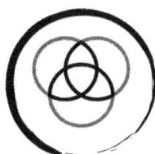

SPIRIT

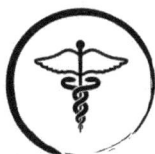

MODERN

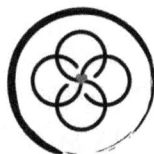

WORK

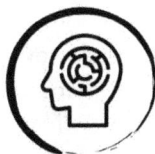

MIND

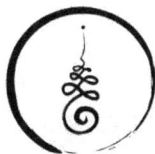

LIFESTYLE

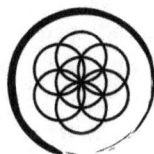

FOOD

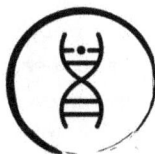

GENES

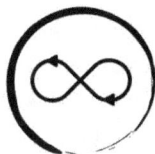

MOVE

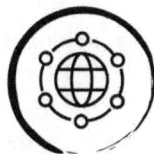

ENVIRONMENT

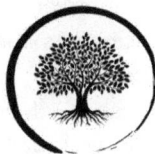

NATURE

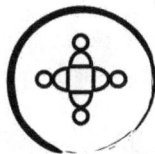

CONNECTION

Dive deeper – (Selfcare.global/12medicines)

START YOUR OWN NATURAL REVOLUTION

We now come to the essence of the SelfCare revolution. How do you start to reach that overflow of joy and good health? By embodying these **12 Medicines of SelfCare** of course. Integrate this framework into your own life!

Since that moment of exhaustion and dysfunction so many years ago, I have extensively researched and developed 12 Medicines that encompass each perspective of our lives. When I stepped out of the current systems of healthcare, I was able to reflect on people's state of being from both a bigger vantage point and also a more intimate one. It saved me in many ways.

I have drawn on my experiences and the expertise of many scholars, scientists, researchers and philosophers, conservationists and campaigners to illustrate the connectedness and SELFCARE balance between humanity, nature and these medicines.

When in harmony these 12 Medicines, that ultimately align human and universal principles, will provide each of us with boundless wisdom of self-care. Remember flowers, like humans are perfectly formed and do not need to be fixed. Unless there is a specific accident, trauma or acute infection, we have all the innate mechanisms within us to survive and thrive, provided that we are connected to nature, nourishing environments and supportive communities. The Medicines are designed to be **EMBODIED**, not just read.

Think of these 12 Medicines as the prevention of disease and dysfunction and the ongoing maintenance of your body's sophisticated systems. They are a powerhouse for natural health and healing, longevity and performance. Three of these 12 Medicines are *external* to our human body and are typically the source of the energy you need to survive and thrive; nature, environments and connection.

Seven Medicines are *internal* and aim to working in sync with each other; genes, mind, food, movement, work, lifestyle as well as our sense of spirituality.

Lastly, there are two important interventional Medicines found in modern medicine and technological advancements that have the potential to enable and empower your unique human experience.

When you read and apply these 12 Medicines you will be in motion, applying all that you have learned to your daily life. You'll be able to reconnect with your intrinsic wisdom allowing you to live and function optimally. But most importantly you will be able to hand this knowledge onto future generations. You will live your legacy!

Start with the 3 external and foundational Medicines.

1. Do you live connected or disconnected from nature's life support systems: fresh air, sunshine and natural spring water that is free of the impurities and toxins?
2. How do your proximity and connections fill or empty your cup: do they fill you up, energize you or drain you?
3. How do the environments you live in enable and empower your wellbeing or prevent it?

Look internally at the 7 Medicines igniting your innate power.

1. How do your daily lifestyle choices and habits positively ignite or negatively inhibit your GENETIC potential and innate wisdom?
2. How does your MIND (beliefs, thoughts, actions) influence your life? Is your default thinking above or below the line?
3. How does your MIND influence your daily lifestyle choices—what types of FOOD you eat, how you MOVE, what do you SPIRITUALLY believe in, how you WORK, and which type of LIFESTYLE you choose.

Look externally to the 2 interventional tools and Medicines:

1. How do you use and leverage technology to stay healthy and promote health?
2. How do you utilize modern medicine to stay in harmony or intervene to keep you well when necessary?

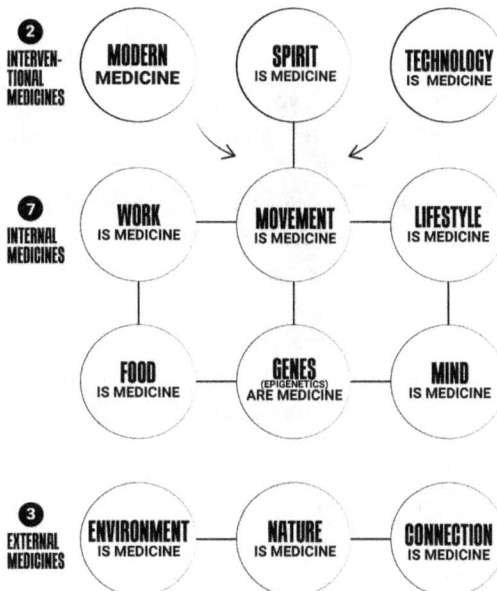

LET'S GET IN MOTION WHILE WE LEARN TOGETHER

The 5 core principles you will learn in this section are how to:

1. Ignite your human potential
2. Empower your experience by taking radical self-responsibility
3. Optimize your human performance
4. Live to longevity, without dysfunction, restriction or disease
5. Live your legacy and be a high-impact human

Selfcare.global/empower

If you would like to take action as you learn each medicine and choose your own lifestyle habits without judgment and comparison, then join "EMPOWER"—our online, interactive, action-orientated course and workbook that will complement your journey and kick you into the action dynamic. You can DIY (do-it-yourself) by following the book or you can do it with some guided support. All energy exchanged with us will be circulated back into helping us have a bigger impact.

We start by welcoming you and igniting your curiosity to dream by asking you: What does your ideal day look like? What does your ideal lifestyle look like, if time, money and resources were not an issue?

8 steps to EMPOWER your own SelfCare revolution

1. Be evidence-based, solutions-focused: Blue Zones
2. Start with your *why*, an inspiring future vision: your True North
3. Create a personal and meaningful goal: What by When
4. Align your internal compass with your True North
5. Choose your normal; minimize self-harm and find a balance of healthy moderation
6. Master SelfCare and the 12 Medicines
7. Fill your cup each day and serve from overflow
8. Self-mastery, power of small and 1% growth per day.

By the end of this book and course you will already be in motion with your own self-care, creating a unique and personalized 3 pillar morning program, where every time you do something good for yourself, something good happens in the world!

4 STEPS TO GET STARTED: FIRST, SELF ASSESS

ASSESS → SHARE

Selfcare.global/assess | Selfcare.global/community

Step 04

ONE PERSON CAN MAKE A DIFFERENCE

GLOBAL
LOCAL
FAMILY
GO FIRST
FRIENDS
COMMUNITY
BLUE ZONES

"RIPPLE EFFECT"

Step 01

HOW FULL IS YOUR CUP?

85%+
70-85%
50-70%
<50%

Step 03

FOOD / MOVE / SPIRIT / WORK / LIFESTYLE
MIND
GENES
ENVIRONMENT
NATURE
CONNECTION

Step 02

STEP 1: WHICH OF THE 4 ZONES ARE YOU STARTING IN?

HOW FULL IS YOUR CUP?

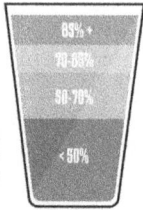

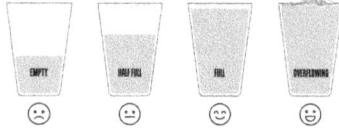

85%+	
70-85%	
50-70%	
<50%	

EMPTY ☹   HALF-FULL 😐   FULL 🙂   OVERFLOWING 😊

4 ZONES	100 PEOPLE
BLUE ZONE	1
GREEN ZONE	4
ORANGE ZONE	45
RED ZONE	50

VESSEL   *PATH*   DESTINATION

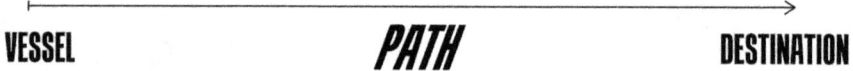

START WHERE YOU STAND.
Which zone are you in right now? Tick only ONE box.
- O Red Zone
- O Orange Zone
- O Green Zone
- O Blue Zone

Why do you feel that you are in this zone?

WHERE ARE YOU MOVING TOWARDS
Which zone are you inspired or desperate enough to move to next? Tick only ONE box.
- O Red Zone
- O Orange Zone
- O Green Zone
- O Blue Zone

How would it FEEL to move out of the zone you are in and be living in another zone?

WHY is it important to be courageous enough to make that change now? (for you, for others, for family, for purpose?)

STEP 2: SELFCARE INTEGRATED WELLNESS WHEEL

*Take the Medicines quiz, then fill it out the Wellness Wheel below.

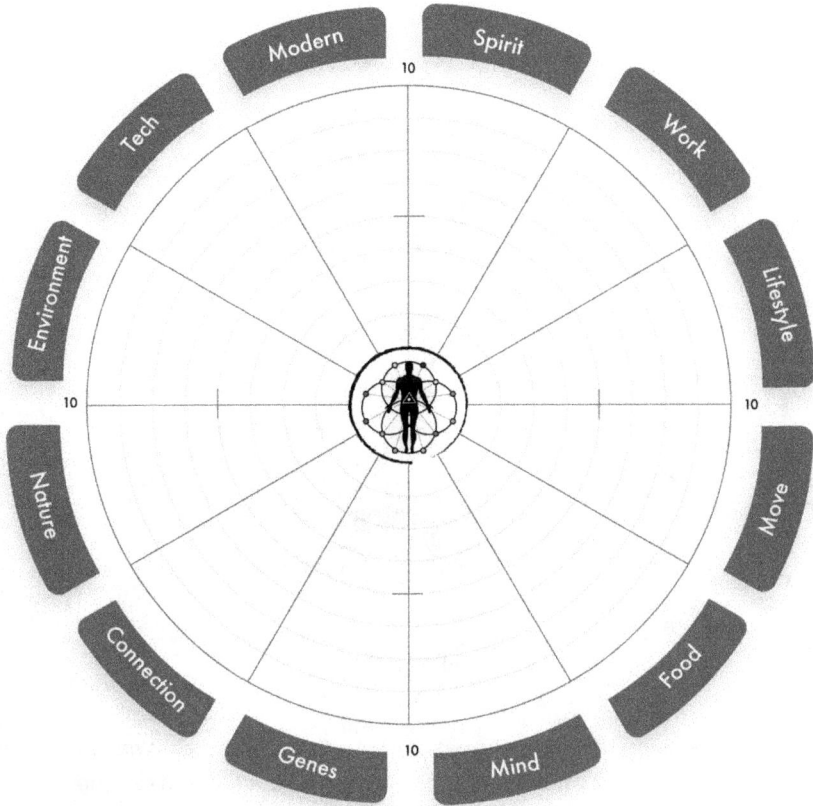

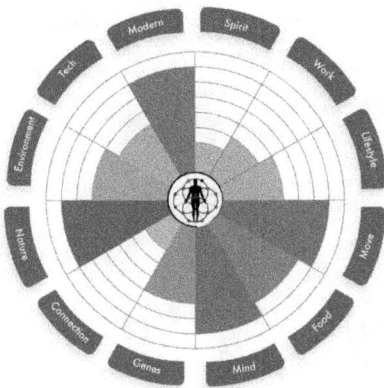

	OUT OF 10
Nature	9
Environment	5
Connection	3
Genes	6
Mind	9
Food	8
Move	9
Work	4
Lifestyle	5
Spirit	3
Modern	9
Tech	4

STEP 3. FILL YOUR CUP AND SERVE FROM OVERFLOW

Take your health and wellbeing "cup" assessment and draw your results below!

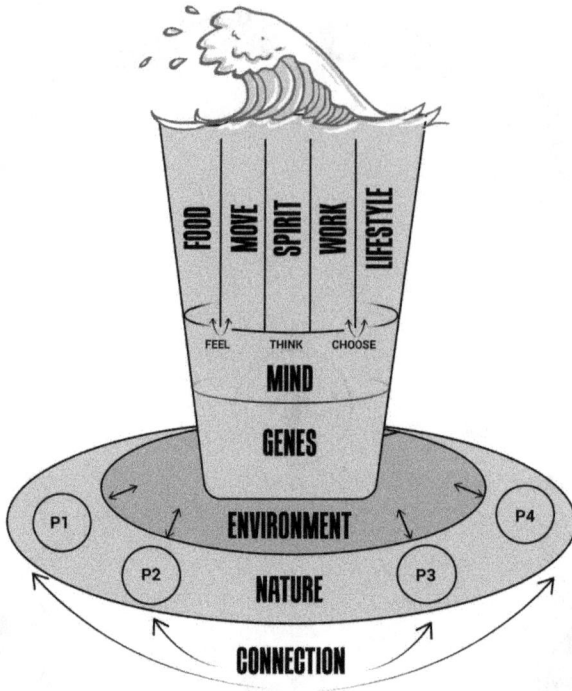

Once you have taken the 12 Medicines quiz, it will become clear which medicines you are nourishing (FULL) and neglecting (EMPTY) in your life. You can then arrange them into your own health and wellbeing cup to see how each medicine integrates and influences you.

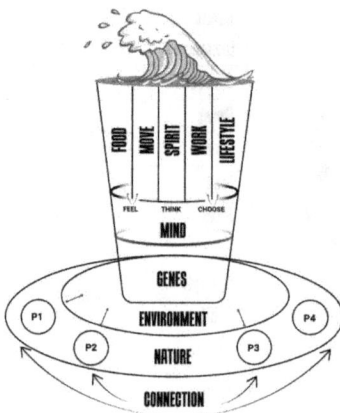

	OUT OF 10
Nature	9
Environment	5
Connection	3
Genes	6
Mind	9
Food	8
Move	9
Work	4
Lifestyle	5
Spirit	3
Modern	9
Tech	4

STEP 4. WHAT LEVEL OF POSITIVE IMPACT HAVE YOU MASTERED?

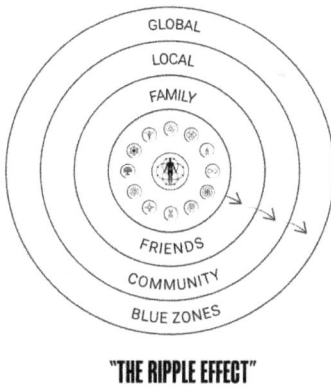

"THE RIPPLE EFFECT"

IMPACT SCALE

10,000 +	GLOBAL COMMUNITY	
1000	NATIONAL COMMUNITY	
100	LOCAL COMMUNITY	IF WE ALL DID JUST THIS! TOGETHER WE COULD MAKE THE WORLD WORK FOR ALL OF US!
10	FAMILY COMMUNITY	
1	YOU, GO FIRST	

ONE TO MANY

Along the journey, you may have heard of expressions like "You can't pour from an empty cup" or "Put your oxygen mask on before assisting others."

When it comes to impact, many of us want to save the world or serve others before serving and saving ourselves. I too have lost my health in the service of others. I have been left drained and empty mentally, physically, emotionally and even financially, wondering how I ended up there again and again.

It is also true that we all deserve to be filled in the same way that we pour. However, many of us are operating from an unconscious desire to have our needs met, with no intention to circulate that energy to others. I'm sure you have woken up one day to find that your job, your partner or even friends have been happy to receive your energy, time and guidance, only to find that they are not there when you need them.

Hopefully this section will help you realize whether you are in a position to impact others, or whether you are in a position to seek support and help to first impact yourself. The truth is that we can serve from an empty, half-full or even overflowing cup. The paradox is that our true purpose is human and sometimes helping someone else, energetically fills you up too!

Your IMPACT LEVEL (Tick just ONE box)

O 1: Your cup is empty or half-full—energetically YOU need support.

O 10: Your cup is relatively full—YOU can positively impact your family and friends.

O 100: Your cup is full and overflowing at times—your front doorstep is in harmony and you have the ability to positively impact your local community.

O 1000: You have mastered the above and can have a positive impact on a national level.

O 10,000: You are in a position to have a positive impact globally.

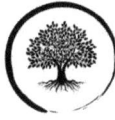

1

NATURE IS MEDICINE

"The art of medicine consists in amusing the patient while nature cures the disease."
— *Voltaire* —

REWILD YOURSELF

In 1979 a teenage boy in northeast India single-handedly began a conservation legacy that the whole world would come to admire. One day after a storm, the young Jadav Payeng came across dozens of dead snakes on a barren sandbar along his island home of Majuli on the Brahmaputra River.

The snakes had been washed ashore in the squall and subsequently died from exposure on the harsh eroded expanse of shoreline. His home was constantly under threat of disappearing due to soil erosion along its riverbanks from the affects of deforestation and severe flooding.

Payeng's compassion for the snakes and his distress at the cause of their suffering motivated him to plant 20 bamboo shoots along the deserted shore. Every day he planted more trees, bringing in seeds from the outer forest until the plantings on the sandbar reached maturity to germinate themselves.

For forty years, Jadav Payeng has been planting trees along his island in the Brahmaputra River. He has become known as The Forest Man of India because his dedication has created an incredible forest reserve covering 1,360 acres![1] The forest even attracts Bengal tigers, rhinos, deer, and a seasonal herd of elephants that come to birth their calves. Today he is extending his forest project into other degraded areas of the island region.

Payeng has become a shining example all over the world, how one person's committed actions can mitigate the actions of many. Today he says the forest feels like his family—what an amazing connection with nature.

WE *ARE* NATURE

We are not separate. The elements in the soil, the plants, the oceans and even the stars are the very same elemental building blocks that make up our human body. Somewhere along life's beautiful and chaotic journey, we collectively lost our way. We have forgotten that the natural world is our primary life support system, nourishing us with every breath of air, every sip of water, every bite of food and every ray of sunlight. We have forgotten that nature is our foundational medicine. Not complementary or alternative; foundational.

Nature designed the human body and its systems to perfection.

This chapter will remind you of the innate knowledge that deeply connects nature and us as one; that we must plug into this connection to fuel our health and longevity. The symptoms, signals, dysfunctions and diseases that plague the modern human being are a reflection of our current disconnection from the natural world, from our biological support system. We built empires, concrete jungles and modern lifestyles at great expense to our health and the natural world. And now we are paying the price.

We are drowning in isolation in concrete cities, swamped by technology at every turn, breathing air fowled by pollution and swimming in oceans and rivers that make you feel dirtier coming out, than when you went in. The sooner we start reconnecting and nourishing the natural environments that support us, the sooner our health and wellbeing will elevate and our human potential will be truly ignited.

To understand how **Nature is Medicine**, let's consciously link ourselves back to nature—right now! Take a deep breath and feel the oxygen saturate your lungs, flooding your bloodstream with life force. It is from nature that the elemental building block of oxygen ignites life, healing and regeneration within every cell of our human body.

I felt this first hand when I was rebuilding my health; every moment I spent in nature left me feeling better than when I'd arrived. We are designed to renew and replenish from the stocks of nature.

Though we are interconnected as one giant web of life, nature can survive just fine without us. However humans cannot survive without nature. We must maintain our support system. If we can build and co-create environments that are integrated with the natural world then we can learn to thrive together in balance with nature, not separate from it. When we live in harmony and connection with the natural world and allow for regeneration of what we consume, then both nature and humans can thrive. Let's begin.

WHAT IS YOUR ECOLOGICAL FOOTPRINT?

Along with our ingenuity comes humanity's insatiable demand for natural resources to maintain the onslaught of "progress." Dr Jane Goodall, from her unique experience with endangered primates and her passion for conservation, poses the question that we have all been avoiding:

"Here we stand, the cleverest species ever to have lived. So how is it we can destroy the only planet we have."

Are we a parasite on the Earth? Living at the expense of our own support system?

To understand the answer we need to reframe the question; how many Earths do you think it takes to sustain our current habits as humankind? According to the Global Footprint Network, "Today humanity uses the equivalent of 1.75 Earths to provide the resources we use and absorb our waste. This means it now takes the Earth one year and eight months to regenerate what we use in a year."[2] This is known as the world's ecological deficit, which has been growing since the 1970s. Each year, human demand on resources surpasses what Earth can regenerate in the same period.[3]

Now, we could take this as a reason to spend trillions of dollars finding ways to inhabit Mars but that's like asking people to go and live in the desert! It seems far simpler to spend trillions of dollars in sustaining this amazing living planet we have been gifted! Understanding the importance of our individual and community ecological footprint is vital in determining how we can learn to live sustainably at 1.0 Earths or, even better, to function in ecological reserve.

Every choice counts.

Before we blame governments, industries and others for the way the world is today, let's take a good look in the mirror. Let's look at every choice we make as a consumer and ask ourselves does it feed into systems that promote *connection* or *disconnection* with the natural world? Let's raise our awareness of our part in everything.

As an example, you may celebrate the fact that you stand up against animal cruelty, but do you still eat factory-farmed animal products—eggs, meat or poultry? I ask this without judgment because I too, am conscious that as the author of this book I have expended trees to print this, used computers and electricity to write this and I have consumed food from multiple sources along the way. It was only when I understood my personal ecological footprint based on my choices that I could take ownership for my role in our ecological overshoot!

It's all about balance. Through our partnership with B1G1, ten trees will be planted for every copy of this book sold, supporting a circular economy as well as the bees![4] Your impact will be visible on **selfcare.global** and we can measure the ripple effect of meaningful change we have in the world together.

Firstly though, how do we find balance and harmony with nature when the hard truth is that 8 in 10 of us live beyond our means? "More than 80% of the world's population lives in countries that are running ecological deficits, using more resources than what their ecosystems can renew."[5]

To determine this number, each person, city, state or nation's ecological footprint can be compared to its biocapacity. If a community's ecological footprint exceeds the region's biocapacity, that region is out of balance and runs an ecological deficit. The community's demand for goods and services that its land and seas can provide—fruits and vegetables, meat, fish, wood, cotton for clothing, and carbon dioxide absorption—exceeds what the region's ecosystems can renew.[6]

We need to share and circulate resources, living within our means for the benefit of future generations. We must listen to the Earth's message by questioning our old beliefs and choices, making real change and connection. Our children will feel the results of our actions, firstly by the state of the environment that they will inherit and secondly their role in the balance of nature that we will have shown them.

> *"Human use, population, and technology have reached*
> *that certain stage where mother Earth no longer*
> *accepts our presence with silence."[7]*
> *— Dalai Lama XIV —*

THE SUPREME BALANCE OF NATURE

Look around and you'll find balance exists everywhere within the natural world. Often it is a quiet and subtle exchange of energy between organisms while other examples show a clear and direct symbiosis. "You scratch my back, and I'll scratch yours" is a common synergy in the animal kingdom. Different species often help each other out in the wild, using their distinct skills to get things they both want.

Some of the coolest animal friendships in the natural world include; gray wolves and striped hyenas hunting together, utilizing their different hunting specialties when prey is particularly scarce. Urchin crabs carrying venomous sea urchins on their backs as a form of protection while the urchin gets a lift to new feeding grounds. Honeyguide birds of Africa leading people to beehives who in turn leave behind the wax combs for the birds to feed on. And we see oxpecker birds eat ticks on zebras' and hippos' coats, relieving them of pests and getting an easy meal.[8] There is no take without providing something in return.

The whole natural world has evolved into a beautiful act of balance; Earth is its own biome and integrated system. Initially we were a small part of this system. Human evolution however, particularly our expanding brain size and intelligence, exponentially increased our survival, population and consumption, tipping nature out of balance. Every time we produce drastic change in nature we detrimentally interfere with the whole ecosystem.

An incredible example of this was discovered when the gray wolf was reintroduced to Yellowstone National Park in the US in 1995. It illustrated how a huge integrated system can be significantly affected by one species and in this particular case, by the *return* of that species to an ecosystem, an extremely rare opportunity to study.

The wolves had disappeared from the National Park by 1930. Largely due to hunting from the success of government predator control programs![9] After much research and 70 years without the top predator in the Park, the US authorities relocated 31 wolves (from Alberta, Canada) back into Yellowstone in 1995.[10] Within a few years of their reintroduction, something positively significant happened to the biodiversity of the whole Park's ecosystem.

The wolves not only brought down the resident elk population, their presence changed the behavior of the elk. From decades of grazing unhindered all over the Park, the elk moved back into more secluded areas, thus protecting the open valleys from overgrazing. The elk no longer meandered along the riverbanks with their heavy hooves, but kept moving quickly. Vegetation returned and stabilized the riverbanks.

Beavers spread out again and built new dams and ponds, these changes had multiple positive effects on stream hydrology as well as enticing other species to return. The willow saplings could now grow tall again and many bird species also returned. The environment started to regain its balance through "top-down control," whereby the top predators regulate and control the structure of particular ecosystems.[11]

Yellowstone has not been fully returned to its original state, there are still ongoing studies into small areas that haven't responded as overtly to the wolves' presence but that's evidence of a human mind looking for linear solutions in this story. Nature does not work that way; it is circular, adaptive, regenerative and forever changing. During the pandemic of 2020, humans were removed from nature...nature thrived and regenerated. When we re-wild ourselves, let's carry this mindset of sustaining balance and harmony with us.

IT'S A WILDLIFE EMERGENCY

You may have tuned in by now to the global movement, "Extinction Rebellion," evidence that human beings are becoming increasingly aware of and concerned about the collateral impact we are having on the natural world.[12] However many people couldn't even guess at the true extent of man's impact on wildlife numbers.

Despite only making up 0.01% of Earth's biomass, the rise of humanity has caused the loss of more than 80% of all wild animals and 50% of plants![13]

A biomass census in 2017 by PNAS (The Proceedings of the National Academy of Sciences USA) finally quantified human impact with these real and shocking numbers. The study's authors declare that, "Over the relatively short span of human history, major innovations, such as the domestication of livestock, adoption of an agricultural lifestyle, and the Industrial Revolution, have increased the human population dramatically and have had radical ecological effects."[14]

The findings of the *Living Planet Report 2018* produced by the World Wildlife Fund (WWF), reinforced the shocking truth of global wildlife loss. The report states that populations of mammals, birds, fish and reptiles reduced by 60% between 1970 and 2014, a stark decline attributed mainly to habitat loss, degradation, and overexploitation of natural resources; all the affects of "exploding human consumption."[15]

We saw the implications of the absence of just *one* species from the Yellowstone National Park ecosystem. It is confronting to conceive the affects of removing 60% or more of the species from the vast and immeasurable ecosystems around the world, and yet that is the harsh reality.

Following the report, Mike Barrett, Executive Director of Science and Conservation at WWF put it bluntly,

"We are sleepwalking towards the edge of a cliff...The shocking truth is that the wildlife crash is continuing unabated. This is far more than just being about losing the wonders of nature, desperately sad though that is. This is actually now jeopardising the future of people. Nature is not "nice to have"—it is our life-support system."[16]

We are both the problem and the solution.

If we can re-wild wolves, then perhaps we can re-wild ourselves and reconnect with nature's life support system. Marco Lambertini, Director General of WWF International believes, "We can no longer ignore the impact of current unsustainable production models and wasteful lifestyles."[17] The fact that we created these systems that guide our daily consumer decisions, means we can change it. That's promising. But where do we start?

The need for natural resources will long continue so we must make a collaborated commitment to sustain the natural world so it can continue to sustain us, and the countless generations to come. The pivot is simple; create tools, build cities, consciously engineer businesses and build homes—just make sure that they are connected with nature's circular "economies"; ensure we are restoring the balance of what we take and allowing for regeneration; ensure we are consuming mindfully and consciously, for the sake of our children and theirs.

WE NEED *NATURE* TO SURVIVE

If oxygen is life then so is the Amazon Rainforest. Often referred to as the "Lungs of the planet," it is the largest, most diverse tropical rainforest on Earth and home to more than half of all plant and animal species in the world. It is unique, irreplaceable and plays an essential role in cleaning the air we breathe. This huge carbon sink absorbs an essential amount of the world's carbon emissions, invisibly helping to regulate the world's climate.[18]

Elon Musk tweeted in 2020 that he will be donating $100 million towards a prize for best carbon capture technology. My heart was elevated when I saw most of the replies said, plant a tree! Knowing that a fully grown tree can absorb up to 21kg of carbon dioxide per year, not to mention supporting plankton in the sea by protecting our whale friends. This is a beautiful example of the mind's ability to make the simple, complex.

The shortsightedness of humans is staggering considering this unique natural asset has been destroyed by deforestation at an unsustainable rate. Clearing of the Amazon began in the 1960s and reached a peak in the 1990s when an area the size of Spain was felled, primarily to clear land for cattle and soybean production.[19] As global concerns have grown over the last few decades, deforestation rates have fallen overall however it's a tenuous feat given the menace from consumerism, capitalism and political agendas is still real. The Amazon is still disappearing at a shocking rate, reducing the region's scale and unique biodiversity.

Recently, in 2020, we have witnessed Amazonian Shaman elders like Davi Kopenawa Yanomami and others as they have come out from under the forest canopies to warn modern civilizations that we are moving past a point of no return. Will we listen? Will we understand that every time an elder dies, a library is burnt. It's time to listen.

Indigenous people of the Amazon feel this loss acutely. In 2014, in a protected area deep in Peru, members of the Harakmbut communities embarked on a pilgrimage into the Amazon to reconnect with a long-lost and sacred place known as "Harakmbut Face." Their journey is documented in a short film *The Reunion*, which reveals the extent of the cultural challenges they face in modern times but even more shocking was the scale of the environmental degradation they saw; huge abandoned wastelands created by mining and logging in the heart of their so-called reserve.[20] Unfortunately this scenario is not isolated and there are many satellite images capturing before and after pictures of such sites in the forest, exposing the enormous scale of the devastation.[21]

To understand the importance of forests like the Amazon, ask yourself what fundamental element do we consume hundreds of liters of each day to sustain our life? Oxygen. What do trees and plants release as a by-product of photosynthesis? Oxygen. If there were no plants and no trees, there would be no oxygen, no human life. This might help you appreciate that 100-year-old tree in your backyard, or motivate you to stand up for those wetlands and trees in your local community.

When we destroy our natural assets, we are indirectly destroying ourselves. It's a form of unconscious suicide. What will it take for each of us to realize this and change the way we interact with the world around us?

Albert Einstein summed up the challenge and paradox for future generations when he said, "Only two things are infinite, the universe and human stupidity, and I'm not sure about the former."

WE NEED *ANIMALS* TO SURVIVE

We've established that our survival is dependent on nature and each other, but more than that it depends on our connection to *all* living beings. To truly acknowledge and embrace the role that each living animal plays in our collective health and well-being, we need to fully understand their significant function in balancing entire ecosystems.

The huge wolves of Yellowstone are one example of rebalancing an ecosystem but ecosystems can also rest on the lives of the smallest inhabitants, right down to the simple bee. A seemingly small and insignificant insect, yet it's function as a pollinator cannot be overstated—playing a massive role in our human survival.

Maurice Maeterlinck, a Belgian Nobel Prize winner, playwright and essayist, wrote his classic book *The Life of the Bee* back in 1901 and declared, "If the bee disappeared off the face of the earth, man would only have four years left to live."[22] Maeterlinck may not have been a scientist but he was an expert beekeeper who identified the intrinsic role bees play in every local ecosystem around the globe.

Certain animals also directly impact the *global* earth biome. It is now understood that whales play a crucial part in our global ecosystem, both in the health of the oceans and our atmosphere too. You're probably wondering—how can a whale down in the ocean, impact something up in the atmosphere? Let me explain.

We all know that whales eat krill but as whale numbers began to decline from overhunting, surprisingly so did the numbers of fish and krill. Killing whales led to *less* food in the oceans, which seems the opposite of what you'd expect right? However scientists actually discovered that whale habits are vital in the life cycle of krill and fish, so their decline immediately and detrimentally impacted other species. Whales help to sustain the entire living system of the ocean—more whales means more fish.

Even more amazingly, plankton, which also grows more profusely due to whale habits, absorbs carbon dioxide from the atmosphere while in the topmost layers of the ocean. The remaining plankton not consumed in the food chain, sinks to the bottom of the ocean and in effect, stores large amounts of carbon dioxide, keeping it out of the atmosphere. The simple conclusion is more whales equal more fish and less carbon dioxide in our atmosphere. What would you prefer promoting? Paying for a carbon offset or co-creating a world where nature and humans are intricately connected as one?

HEALING POTENTIAL OF NATURE

Industrialized communities, concrete jungles, time spent on technology and living in a virtual reality have been shown to negatively impact not just our physical health, but our mental health and well-being. A lack of time in the natural world has been associated with reductions in physical health and a rise in mental health issues such as anxiety and depression. Excessive screen time has also been associated with loss of empathy and lack of altruism.[23] Which is the very thing Dr Goodall concedes is her biggest fear for humanity; apathy and a disconnection from the natural world around us.[24]

Perhaps technology can be medicine, but it may also be driving our rising epidemic of mental health issues. Technology can enable humanity, but in this Medicine I want to emphasize its potential to disconnect us from each other and the natural world in the process. We need to find the balance. Connecting back with nature, whether walking, surfing, trekking, camping or simply being in nature has been shown to reduce our anger, fear, and depression and improve our mood and psychological well-being. This not only increases our happiness, it makes us feel better physically.

For the rationalists out there, what does the science say? On a human level we all know that we feel better when we're surrounded by nature. Having plants in our offices makes us feel better and promotes clean air where we work. With that in mind, why couldn't allied health professionals prescribe nature as a treatment? Well—some now do!

PRESCRIBING NATURE AS MEDICINE

In 2019, the government health board for Shetland in Scotland authorized their GPs to prescribe nature to their patients![25] Various nature activities can now be prescribed to supplement normal medications and therapies for chronic and debilitating illnesses. Surprising to some, but it is working! The mounting evidence for the benefits of nature on mental and physical health is extensive.

Spending time in nature can reduce blood pressure, anxiety, aggressive tendencies, ADHD symptoms, improve pain control and the immune system while also increasing happiness! "If you spend 90 minutes of your day outside in a wooded area, there will be a decrease of activity in the part of your brain typically associated with depression."[26] So you see what I mean by saying nature is literally medicine? Just 90 minutes in nature a day can be great medicine.

In support of this have been studies by psychologists who investigated how people cope with isolation such as solo explorers and mountaineers. They found that despite being alone for an extended period, these adventurers found immense spiritual comfort and mental strength from the majesty of the natural world surrounding them.

According to Norwegian psychologist Gro Sandal at the University of Bergen in Norway, transcending the reality of their situation was a common coping mechanism that, "...made them feel safer and most interesting of all, less alone."[27]

They bridged the isolation with nature because human beings were not designed to be alone. We can connect with nature in the same way we connect to each other. It may even enable us to connect deeper within ourselves so that we can feel the interconnectedness of all things as one.

WE MUST RECONNECT AND PIVOT

So what's next? How do we reconnect humans with nature? How do we reduce our personal and global ecological footprint so that we can live and function with ecological reserve? How do we live under 1.0 Earths individually and collectively as 10 billion people in the coming decades?

Let's hear from NASA scientist and astronaut Piers Sellers, who dedicated his final years to science and the humanity of climate change. He appeared in Leonardo Di Caprio's documentary, *Before The Flood*, and left three simple solutions to us before he died;[28]

Solution 1: "If we really want to reduce the human impact on the environment, the simplest and cheapest thing anyone can do is to eat less meat. Behind most of the joints of beef or chicken on our plates is a phenomenally wasteful, land and energy-hungry system of farming that devastates forests, pollutes oceans, rivers, seas and air, depends on oil and coal, and is significantly responsible for climate change."

Now you can still remain a compassionate carnivore, just remember the most climate-friendly meat is pigs and poultry. They only account for 10% of the livestock gas emissions and yet they produce three times more meat globally than cattle, while needing five times less feed to produce the same weight in meat than a cow![29]

Solution 2: "Promote Green Energy. Model Iceland, they are the greenest country in the world according to the EPI (environmental performance index). Interestingly, Iceland is also among the happiest nations in the world."

Solution 3: "Take ownership of your local environment. Start local, then we can impact global. Think global: act local. Look after your front door step. Only then will we change the world, one community at a time."

You don't need to set out to save the world. Concentrate on improving your own personal ecological footprint and then get to work on sustaining your local environment. Empower others to do the same and show respect and empathy for the environments of all other living things. Another free solution to Elon's 100 million dollar prize.

"Even if I knew that tomorrow the world would go
to pieces, I would still plant my apple tree."
— Martin Luther King Jr —

Start Now!

There is a simple philosophy to live by that encompasses the guiding principles behind Nature is Medicine. Dr Jane Goodall inspired this message in her address to the world on International Peace Day in 2017.

"On this International Day of Peace, during the minute of silence after the ringing of the Peace Bell, let us make a solemn vow to do our best to live according to the **Golden Rule.** *This rule that is shared by all the major religions, urges us to* **'Do to unto others as we would have them do unto us.'** *And we should include animals in this vow, knowing they too have emotions and know fear and pain...Every day you make a difference and you must decide what kind of difference you want to make...Let us send up our prayers for greater understanding and make a commitment to do what we can, however little, to promote peace and harmony around us. To actually take action—and to take action every day—* **not** *make a promise that is just words."[30]*

Our opening story about the Forest Man of India embodies this simple yet masterful message for every one of us; Payeng took real and consistent action as a result of the snakes' suffering. This vow to create harmony and peace amongst all living organisms will trigger empathy, motivation and collectively engender positive action!

I want to leave you with one final practical rule to follow every day for Nature is Medicine. I call it the "30/30/30 Rule." Whether meditating for 30 minutes in your garden as the sun rises in the morning, spending 30 minutes looking after that small permaculture garden during the day, or simply taking the dog for a 30 minute walk in the afternoon at the beach as the sun sets. Doing these activities each day, tunes you into nature's energy to replenish and reconnect for health and longevity. Fill your lungs and get going!

🌳 NATURE IS MEDICINE PRESCRIPTION

» Spend 90 minutes in nature. You can use the **30/30/30 rule** but I encourage you to simply start wherever you can. Even 30 minutes per day is great! You'll feel a cascade effect of wanting more which will motivate you to make time for it!

» Use the Ecological Footprint Calculator[32] (**selfcare.global/tools**) to see how many Earths would be needed to sustain your lifestyle.

» Name two ways in which you can work towards living at 1.0 Earths

1. ....

2. ....

» Plant a tree! Hug a tree! Develop your green thumb! Yes, it may seem a hippie thing to do but science has now validated the health benefits derived from a little tree cuddling and having a green thumb.[33]

To learn more about this medicine, or to contribute to this medicine, visit **selfcare.global/nature**. Here you will find blogs, videos and podcasts.

Selfcare.global/nature

NOTABLE EXPERTS IN THIS CHAPTER:
Voltaire, Jadav Payeng, Dr Jane Goodall, Dalai Lama XIV,
Mike Barrett, Marco Lambertini, Maurice Maeterlinck,
Gro Sandal, Piers Sellers, Martin Luther King Jr.

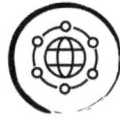

ENVIRONMENT IS MEDICINE

"When a flower doesn't bloom, you fix the environment
in which it grows, not the flower."
— *Alexander Den Heijer* —

When tuning into this section remember the story of the flower that didn't bloom and the rat park experiment.

Environment is a potent medicine Dr Julian Baginni is a founding editor of the Philosopher's Magazine and author of the brilliant book *Freedom Regained: The Possibility of Free Will*.[1] He shares the story of identical twins Ann and Judy, who have 99.99% the exact same genes, you couldn't get more identical—yet their environments created big differences in their health, happiness, connection and abundance they attracted in their lives.

Ann and Judy were born in Wales in 1940, a particularly challenging period after The Great Depression and the beginning of The Second World War. They were born into a working class family who already had five children and couldn't cope with any more. The tiny babies were sent to live with separate aunts. Judy's placement did not work out and she returned to her biological mother at three months old. Ann's placement continued on and she stayed with her aunt and uncle as their only child.

Even though their geographical and cultural environments were similar, the two households in which Ann and Judy grew up were very different. Judy's family were a tough grass roots family and she recalled that, *"she was a street kid, always out."*

While Ann's uncle worked in the same steelworks as her biological father, he had managed to get ahead being careful with money and partly because they only had the one child to care for. Ann said she always had her *"nose in a book because I was on my own."*[2] Ann then passed the 11-plus exam and was accepted into the local grammar school before entering a white collar job. Judy ended up at the local secondary school before leaving early to work in a furniture shop.

The next stages of their lives followed similar paths yet the consequences were very different due to their **social environments**. Within six months of working, Ann became pregnant and quit her job. Interestingly, only two months later, Judy became pregnant and quit her nursing course. There was also a parallel in the men they married; both men were violent. Ann didn't stay married for long. *"I left and went back home* **(environment)**, *and they were very supportive when they found out what was going on."*[3]

Judy, however, stayed married for 17 years and didn't leave her husband because she lacked support. She had three children by age 21. Her mother was no help with the attitude of "you made your bed, you lie on it."[4]

While Ann was able to rebuild her life, Judy stayed in a stressful environment for two decades. By the time the twins rekindled their sibling relationship at the age of 48, the health differences were apparent. Judy was battling high blood pressure, a problem with her kidneys and had had a hysterectomy. Ann had a supportive environment and always had access to money and resources; Judy did not.

Tales of identical twins like Ann and Judy show us that we are much more than the sum of the genes we are born with; our human potential is ignited (or otherwise) by the environments in which we spend the most time. Ultimately, various options are penciled in by our genetic blueprint but nourishing environments also need to be considered. This story is not to trigger the old and long-standing Nature versus Nurture debate, but to see that environment does play a role in our growth.

Think about what environments restrict your potential for health, well-being and success. Do they support you? Can you support others looking for their nourishing environments?

Every moment is an environment to connect and nourish yourself or someone else.

CO-CREATING NOURISHING ENVIRONMENTS

For some of us, not all environments in which we live and grow are nourishing. Perhaps its luck of birth right, fate or simply the hand we were dealt in life. So how do we co-create environments that allow everyone to be nourished irrespective of social, cultural or geographical starting points?

The health of any living organism depends on its environments. They provide energy, connection and support for it to thrive.

Generations of artificial environments have conditioned us to be passengers in our own human journeys, accepting that everything in life "is just the way it is." We seek passive interventions for the signals and symptoms that our bodies have been showing us for decades. Dysfunctions that tell us we've lost our way, lost our harmony and our balance between our internal and external environments. Sure, you can try to adapt to any environment like a fish surviving in dirty, polluted water or a stubborn plant determined to try and bloom in the crack of a concrete jungle.

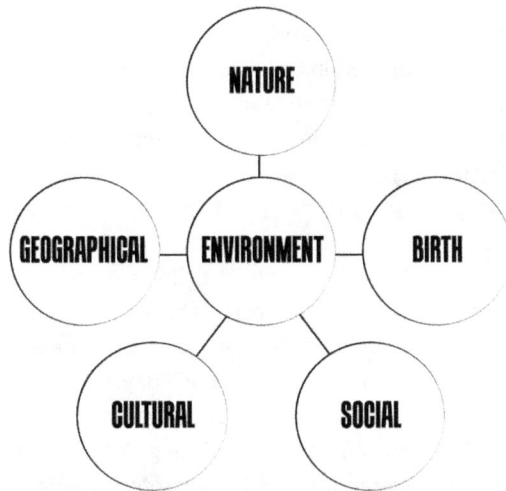

NATURE

GEOGRAPHICAL — ENVIRONMENT — BIRTH

CULTURAL   SOCIAL

Or—you can choose differently. You can seek environments that nourish and support you to reach your potential and longevity of your journey, allowing your cup to stay full. This chapter will deconstruct the idea that we need to be fixed by paying for passive solutions.

Delving into the significance of our environments; geographical, social, cultural and natural, will help you step back and observe your environments and if they are right for you. Whether it be the new house you walk into that feels just right, the country or place that you most love, the work colleagues that you enjoy spending time with or the partner who builds you up rather than brings you down. You will feel which environments nourish you and those that do not.

This paradigm shift will help you break through social barriers and cultural constructs to empower you to actively seek nourishing environments and solutions to live in a state of good health, wellbeing and towards longevity. Anyone you care about can find a nourishing environment within the context of their own life right now. However, it cannot happen without some hard truths, deep reflection and a courageous internal pivot in the way that you live.

FROM SCARCITY TO ABUNDANCE

Today, we have created modern medical and healthcare systems that are focused on "fixing the flower." Nowadays it is "normal" for one in two people to develop uncontrolled cell growths—cancers—in their bodies, and it is statistically accepted that seven in ten people will die from the effects of their lifestyle choices that lead to heart disease.[5] We are well conditioned to these maladies of 21st century living but with the SelfCare revolution, it does not have to be "normal."

Our innate knowledge and internal mechanisms have been forgotten in favor of becoming patients looking to be "fixed" and jumping from one doctor to another, from different specialists, healers and coaches onto the next. Hoping for a quick check-up and monetary solution in order to return to busy, artificial environments from where the dysfunction will reappear and begin the cycle again.

The challenge now is to deeply question these artificial environments and systems that foster modern stress. Stress that is often related to work or financial pressures from living beyond our means or the physical strains of our sedentary lifestyles sitting in offices or traffic for most of our day!

I want you to ask yourself if it feels like life is working with you or against you. Is it so hard to get ahead that you're constantly battling dysfunction and disappointment? Answering yes to these questions means you are living in scarcity, trying to serve from an empty cup each day.

What does it mean to be living in scarcity? It means your natural sources of energy, connection and support are missing. You are the flower trying to struggle through the pavement of a busy street. Living this way can bring out resilience in your human vessel's ability to survive; you are one tough cookie that can put up with a lot and humans often find remarkable strength against adversity, I grant you. But what physical, emotional and mental cost does this kind of survival demand? It can be difficult to acknowledge the pain, pressures and dysfunctions that your current environments promote. It is difficult to let go of what you thought you knew, these habits promoting scarcity are probably deeply ingrained in your definition of a "successful" life. I know because I had to stare at myself in a mirror and question this myself too. Not easy to always swallow the truth.

However, this is the powerful realization that moves you to the driver's seat of your own life. The choice of choosing an abundant environment is waiting for you. You can join a whole community of people to nourish each other and thrive together as one. I'm not saying you shouldn't choose a city lifestyle, but I am saying choose the energy of your environments carefully.

You might:
- Create more space for nature in your home or backyard
- Cut back your work hours
- Volunteer doing something you love
- Join that book club or Tai Chi class
- Change employers or start a business you love
- Look for more spiritual connection in your neighborhood
- Get new friends or people you spend the most time with
- Move home or travel to a new geographical location
- Look for new experiences in the world

These are empowered choices that create abundant environments and mindsets that lead you away from an unhappy, unhealthy, disconnected and unfulfilled life! These choices are our defenses against the burden of chronic preventable disease.

You might feel some resistance with this growth at first, in the same way that a plant's roots must use oppositional force to infiltrate deeper into the soil, strengthening its foundation for every inch that it grows. Self-care is that growth, so stay strong in your new convictions. Be courageous enough to seek nourishing environments where you are loved and appreciated as you are! For people following my story, you will see that I left the comfort of Australia and moved to Indonesia during the pandemic. I voluntarily liquidated my Australian business and moved it to Singapore. I surrounded myself with a culture of karma, self-governed communities, inspiring entrepreneurs seeking a similar lifestyle and set up my businesses in systems that were positively geared, not negative sum.

ABUNDANCE FOR SOME, BUT WHY NOT ALL?

Abundance and scarcity must be considered from another simple yet powerful perspective. Perhaps you've experienced this first hand while traveling and already seen the dual nature of our world; the uneven scales of abundance and scarcity.

Global platforms such as the United Nations Sustainable Development Goals, World Health Organization, UNICEF, Oxfam, World Food Programme and every other organization serving their local communities report the same evidence of inequity.

I highlight these figures so they may instill a sense of humility and gratitude for all that we have through fortune of birth. Firstly, we must see the world around us as it truly is before we can change it.

- If you have access to **clean water** that won't make you sick, you have access to an essential element that more than 750 million people do not have.[6]
- If you have access to **food** today and didn't go to bed hungry last night, you have more abundance than 805 million people worldwide who do not have access to enough food to eat today.[7]
- If you have access to **electricity** to turn a light on or charge a mobile device, you have access to something that a quarter of all humans live without; electricity—approximately 1.6 billion people.[8]
- If you can buy your daily coffee or juice and still have more than $3 in your pocket, that is more than 3 billion people who live on less than $2.50 a day. 1.3 billion live in extreme poverty and live on less than $1.25 a day.[9]
- If you made more than $10 today, you are more abundant than 80% of the world's population that lives on less than $10 a day.[10]
- Even with inefficient agricultural practices and modern farming methods we have enough food to feed over 10 billion people. The World Food Programme says, *"The poor are hungry and their hunger traps them in poverty."* Hunger is also the number one cause of death in the world, killing more than HIV/AIDS, malaria, and tuberculosis combined.[11]

GRATEFULNESS NOW

What has your abundant environment enabled and empowered you to do and be?

What are three things about your environment that you are grateful for right now?

1. ....

2. ....

3. ....

Think about how you can help co-create abundant environments for the 80% of the world that may not have access to the opportunities that you are fortunate enough to have.

Close to every country in the world has marginalized people that need help. Little lifestyle changes can impact the greater whole; backyard composting, community gardens, social programs connecting youth and the disenfranchised, community recycle, waste and sanitation programs, using clean energy, standing up for increasing parks and gardens. Supporting these actions snowball into wider awareness and action for everyone.

SAME GENES, DIFFERENT ENVIRONMENTS

Even in a scarce environment, any child with parents or carers who give them unconditional love, access to education and whatever other opportunities and means they can find, can go from the slums to the presidential palace if they choose. In the same way Indonesian President Joko Widodo "Jokowi," a 53-year-old former furniture exporter, rose from the slums of Jakarta to the presidential palace![12] Many of his early environments were lacking but others supported and helped his chances at success.

As empowering as it is to take control of your environments, there is one that nobody gets to choose; where they are born. Your access to living in good health and wellbeing would be very different if you were born in Sierra Leone, Chad or Nigeria versus being born in Hong Kong, Japan or Sweden.

If you were born in any of these African countries you would be lucky to live beyond the age of 55, where as, if you were born in any of the Top 10 countries for life expectancy such as Japan, you could likely live beyond 85 years of age![13] How can the world have two birth environments with a 30-year variation in life expectancy?!

Conflict, hunger, poor sanitation and lack of healthcare are some of the factors behind communities with lower life expectancies around the world. These environmental barriers are enormous hurdles to overcome in helping each child reach their potential.

The Human Development Index calculates data based on a country's life expectancy and standard of living and it reveals that our geography and health are intrinsically linked. *"Where we are born, live, study and work directly influences our health experiences: the air we breathe, the food we eat, the viruses we are exposed to and the health services we can access."*[14] It is alarming to think of the pre-determined projections that millions of children are born into.

Imagine you are the parent of a child born into these circumstances, how far would you go to escape danger and disease for your child and create better environments? The refugees you see on the news are simply other human beings like you, fathers, brothers, mothers and sisters; people with a different "luck of birth." For whatever reason behind it, their basic human needs are not being met (food, water, safety, shelter) and they are simply looking for their right to obtain these basic elements. Like you might be, my European ancestors were immigrants to Australia after the second world war. They too were seeking safer environments to raise their families, creating a legacy for future generations. Without their courage, this book would not be here for you to read.

According to the World Economic Forum, more people are moving around the world than ever before. In fact 258 million people are far from their home country. Yet the families they leave behind are not forgotten because as these migrants settle into their new country, gaining different employment skills and knowledge of their new home, they also contribute to their families and communities by sending money back home. So much so that migrants have become a global economic force—sending an estimated $466 billion to families in developing countries![15] Sharing the wealth as it were!

What if the top 50 most abundant countries, helped the bottom 50 countries that lacked abundant environments to raise their children in? What if all children could be born into environments that had life expectancies of 80 years or more before they took their first breath, let alone start to make choices?

EDUCATION AND HEALTHY ENVIRONMENTS

There are no borders from space; only human rules that strike division and inequity. Imagine being born in Myanmar rather than Australia, Palestine rather than France, or being born south of an artificial line that meant you were Mexican rather than American? A harsh reality that means your predetermined geography will govern your access to healthcare and education in your foundation years.[16]

On the whole, people are healthier, doing better financially and living longer today than thirty years ago.[17] If you were born in France, you would have access to a fully integrated system, the best in the world and free! If you were born in war stricken Myanmar, you would not have access to much at all, even struggling for clean water and sanitation. It's confounding to think that an 8,500km distance can influence so much in the lives of two children born on the same day on the same planet.

There are also huge differences in health care expenditure between countries. While the WHO estimates US$44 provides basic life-saving services per person per year, poor countries' expenditure can be as low as US$12 per person per year![18] For high-income countries, the average is over US$3,000.[19]

The past thirty years have seen endless challenges amid rapid population growth and urbanization, growing rates of chronic and infectious diseases and continuous political and regional conflicts that affect the lives and opportunities of millions of people. The next thirty years will require a more agile and flexible universal healthcare system that empowers self-care and supports self-governance within each community.

Using global blue zone communities as a model for us all to learn from and apply in the context of our own lives, families and communities. Every child irrespective of birthright, deserves access to the basic resources needed to survive, and ultimately the same opportunities to thrive and create their own positive impact on their community.

EDUCATION AS A BIRTHRIGHT

Despite wi-fi reaching practically every corner of the globe, smartphones and rapid technological advancements, it's hard to believe in 2020 that every child does not have access to education. Unfortunately, disconnection and war from past inter-generational grudges is hindering the development of so many children's futures. Over 50% of out-of-school children of primary school age live in conflict-affected areas. This suggests that connection, compassion and peace NOW is the recipe for the health of future generations.

The "access to education" ripple effect is profound. Planting seeds of development that give children access to education in one generation perpetuates socio-economic stratification for many generations to come. There is always that one person in any family that changed the course of that family's history.

As Malala Yousafzai shared in her impassioned speech when she addressed the UN as a girl of 16, *"One child, one teacher, one book, one pen can change the world."*[20] Her powerful words are generating action all around the world.

Investing in education for girls and women brings multidimensional benefits. For example, if all girls in developing countries were to complete secondary education, the under-five mortality rate would be halved.[21] Improving education for girls and young women not only saves lives, it lowers birth rates, improves nutrition, increases their employment and narrows the pay gap between men and women.[22]

Even more interestingly, a UN report reveals that, "Girls and women spend 90% of their earned income on their families, while men spend only 30–40%."[23] This suggests educating and employing women in developing countries from marginalized communities is an important step in growing the economies of small communities everywhere and increase opportunities for the next generations.

Access to healthcare and education are fundamental for our growth and development in the modern world. Having access to free education growing up is like winning the opportunity of life lottery. What we do with that opportunity is up to us as the individual.

SHAPING OUR SOCIAL ENVIRONMENTS

We've established the roles our birth and geographic environments play in our lives. The factors of these fundamental environments give rise to our social environments. And amazingly, our *social* environments are even more strongly associated with our health! Our neighborhood, our education, our work, our income and our social groups (known as social determinants) all contribute to our abundance and longevity over our lifetime. The reality is that these social determinants *"...are shaped by the distribution of money, power and resources at global, national and local levels."*[24]

Social determinants are extremely relevant in regards to rates of disease, both communicable and non-communicable.[25] This tells us policy makers need to look at a broader approach at improving human services not just aimed at healthcare. Being born into a lower or higher socio-economic community can pre-determine your life expectancy. This explains why life expectancy in Japan is double that of Sierra Leone, or why sadly indigenous Australians have a ten-year lower life expectancy than non-indigenous Australians.[26]

In the US the Robert Wood Johnson Foundation showed how zip codes either positively or negatively impact your health and even your life expectancy. They found that people living just a few blocks apart had vastly different opportunities to live a long life, depending on the social factors of the neighborhood they grew up in.[27] Imagine learning to survive on the streets of Chicago, versus the streets of San Francisco.

On a community level we can start to understand why groups of people are living in a different zone of health and wellbeing, even when they are only suburbs a part! We mimic the behaviors and rituals of the people we spend the most time with (mostly unconsciously). Our parents have been conditioning our thoughts and consumption habits long before we became consciously aware of our own choices. Even to the extent that we sometimes disconnect from certain groups of people that challenge our way of living and being. It is challenging to recognize this behavior in ourselves.

An example of the affects of conditioning was seen in a 2017 study showing, "Children from families with obese parents were at a significantly higher risk of obesity compared to children with normal-weight parents."[28]

Similarly, research also shows mental health disorders can be affected by social factors and not necessarily related to genetic causes as is often touted.[29] For example, according to psychiatric epidemiologist Myrna Weissman Ph.D., "Americans born before 1905 had a 1% rate of depression by age 75.[30] Among Americans born a half century later, 6% became depressed by age 24! Similarly, while the average age at which manic-depression first appears was 32 in the mid 1960s, its average onset today is 19."[31] Only social factors can produce such large shifts in incidence and age of onset of mental disorders in a few decades.[32]

"MY GENES MADE ME DO IT!"

How much freedom each person has to develop, returns us to the issue of whether nature and nurture can be separated. Thinking of traits as being either environmentally or genetically caused, cripples our understanding of human development.

We all like to think that we make choices on the basis of our own conscious deliberations. What would it mean for humanity if our decisions were already written in our genetic code, or perhaps our external environment? The whole concept of personal responsibility would cease to exist.

Professor Jerome Kagan, studies close up the interaction between nature and nurture and how it plays out in our lives. He is worried that we are too quick to blame our personal behavior on factors outside of our control. To put it more eloquently he shares that, "To ask what proportion of personality is genetic rather than environmental is like asking what proportion of a blizzard is due to cold temperature rather than humidity."[33]

As an example, do you think someone could get out of a murder charge by blaming their genes? Stephen Mobley desperately tried to avoid execution by saying that the murder of the Domino's pizza store manager was due to a mutation in the monoamine oxidase A (MAOA) gene.[34] The judge declined the appeal suggesting that the law was not ready to accept such evidence.[35]

So did, *"My genes make me do it?"* Did I consciously choose to do it, or did my environment unconsciously guide me to this point and this choice? Is environment stronger than nature's genetic blueprint? Fortunately, Tim Spector a Professor of Genetic Epidemiology believes so. He told *The Guardian*,

"The environment is almost always more influential than genes and is clear in the case of Ann and Judy. The sisters shared the same genes but with a middle-class background Ann did better at school, earned more money and enjoyed better health. Too much attention to genes blinds us to the obvious truth that access to financial (abundant resources) and educational resources remains the most important determinant of how we fare in life."[36]

IS ENVIRONMENT STRONGER THAN PERSONAL WILLPOWER?

Imagine that you were born in a low socioeconomic family and your parents had passed away due to the war that you were born into. What chance do you have of finding health, happiness and connection in this lifetime? It is plain to see that individuals born into disadvantage have few strategies available to better their conditions.

Poor people and environmental damage are often caught in a downward spiral. Not necessarily the cause of past resource degradation but they often bare the brunt of it, deepening their poverty and environmental decay as they are forced to deplete resources to survive on the fringe of an integrated world—human rights require global justice.[37]

Some people risk everything to leave their home environment and community in search of more physically and economically secure environments. This is a huge step and not everyone is brave enough to take it. When we look back into our own family history however, it is very unlikely that any of us are living in our family's country of origin. One of our ancestors took courage and left!

This perspective actually sheds love and light on the concept of one global family, we are global citizens. The essence of humankind is survival and seeking more abundant environments, seeking to be the *one* person that changes the trajectory of their family's fortunes for generations to come.

ENVIRONMENT IS MEDICINE PRESCRIPTION

» Immerse yourself in empowering & enabling environments.

» Birth; Where were you born? Make a list of all the wonderful things you already have access to and say a quiet "thank you" for everything you have. (The list should be quite long!) e.g., water, trees, schools, healthcare, education, electricity.

» Geographical? Name one place on this planet that feels like home, a place that nourishes and enables you, to be the best you and feel bliss often!

» Social? Take stock on the 5 people you spend the most time and ask whether they enable and empower you? Write down two people that you can confide in.

» Work? We spend most of our life working, ask whether it is an environment that you want to be in? Or is there somewhere more nourishing?

» Cultural? Cultures develop over centuries with underlying belief systems and ways of living and being. Does your culture support and nourish you to be free to be?

» Calculate how many of your 168 hours a week do you live in an nourishing environment. Are you spending a substantial amount of time in a loving, supportive, healthy, empowering and enabling environments? (at home, work, socially, geographically etc.)

» List two changes that you can make to enhance your wellbeing in your current environment. More indoor plants? A fountain? A sea change or change of proximity?

To learn more about this medicine, or to contribute to this medicine, visit **selfcare.global/environment**. Here you will find blogs, videos and podcasts.

(Selfcare.global/environment)

NOTABLE EXPERTS IN THIS CHAPTER:

Alexander Den Heijer, Dr Julian Baginni, President Joko Widodo "Jokowi," Malala Yousafzai, Dr Myrna Weissman, Professor Jerome Kagan, Dr Tim Spector.

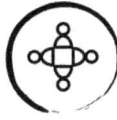

3

CONNECTION IS MEDICINE

*"We are all connected; to each other, biologically. To the earth,
chemically. To the rest of the universe atomically. We are
not figuratively, but literally stardust."*
— *Neil DeGrasse Tyson* —

"I AM BECAUSE WE ARE."

Not long ago, an anthropologist was studying the habits and customs of an African tribe. After he gathered up his research on his last day there, his transport was delayed and so he waited in the sparse shade of the village trees dotted about the dry earth.

The children of the tribe were never far away; he had enjoyed their ready smiles and laughter during his stay. So while he waited the anthropologist proposed a game for the children to play. He carefully wrapped some candy and sweets he had bought in the city and placed them in a basket tied with a ribbon.

He laid the basket under a solitary tree and called the kids together. Drawing a line in the sand he explained to wait behind the line for his signal. When he said "Go!" they should rush over to the basket, and the first to reach the tree would win all the candies.

After he said "Go!" all the children unexpectedly held each other's hands and ran off towards the tree as a group. Arriving together they happily sat down to share the candy with each other. Rather surprised, the anthropologist asked them why they had all gone together, especially if the first one to arrive at the tree could have all the candy.

A young girl replied simply: "How can one of us be happy if all the others are sad?"

The anthropologist finally realized that after all his time spent studying their customs, it was a simple children's game that truly showed him the essence of their beliefs and way of life.

> *"Ubuntu…is about the essence of being human…it is part of the gift that Africa will give the world…We believe that a person is a person through other persons, that my humanity is caught up, bound up, inextricably, with yours."*
> *— Archbishop Desmond Tutu —*

CONNECTION AS MEDICINE

Everything is connected to *everything*; from the cosmic level down to you and I and our morning coffee. Chemically, biologically, energetically and metaphysically everything in this world, is literally connected as one! There is a quiet undertow of flowing energy waiting to be tapped into each day, to ignite your senses and orchestrate your interpretation and experience of the world.

Connection as Medicine refers firstly to the interconnected energy between human, nature and spirit as a whole; everything in life has originated from the same source; so the concept of separation is an illusion, a powerful mental construct. Connection as Medicine secondly refers to humanity's need for collective social connections. Separation and disconnection is the disease modern humanity is battling. We need to deconstruct this concept of separation and reconnect with our innate truth.

Connection as Medicine shines the light on many solutions hidden in plain sight; from the rituals of blue zone communities that thrive together towards longevity, to social relationships that lighten the mental, physical and emotional loads of our lives, and internal reflection that connects us with the deepest parts of ourselves. Including awareness our shadows, fears, insecurities and even past traumas that unconsciously drive our everyday behaviors without us consciously knowing it!

In this chapter, we will explore the origins and importance of our connections to source, self, people, humanity and nature. Even our fates are connected, mine over here with yours over there. I want to see you and your community thrive in life and I hope you feel the same about my community and me.

Optimizing our connections is the way there.

EMBRACE AND ACKNOWLEDGE CONNECTION

Ancient belief systems revered the relationship and energy between all things, both visible and invisible. Over the last few centuries of modernization however, human beings developed rigid, linear explanations and doctrines for our circular, infinite world; rules and boundaries that have created separation.

However a great mental shift is afoot amongst our generation, you may have already begun to sense this reawakening amongst humanity with the bourgeoning of wellness and spiritual movements around the globe that embrace all races and religions. There is growing momentum as philosophers, scientists and curious souls the world over reach the same conclusion about the intrinsic connection between all things.

The famous quantum physicist Neil Degrasse Tyson has hopes that one day people will, "Recognize that the very molecules that make up your body, the atoms that construct the molecules, are traceable to the crucibles that were once the centers of high mass stars that exploded their chemically rich guts into the galaxy, enriching pristine gas clouds with the chemistry of life...It's not that we are better than the universe, we are part of the universe. We are in the universe and the universe is in us."[1]

This concept is both grandiose and humbling; we are universal and miniscule all at once, we are the same matter uniquely formed into different organisms. This source energy flows continuously between all things. There is literally an exchange of matter and energy, of photons and electrons between our forms and those around us; an inseparable wave of relationships.

We can no more be separated from the cosmos as from the air we breathe, the ground we walk on or the bacteria in our stomach that digests our food. The next time you pass someone on the street, remember there is only 0.5% of our evolutionary blueprint that makes us different shapes and sizes and colors. We are one; connected to the same source. Each soul we see becomes a reflection of ourselves. Each feeling is a reflection of something deeper within ourselves. Ultimately we see the world and act according to how we feel it to be. The hard truth to accept is that our external reality; the peace, the chaos, the drama, the abundance and the scarcity is ultimately a reflection of our inner world.

CONNECTION ENABLES SURVIVAL

"From the dawn of our time, ancestral humans who were inclined to form social connections, communicate, work together, share food, and defend and retaliate in the face of violations of reciprocity norms, had a selective advantage to survive and pass on their genes."[2]

Most primates are social creatures. Not just cursory interactions, I'm talking about strong relationships between young and old throughout their life. Young primates have to learn all their survival skills from experienced adults so they become adept at living in their environment, gaining essential social skills along the way.

Banding together in this way helps them to outwit and intimidate predators and control food sources. Like our primate ancestors, humans learned and adapted to be social as a survival technique, which then enabled some breathing space for reproduction and evolution of the species! However, we have to learn that success requires that we thrive together with nature. The 6th mass extinction is underway.[3] This is not a measure for the most successful species.

Matthew D. Lieberman, Director of UCLA's Social Cognitive Neuroscience Laboratory, has spent decades studying how the human brain responds to its social environment. He has repeatedly educated people how our brains aren't just wired to perform tasks and think, but ultimately they are wired to connect.

Socialization has remained a stalwart of our evolution and Lieberman explains each adaptation intensified the connection we felt with those around us, we began to predict the actions of others and ultimately cooperate with them. "This is what our brains were wired for: reaching out to and interacting with others. These are design features, not flaws. These social adaptations are central to making us the most successful species on Earth."[4]

Lieberman defines three major adaptations that have made us so irresistibly responsive to the social world.[5] The first step was developing connection— a capacity to feel social pains and pleasures; a uniquely mammalian trait that forever links our wellbeing to our social connectedness. As an example, from the moment of birth human babies strongly express this deep need to stay connected which can continue throughout their lives (with deviations in some teenage years).

Our next evolutionary step a few million years later was mindreading. Lieberman describes primates as having developed a supreme ability to understand the actions and thoughts of those around them. This improved their strategic interaction and ability to stay connected. In toddlers for example, you will see clever forms of social thinking that are more developed than adults of other species. It enables human beings to form purposeful groups and implement ideas by anticipating the needs and wants of others.

The most recent evolutionary offering Leiberman calls harmonizing, which resulted from our sense of self, which developed a few hundred thousand years ago.[6] Along with distinguishing ourselves from others and a fancy for selfishness, the self is actually an important driver behind social unity. As an example, you may remember your teenage years where an identity crisis ensued. To satisfy this deep need for belonging and connection, we often allow neural adaptations to let the beliefs and values of others to influence our own. We now refer to this as "peer pressure" and let's be honest, some people (and politicians) never grow out of this phase.

Let's be frank...group connections affect your way of thinking, your self-esteem and your decisions. Not surprisingly therefore, your future is actually connected to the people you spend the most time with, whether you like it or not. Motivational speaker Jim Rohn famously proclaimed, "We are the average of the five people we spend the most time with."

CHOOSE YOUR TRIBE WISELY

So connecting with the right tribe could well be the ultimate difference you need to thrive in life. Your health, your abundance, your mindset, your confidence, who you are in this moment and ultimately who you become are all affected by the people you spend the most time with. So choose your tribe wisely! Spend time with people who are happy, healthy and connected and perhaps stop taking advice from unhealthy, unhappy and disconnected people.

Stay connected; stay involved in your local community and try different interests. Finding your tribe is part of your purpose in life to achieve fulfillment and overflow. Think about who you connect with as a group? Aim for active, high-vibing people who are passionate about the same thing as you. Your group's collective energy and passion raises your vibration and well-being, helping to prolong your "functional capacity," an integral part of Blue zone communities!

> *"Without the sense of fellowship with humans of like mind, life would have seemed to me empty."*
> *— Albert Einstein —*

ISOLATION IS THE SILENT KILLER

Isolation and disconnection from others isn't always bad but some people's company can take us down a path that leads away from health, happiness and inner peace. A crowd can energize some people, whilst others find it draining. A bit of breathing space is often needed to escape the demands of our colleagues or the heavy vibe of large groups. It's the reason why meditation and connecting inwards is just as important as connecting socially.

It's good to be alone from time to time, but not "alone" alone. For the vast majority of people, prolonged social isolation is detrimental, particularly mentally. It is also the reason that solitary confinement is reserved for our worst prisoners.

Doctors have known for a while that loneliness and isolation leads to mental health problems like depression, stress, anxiety, and a lack of confidence. But there's growing evidence that social isolation is connected with an increased risk of physical ill health as well.[7]

An BBC Future article by Michael Bond describes how, "Chronically lonely people have higher blood pressure, are more vulnerable to infection, and are also more likely to develop Alzheimer's disease and dementia. Loneliness also interferes with a whole range of everyday functioning such as sleep patterns, attention and logical and verbal reasoning."[8] Bond acknowledges that although the processes behind these consequences are still uncertain, it is clear that social isolation triggers an extreme immune response—a torrent of stress hormones and inflammation that were useful in our ancient past for running like hell back to the safety of our tribe.

Today however the physical risks are no longer there yet our immune response remains the same; surviving alone carries extreme mental, emotional and physical stresses for most people. It goes against our innate need and adaptation to thrive together as one. This research highlights the importance of family, community and the five people we spend the most time with, in supporting our health and wellbeing.

Sometimes we can feel internally disconnected from ourselves even when we're surrounded by people. We can suppress feelings and emotional needs in favor of "rationality" or a busy work schedule dedicated by the environments we choose to live in and the values of our conditioning. These distractions and blockages prevent the flow of energy reaching your internal "real" you. The resulting stress from losing sight of our values and feeling the pressures from work and society have many physical side affects and our human systems start to malfunction.

This is your clue to reconnect! To yourself, your tribe, humanity, nature and to the Source! Take a walk alone, phone your old friend, join that conservation group you've been thinking about, gaze at the stars. These are blue zone philosophies that restore human health and promote longevity.

THE UNINTENTIONAL DISCONNECT

Think about the way you spend your day, the people you see, the words you say, the food you eat, the places you shop, the lifestyle you choose. All these choices support the continuation of the processes that produced that end result. **Every decision you make, whether consciously or not, either promotes connection or disconnection.**

Let's look at the practical connection of our decisions that have consequences so far down the chain we fail (or pretend not) to see them.

My decision to use plastic bags with every purchase at the markets may result in those plastic bags ending up in the ocean you swim in. Those plastic bags break down into micro plastics that can travel great distances on the ocean currents and are then unintentionally consumed by a fish that you will catch or buy for dinner. Your family eats that fish! Those microplastics enter your human vessel and are likely to negatively influence your internal systems and thus your health and wellbeing.

It all started with me saying yes to plastic bags—unaware of the impact it was having on our global family over time. I'm sure that Swedish engineer Sten Gustaf Thulin who invented the plastic bag had no intention to harm the world or future families. He simply wanted to solve a problem, but was unaware of the future impact.

Ask yourself what state of the world do I want to hand over to future generations. We all need futuristic thinking that considers our potential impact on a local and global scale as well as each other.

One of the toughest points of practical disconnection for us to acknowledge is the affect of industry and transport emissions from the burning of fossil fuels. These processes allow for over a billion cars globally to carry us around in comfort yet contribute significantly to air pollution around the world. Unconscious decisions made with good intentions and a good heart yet they unknowingly, negatively impact the natural world and the lives of the people we care about.

One particular heavy metal that is increasing in environmental pollution is mercury; fine in natural trace amounts but hazardous as levels increase. Tuna fish often have naturally high levels of mercury due to their position in the food chain. It's recommended humans only eat small amounts of tuna as mercury is classified as an endocrine disrupting chemical, severely affecting the body's internal system and is even carcinogenic (cancer forming).

Mercury does come from natural sources like volcanoes, but also from many man-made practices that produce air pollution. Once mercury enters the atmosphere it rains down on the Earth's surface where it enters the food web. Eventually landing on our dinner plates and in our children's lunch boxes!

We can no longer consume as if we are separate and have no collateral impact on the world around us. The challenge is negating willful ignorance and to awaken those apathetic characters that do not consider any impact beyond themselves. They morally detach from the reason why they wear masks against air pollution or from the waste and pollution on the side of the road.

I know its hard to relate your decision at the gas pump to fill your fossil-fueled car each week, or the use of electricity in your house, to the endocrine disturbances in someone you love and even cancer forming in a young child. There is no direct, linear A-B-C answer that humans prefer. Yet, simply understanding that everything is connected might help us embody new choices together. I have no desire to harm myself or my family or community and I'm sure you feel the same too. But we need to question what our choices are supporting in everything we do.

TO CONNECT MORE—FEEL MORE

If the greatest danger to our future is apathy as feared by Dr Jane Goodall, then perhaps empathy is the one tool that could connect a disconnected world.[9] Humans have a deep predisposition to feel the emotions of others.[10] Empathy has enabled people to connect and achieve more as a tribe throughout history. Sometimes it is even powerful enough to prevail over the dictates of powerful oppressors.

Fellow primatologist Frans de Waal asserts that, "In principle, empathy can override every rule about how to treat others. When Oskar Schindler kept Jews out of concentration camps during World War II, he was under clear orders by his society on how to treat people, yet his feelings interfered."[11] He made a decision based on being human and being able to put himself in their shoes. What if this was his brother, mother, father or someone he loved? What decision would he make? Listening to his heart rather than social constructs in his mind allowed him to make decisions based on being human. There was no separation.

De Waal sees the way to surpass our evolutionary tribal differences is by using emotion because, "emotions defy ideology." What a game-changing mind-set! Empathy today helps us to reach out and understand someone else's situation. De Waal continues, "If we could manage to see people on other continents as part of us, drawing them into our circle of reciprocity and empathy, we would be building upon, rather than going against our nature."[12]

When astronaut Pier's Sellars looked down at planet Earth from space, he saw no borders, no boundaries; just one planet and humankind. His final message called for all groups, scientists, policymakers, and industrialists to, "Work together towards the common goal of maintaining the Earth as a planet that can continue to support life—including all of us."[13]

The great comedic genius Charlie Chaplin gave an impassioned speech at the end of his 1940 movie, *The Great Dictator*:

> *"We think too much and feel too little. More than machinery, we need humanity; more than cleverness, we need kindness and gentleness. Without these qualities, life will be violent and all will be lost."*[14]

You may find it contrary that such a solemn message came from a comedian. Yet comedians could be our best self-care doctors. They look for the commonality in everyone, emotionally connecting us to the world we live in and each other, breaking down barriers and mental constructs of separation such as racism, gender bias, politics and worldviews. Comedians invite us all to laugh about it together, it's irresistible! Communing in laughter can reach the highest of human vibrations. Anyone that reminds us that we are feeling beings that think could be the best treatment prescription and pattern interruption for a busy world!

Charlie Chaplain was right. We need to think less and do and feel more—connection is that simple. Combat isolation and find your tribe as part of your purpose. Break free from assumptions, someone you meet tomorrow may have better intentions for you, than someone you have known your whole life, and that is okay. Welcome it, receive it and continue to share and circulate that abundance with others who might be looking for someone like you to spend most of their time with. This vibration enables you to serve from overflow, in helping and connecting to others and your community.

Our longevity depends on the strength of our connections and the depth of our social relationships. Imagine what it would feel like to find inner peace, have two people to confide in, surrounded by five high vibing people who support the lifestyle you are inspired to live and the person you are driven to be. The vibration and abundance of our tribes and the communities we live in will ultimately determine our health, well-being and longevity.

On a natural level, find ways to connect, protect and immerse yourself in nature's abundance. On a spiritual or energetic level find a way to continually connect to the source of abundance and amazing human potential we all possess.

Then connect it all as one, reminding your conscious mind of what nature and your human vessel innately knows to be true. It takes a village to raise a child; it takes a community to heal the sick. We can thrive together, but only as one interconnected species with all that is living and non-living. We were never meant to survive or thrive alone.

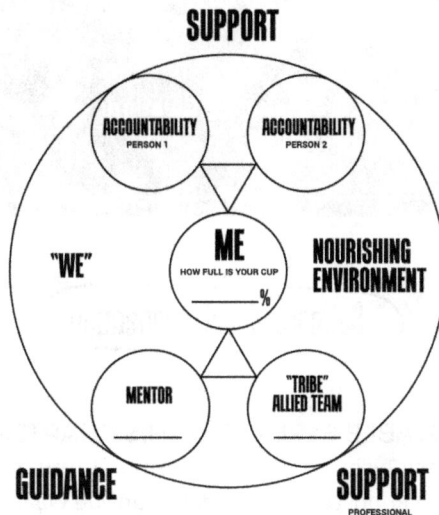

SUPPORT

ACCOUNTABILITY
PERSON 1

ACCOUNTABILITY
PERSON 2

"WE"

ME
HOW FULL IS YOUR CUP
_____%

NOURISHING
ENVIRONMENT

MENTOR

"TRIBE"
ALLIED TEAM

GUIDANCE

SUPPORT
PROFESSIONAL

⚛ CONNECTION IS MEDICINE PRESCRIPTION

» Name 2 people you can confide in

1. ....

2. ....

» Who are 5 high vibing people in your life?

Person 1 ....

Person 2 ....

Person 3 ....

Person 4 ....

Person 5 ....

» Connect with like-minded people, for example, people you meet while surfing or walking your dog.

To learn more about this medicine, or to contribute to this medicine, visit **selfcare.global/connection**. Here you will find blogs, videos and podcasts.

Selfcare.global/connection

NOTABLE EXPERTS IN THIS CHAPTER:
Neil DeGrasse Tyson, Archbishop Desmond Tutu, Matthew D. Lieberman, Jim Rohn, Dr Jane Goodall, Frans de Waal, Pier Sellars.

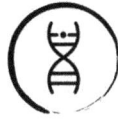

4

GENES ARE MEDICINE

"Only 5% of disease-related gene mutations are
fully deterministic, while 95% can be influenced
by diet, behavior and other environmental
conditions. You are not simply the sum total
of the genes you were born with." [1]
— *Dr. Deepak Chopra and Dr. Rudolph Tanzi* —

NO ARMS, NO LEGS, NO WORRIES!

Fellow Australian and all-round incredible human being Nick Vujicic,[2] who was born with no arms and legs from an extremely rare congenital disorder known as Phocomelia, which is characterized by the absence of legs and arms. At 33, he openly shares how we struggled mentally, emotionally, and physically. He shares how he was bullied at school and attempted suicide when he was just 10 years old. Living as a victim of the genes he was born with.

However one day something changed. He came to terms with the 5-20% outside of his control and decided to accept and really play the hand he had been dealt in life. Eventually he came to terms with his physical condition and something special happened. He decided to become vocal about living with disabilities and finding hope and meaning in life.

Today, he travels the world addressing huge crowds. He has visited more than 57 countries and given over three thousand talks, some of which have attracted audiences as large as 110,000 people. He is a bestselling author and runs a non-profit ministry. He is happily married to his wife Kanae and they a beautiful brood of children.

He is a living example of living fully. A man who shows that genetic factors absolutely do have a say in the way we are born, but they don't always prevent us from living our best lives.

Our genes are in fact, more than medicine. They are the blueprint for our human potential and thus our human experience. Our genetic blueprint is nature's masterpiece, a marvel that science is still trying to wrap its evidence-based head around. By understanding that our genes contain our human potential and that we are the authors of our human experience, allows us to firstly make peace with the things we can't change (like Nick) but also realize that our genes are not our destiny. Wow! That's a massive deal! Why? Because it means that we aren't at total mercy of our genetics, we have some freedom and choice. And choice is power.

Secondly, we can get busy stimulating and nourishing our epigenetic pathways through our daily lifestyle choices to become whoever we dream ourselves to be. Genes are only responsible for 5% of who you are right now. They are not deterministic. Each gene and its interaction with other gene expressions can create billions and even trillions of variant expressions. Ultimately, who you become in the future is within your control.

YOU ARE NOT THE VICTIM OF YOUR GENES

Yep, that's right—you are not a victim of our genes. Now, please don't misinterpret this—I understand that people such as Nick Vujicic are born with a genetic factor that cannot be altered. I am not suggesting that people can change these things. I am saying that everyone is a victim of their lifestyle choices and the environments that support those lifestyle choices. When you understand the potential in your genes **that you have**, you will be open to greater possibilities for yourself and for others. Something that Nick advocates to do.

Being reminded that you are 99.5% genetically the same as the person standing next to you or the person you admire most, will help ignite the human potential hidden within your genes. By empowering you to take ownership of your potential. Only discovering this spark the moment before you take your last breath is something I wouldn't wish on anyone. Don't wait until the end to meet the person that you could have been!

By the end of this chapter, you will have better context to embody these changes in your own story. The power of your genes comes down to how you think (thoughts can change your DNA), the lifestyle choices you consistently make and the environments that you spend the most time in. You have the pen; you have the paper, be your own director in your life's script. Simply match your daily lifestyle choices with the character you wish to be and you can manifest any future for yourself. I'm not kidding.

By going first, taking control of the 95% within your hands you will give others the inspiration to do so. Be courageous in this knowledge and embody it each day, feeling deep down that nature had your back long before we wrote a book about it.

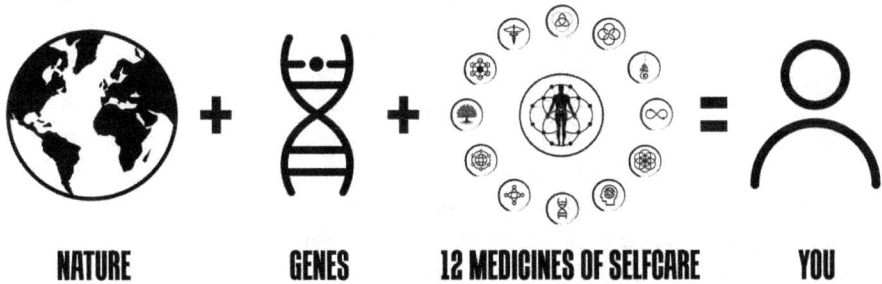

NATURE + GENES + 12 MEDICINES OF SELFCARE = YOU

DEFINE GENES AS MEDICINE

Our genes are the stretches of coding sequences within our DNA. Each gene contains instructions that determine your features or performs a molecular function such as create insulin in the body. This process is known as gene expression. Too often this process is mistaken as an absolute, that genes "will" cause x, y and z. However;

Genes are the hardware (5%); environment and lifestyle are the software (95%).

When you're born, your genes determine who you are in that moment, but you get to start your life with a blank canvas. This is known as tabula rasa, a Latin term which translates to "empty slate,"[3] suggesting that we can't draw water (experiences, knowledge) from an empty well (blank mind).

Individuals are born without built-in mental content therefore all knowledge comes from experience or perception. The meaning we make from our life experiences and our senses ultimately determine who we become and our success (or otherwise) to thrive.

Stimulus rich environments, positive mental constructs and environments where you can model the success of others will help you develop ways to express the best version of a dormant genetic blueprint waiting for the right stimulus, and a chance to dance and connect with the external environments of your lifestyle choices.

The Human Genome Project[4] began in 1990 and was a history-making research project to map and understand all of the genes of human beings—together known as our "genome." This international scientific journey took 13 years, and is a blueprint and manual for life on Earth. Upon its publishing, Francis Collins, Director of the National Human Genome Research Project stated:

> "It's a history book—a narrative of the journey of our species through time. It's a shop manual, with an incredibly detailed blueprint for building every human cell. And it's a transformative textbook of medicine, with insights that will give health care providers immense new powers to treat, prevent and cure disease."[5]

Genetically, the key message from The Human Genome Project is that as humans we are more the same than we are different. Our closet living animal cousin—the chimpanzee—shares 98% of our human genes. Vastly different looking mammals still share 92% and even plants share up to 18% the same genes as humans![6] So when you look at another living organism, animal or plant, realize that it too shares pieces of what makes you, you.

Individual human beings however, share 99.5% the same genetic blueprint.[7] This mind blowing statistic means that all the "differences" we see in other human beings separating "us" from "them," are simply mental constructs conditioned to focus on the 0.5% that makes us different. When we are born, our uniqueness, whether skin or hair color, height and any other perceived differences are all due to that small 0.5%.

What if we condition the mind to create a mental construct to focus on the 99.5% that makes us all human—true global citizens? Let's celebrate our individuality and focus on what makes us collectively human. Really understanding this, would allow all the mental constructs of separation to dissolve overnight, or even in this moment. Look and smile at the person next you see. Focus on the 99.5% that makes us human; surrender and let go of focussing on the 0.5%.

GENES ARE NOT YOUR DESTINY

Hypothetically, let's say one day in the future you decide to get a genetic test to assess whether you have the gene for certain health challenges, diseases, dysfunctions or conditions. Imagine the results come back positive; you have the gene for disease X!

How would it make you feel? A helpless victim? Would you become anxious and fearful of your impending mortality? Or would you change your lifestyle behaviors? Do everything you can to reduce your risk? Would you rationalize it amongst all the other information out there and come to peace with the fact that this is just a test and does not determine your life?

There are in fact genetic superheroes out there who, *"...stay healthy despite profound genetic defects."*[8] This extremely impressive paper published in *The Nature Research Journal* by Daniel Macarthur[9] confirmed something that researchers have long known. Our genes are not completely deterministic.

The refreshing perspective about the study Macarthur refers to is that rather than it focusing on people with the disease, the defect, the challenge. The study focused on the people with the genetic mutation that did not get sick, to learn from the health and wellbeing of the individual.

Led by researcher Stephen H Friend, he and his team conducted a comprehensive screen of 874 genes in 589,306 genomes leading to the identification of 13 adults harboring mutations for 8 severe Mendelian conditions, with no reported clinical manifestation of the indicated disease.[10]

Consider that these 13 adults who carried the exact genetic mutations that cause diseases such as cystic fibrosis, which severely affects the lungs and digestive system, had not developed these diseases, despite the mutations. These genes are extremely rare (13 in nearly 600,000 genomes tested) and even if you do have the genetic risk, this does not mean that these genes ever get a chance to express themselves (epigenetics!).

As Drs Chopra and Tanzi state, we are not simply the sum total of the genes we were born with—we are the authors of our own biological story. The presence of the gene in our genome is not fully deterministic of the disease occurring, it can remain dormant. Other genetic pathways, perhaps healthier ones may express themselves.

This means that genetic screening is a limited avenue; it provides lots of information but also no firm answers. Just because you marry a person who carries the red-headed gene, it is not deterministic that your child will have this gene. It can be recessive and perhaps even suppressed. If you have a child with someone who has the gene for cystic fibrosis, it is not deterministic that your child will be born with this genetic defect. Especially if the parents focus on expressing their ultimate human potential and focus on their health and wellbeing. What an amazing relief!

Human beings love seeking a linear answer from A to B, but nature does not work that way. It never has. Your genetic blueprint is malleable and can change its expression through epigenetic pathways! Your lifestyle choices in this lifetime may be impacting the genetic expression of children in future generations. To show how much you really value your family, make better lifestyle choices today and focus on igniting your human potential and focussing on the health and wellbeing of your human vessel in the context of any environment.

GENES ARE INFORMATIVE, NOT DETERMINISTIC

The Human Genome Project is expected to produce a sequence of DNA representing the functional blueprint and evolutionary history of the human species. However, only about 3% of this sequence is thought to specify the portions of our 50,000 to 100,000 genes that encode proteins.[11] Pioneer of the Human Genome Project, J. Craig Venter reported in their genome manuscript: *"A single gene may give rise to multiple transcripts, and thus multiple distinct proteins with multiple functions."*[12]

One gene is not deterministic of your future. Neither is it up to one gene to create the full human expression. Paul H. Silverman, an early advocate for the Human Genome project, shares that, *"A combination of just three genes, each with a thousand possible variants, offers a billion possibilities for natural selection; 10 genes each with 100 variants offers the evolutionary process infinitely more responsive combinatorial possibilities."*[13]

Now, imagine what it means to have 50,000 to 100,000 genes creating proteins for human function. As each gene interacts with each other, these expression variants increase, by a million fold or more; the raw material for evolutionary development is endless. Your genes suggest infinite possibilities for expression; you influence how those genes express themselves with nearly an infinite number of potential expressions.

When you consider the role of epigenetics—the study of genes being switched on and off by external factors—this suggests that your lifestyle choices are stimulus to trigger these limitless genetic pathways. Your lifestyle choices; diet, fitness, stress etc. will determine how your genetic blueprint expresses your ultimate human potential! Not forgetting that your lifestyle choices will be influenced by the environment you live in and the people with whom you spend the most time. We influence our own human potential and the potential of those around us.

This all means we might never be able to run as fast as Usain Bolt or change our physical image overnight. However, within the constraints of our genetic blueprint, we can get faster, fitter, stronger and transform our physical, mental and emotional body to overcome many challenges. We have all read or known about inspiration "disabled" athletes who have overcome their physiological constraints to do the seemingly insurmountable—win gold medals, climb epic mountains and reversed chronic preventable diseases like type 2 diabetes. Ultimately, beyond birth our lifestyle choices and epigenetics determine how our genes truly express themselves.

EPIGENETICS: *"GENES LOAD THE GUN, THE ENVIRONMENT PULLS THE TRIGGER"*[14]

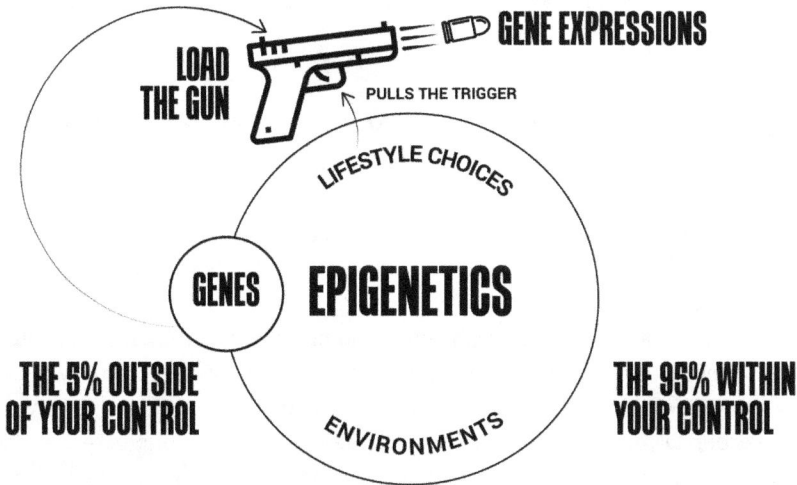

It's clear that the environment, lifestyle and behavior determines health outcomes and performance more than genes and other factors, but what does this mean for you?

It gives you greater control and means that you can influence the expression of your genes more than you perhaps recognized. You can influence the sleep you get, the stressors you allow into your life and the health practices you take part in. You can minimize the amount of toxins you are exposed to and maximize good nutrition, fresh air and exercise.

It helps to know that you are not at the sole mercy of your DNA. When we understand our power and realize that we have the ability to create a personalized plan for ourselves, it then begs the questions:

1. What type of old person do you want to be?
2. What type of blueprint expression do you want for future generations?
3. Perhaps more importantly, what type of lifestyle do you wish to live, to hand over the habits and behaviors that will best serve others and their genetic expression for their own longevity?
4. Lastly, how good could it possibly get? Can we live to 142 with both length and quality of life?

The future of health and wellbeing and, *"...precision medicine recognizes that we as individuals are each unique, that accordingly we have different health needs and health risks, and that we will respond differently to various treatments and medications."*[15] In the future, we will be treating the unique individual within the context of their lifestyles and their vision for themselves, to achieve the best health and wellbeing outcomes for them.

NEWSFLASH: THOUGHTS CAN INFLUENCE YOUR DNA!

Yes it's true! While our thoughts cannot change our genetic hardware, they can change the *epigenetic expression* of our genes with virtually unlimited potential relative to what we "think we know" and are capable of. According to cellular biologist Dr. Bruce Lipton, our thoughts and emotions can literally change our DNA, and by extension, our health![16]

This for me was the most astonishing finding, that our thoughts can literally change the expression of centuries, if not millennia of evolutionary biology. Knowing and believing this as a truth is so powerful, because if internally we can influence our DNA, then imagine what we can manifest in our external reality through our thoughts and by extension, our actions!

To paint a picture for the endless opportunity of knowing the power of our thoughts and lifestyle choices, Martin Fussenegger a Professor of Biotechnology and Bioengineering is excited that,

> *"For the first time, we have been able to tap into human brainwaves, transfer them wirelessly to a gene network and regulate the expression of a gene depending on the type of thought. Being able to control gene expression via the power of thought is a dream that we've been chasing for over a decade."*[17]

Anything is possible from here! We all just need to think differently with a common future vision for all in the back of our mind: health, happiness and connection in a unified and sustainable community.

THE FUTURE OF GENETICS?

Could it be possible to one day adapt our genome to develop cancer and tumor suppressing mechanisms? Nature has some incredible insights that suggest perhaps in the future we can. One would assume that animals and organisms that are larger and live longer than us would be more prone to uncontrolled cell growths—cancers—over that time. However, it is not so. In fact one of the oldest living whale species, the bowhead whale has an average lifespan of 200 years and doesn't get cancer. Joao Pedro de Magalhaes at the University of Liverpool shares that, *"They live a lot longer than human beings, yet they are living in the wild, without going to the doctor or any of the perks of human society, so they must be naturally protected from age-related diseases."*[18]

Perhaps we simply need to learn to adapt like whales. It's been investigated that based on human rates of cancer, large whales should be cancer-ridden by the time they reach maturity. But they don't become riddled with it like humans. In fact, they live for at least another one hundred years. This interesting and provocative whale fact suggests that whales have some evolutionary capabilities when dealing with aging and cancer mutations.[19]

Vadim Gladyshev[20] at Harvard University agrees. *"This is the most important biological question, because the majority of chronic human diseases are the consequences of ageing. The way biomedical science is organized, it has mostly focused on particular diseases, like cancer, Alzheimer's, or diabetes. But if we flip our approach and focus on delaying ageing we could delay the incidence of all these diseases at once."*[21] This would be an enormous benefit to humankind! Perhaps, rather than focusing on reversing ageing. We each realize that we are dying each day as our biological clock ticks. Healthier people, who value self-care and make better lifestyle choices, simply age slower. Others simply accelerate the natural aging process through more self-harm.

Scientists like de Magalhaes and Gladyshev have shown how natural selection has somehow pushed certain creatures to evolve their own elixir of life[22]. Developing tumor-suppressing mechanisms that we lack. Which means that perhaps we can too! What an inspiring thought.

SOLUTIONS

I believe that we are entering a new era where our scientific discoveries and innate knowledge and wisdom will transform our definition of health and allow us to revolutionize the human condition at large and apply better health practices across the globe. We will undoubtedly open up new vistas of exploration.

When you shift your awareness to truly know that you're not at the mercy of your genes, the world opens up for further possibilities. Scientist, Dr Bruce Lipton explains that this new perception of your own biology moves you out of victimhood and into mastery—mastery over your own health.[23] He is referring to using thought and emotion to alter gene expression; you can't get more self-control than that!

> *"We are still masters of our fate. We are still captains of our souls."*
> — **Winston S. Churchill, The Crisis** —

We *are* victims of our individual and collective choices. We are victims of the environments we create for ourselves to live in. To create the ultimate human expression of who you are and who you were born to be, cast a vision in your mind, hold it to be true and bring it into your reality.

If your thoughts can change evolutionary DNA, then why not let them positively influence who you are, who you become and the ideal life that you live! Nature has your back—environment will help you thrive. The 95% of who you are and who you become is in your hands.

So, how do you do this? In many easy ways.

Knowing that our thoughts, feelings and emotions drive our actions and behaviors, helps us realize that we are feeling beings that think and we ultimately become what we feel and think about most often! Who we are today is a result of past feelings, thoughts, actions and repeated behaviors. It suggests that to change our future external reality, we must start by harmonizing our internal reality. The deeper work that many of us avoid.

When pain arises on your path, learn from it. Using it as a whisper or a hammer from the universe to address underlying feelings, insecurities, traumas, shadows and thought patterns that have led to the behaviors you have today. When you feel bliss, or notice when time stands still in a place, with a certain person or when doing something you are passionate about; note that down and follow that energetic path.

We are victims of our individual and collective choices. We are victims of the environments we create for ourselves to live in. To create the ultimate human expression of who you are and who you were born to be, cast a vision in your mind, hold it to be true and bring it into your reality. If your thoughts can change evolutionary DNA, then why not let them positively influence who you are, who you become and the ideal life that you live! Nature has your back—the environment will help you thrive; 95% of who you are and who you become is in your hands.

Name 3 factors that negatively impacts your genes and thus your human potential (e.g. processed foods, negative beliefs, toxins)

....

....

....

Name 3 lifestyle changes you could make to protect and empower your innate genetic potential

....

....

....

Name one person that inspires you that anything is possible for you too!

🧬 GENES IS MEDICINE PRESCRIPTION

» Protect and co-create healthy of the environments around you; home, work, nature.

» Minimize the toxic burden on your body and mitigate the impact of endocrine disrupting chemicals entering your body from the industrialized world we have created for each other.

» Promote lifestyle choices that minimize internal harm and ignite your human potential.

» Support each other as collective communities.

» By doing all the above you ignite an epigenetic pathway with amazing potential! Be inspired by someone who has gone first!

To learn more about this medicine, or to contribute to this medicine, visit **selfcare.global/genes**. Here you will find blogs, videos and podcasts.

Selfcare.global/genes

NOTABLE EXPERTS IN THIS CHAPTER:

Dr. Deepak Chopra, Dr Rudolph Tanzi, Dr Joe Dispenza, Dr Bruce Lipton, Nick Vujicic, The Human Genome Project, Francis Collins, Daniel Macarthur, Stephen H Friend, Paul H. Silverman, Dr Scott Kahan, Martin Fussenegger, Joao Pedro de Magalhaes, Vadim Gladyshev.

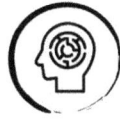

5

MIND IS MEDICINE

"Watch your thoughts, they become your words; watch your words,
they become your actions; watch your actions, they become
your habits; watch your habits, they become your character;
watch your character, it becomes your destiny."
— *Mahatma Gandhi* —

CONTROL YOUR THOUGHTS, CONTROL YOUR REALITY

Russel Brand knows a lot about addiction. His acting and comedic wit led him to fame and fortune. Along the way he succumbed to more than one addiction; alcohol, heroin, sex, food and even technology. Now he is using connection and spirituality to continue to beat his addictions.

Addiction is much more than a personal choice; it is guided by the modern day reality and symptoms of a disconnected world that we have unwittingly co-created for each other; dragging along the baggage from our upbringing while we try to conform to the cultural environments of modern life. Brand remarks, *"You are the person you were told to be."*[1]

In his book[2] he reveals how to overcome addiction and truly recover. That it is not about avoiding pain; after all what we resist persists. Allowing yourself to feel pain, to stop and feel the emotion, might actually be the internal driver that pivots any human being back into alignment, inner peace and living in harmony with their internal and external world.

Brand found a community and support in Alcoholics Anonymous and their 12 Steps program. He began to crave real connection; internally with himself, with others, with humanity and even a deeper spiritual connection to the source of it all. To awaken this connection he had to disengage from the isolation of watching mind-numbing TV and technology devices. He found that meditation stilled his mind and created space to really feel and re-examine old narratives and memories, learning from them and releasing them from his negative mindset to create a new, positive future narrative.

Stillness in his mind let him really *feel*, finding bliss in everyday moments without the need for mind-altering substances. Brand's story shows us all how we can deconstruct our mental roadblocks and realign internally, discovering the right energy and behaviors that move us up the health spectrum.

OUR MIND IS SUPREMELY POWERFUL

As Buddha said "we become what we think." Our mind can achieve brilliance but it can also hold us back. Every day we are fighting an internal war in our mind, between our 3:1 negative bias that seeks safety and survival, with our inner voice and positive bias that reminds us that the world is abundant, safe and that anything is possible. So much of our potential never sees daylight because of the conscious and unconscious blockages and apprehensions we develop as we grow up and live our adult lives.

Every action starts with a feeling (a sensation) and a thought, a chemical reaction in that beautiful brain of yours! It's a never-ending energy exchange that tunes into the mind stream of our external environments. However the collective unconsciousness of our environment often proves greater than our personal ability to make our own decisions and choices.

Many of our actions and decisions are made without conscious thought; these are constraints we must break free from. Separating the thoughts that are willfully ours, from those that have been unconsciously embedded into our psyche is the most challenging part.

FROM POWERLESSNESS TO REALIZATION

Your mind is your tool to learn how to "think different" and "choose different" as you tune into a higher vibration of awareness. Observe your own thoughts and decisions; observe your reactions to events and question where they came from. Do they serve you well? Or take you to a lower vibration?

This very moment could be *the* moment of your awakening.

To take control of your mind means no more blame and victimization and more acceptance, gratitude, courage, forgiveness and seeking opportunity. Learning to use your mind to its ultimate compacity takes education, learning, exploring ancient wisdom, asking courageous questions and simply being curious. Understanding the dynamic between our thoughts, choices and our environments is fundamental when learning to live our ultimate human experience. You have the freedom to think differently and create accordingly.

Mind as Medicine will show you how the power of your thoughts determines your life's perspective and sense of abundance. When your high-vibe thoughts and external actions are in alignment—then you are living in harmony. Whether it's trekking mountains or simply planting your garden, the longer we can spend in alignment, the more you will feel inner peace, bliss, happiness and activate your ultimate human potential.

DEFINING YOUR MIND AS MEDICINE

Let's consider more deeply the chemical reactions within our brains known as thoughts. How do we know they are even our own? Are they inherited from past generations handed down unconsciously as "truths," "beliefs" and other streams of consciousness?

On the surface you would probably disagree and answer that of course your thoughts are your own. However we actually have at least three minds[3] that are constantly working together, mostly without our conscious awareness. Understanding why you think the way you think, do what you do and live the way you live requires unraveling these three minds to uncover constructs and biases that have been implanted in your mind since you were born or even earlier.

In addition there is an energetic mindstream of collective consciousness and unconsciousness in the world around us, imperceptibly influencing our thoughts and actions as individuals and as a species. Added to this is our virtual mind or our virtual consciousness known as artificial intelligence (AI) that is even starting to create a whole new virtual reality and virtual mind stream!

In James Justin's book *Mindset: How To Transform Your Life From Ordinary To Extraordinary*, the life coach and speaker uses the "iceberg" model to explain how our three minds work.[4] Justin relates our conscious mind as similar to a ship's captain standing on the bridge giving orders. It's "the surface crew" on the deck (the subconscious) and "the deep crew" in the engine room below deck (the unconscious) that actually implement his orders; our actions. The captain may command the ship, but the collective crew actually guide the ship according to the level of training they have had over the years.

We all know that calms seas never made great sailors. The sailors that succeed have experienced storms and tempests in their life experiences and have practiced how to act and react with character, keeping their internal compass in check and true north in sight! The ship, the crew and the vessel can work in harmony together to survive and thrive, or they can fight amongst themselves creating a disconnect between the inner workings of the crew and what the captain sees and commands. This can cause the vessel to run in circles, stop completely and potentially even sink!

Finding harmony within is the key to finding harmony in our external world. Imagine the "conscious" captain in your mind casting a future vision and direction that the crew are internally aligned with and commit to persevering against all weather. This creates a vessel that is resilient to go the journey, no matter what storm it faces!

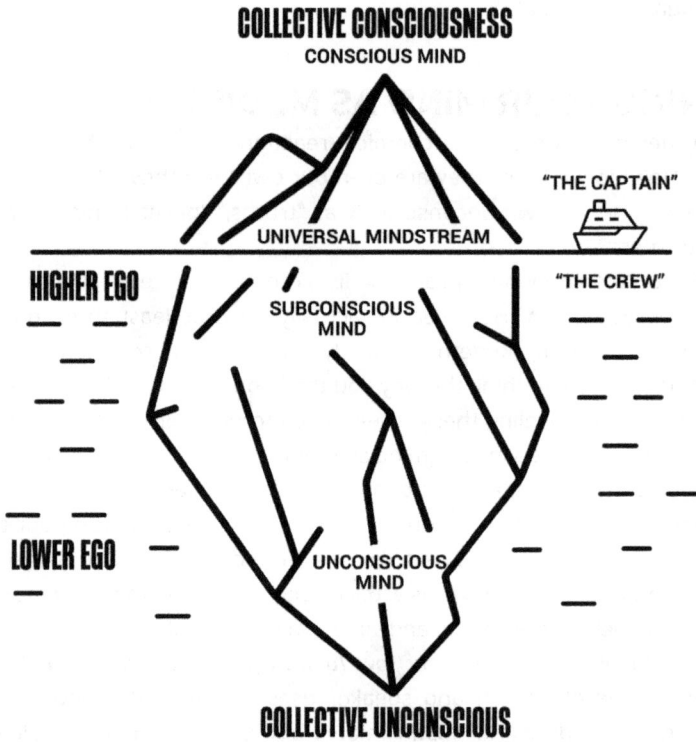

COLLECTIVE CONSCIOUSNESS
CONSCIOUS MIND

UNIVERSAL MINDSTREAM

"THE CAPTAIN"

HIGHER EGO

SUBCONSCIOUS MIND

"THE CREW"

LOWER EGO

UNCONSCIOUS MIND

COLLECTIVE UNCONSCIOUS

THE THREE MINDS THAT STEER YOUR LIFE

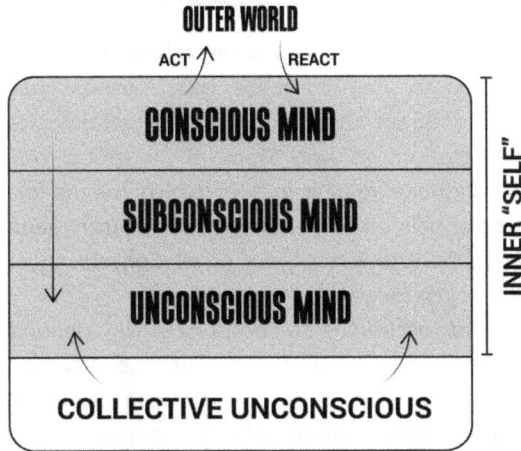

3 HUMAN MINDS

MIND 1
The Captain—*The conscious mind* communicates to the outside world and the inner self through speech, pictures, writing, physical movement and thought.[5]

MIND 2
The Surface Crew—*The subconscious mind* is responsible for our recent memories and is in continuous communication with the depth and beliefs of the unconscious mind.

MIND 3
The Deep Crew—*The unconscious mind* is the storage center for memories and past experiences, these memories and experiences can be forgotten, sifted out as "unimportant" or even repressed due to trauma. This library of memories and experiences form our beliefs, habits, and behaviors.

When considering The Captain's choices we need to remember something bigger is at play. There is a collective consciousness and energetic mindstream in the world around us that is influencing our crew and even our captain's conscious thoughts.

The Collective Mind (or the collective consciousness) is a fundamental sociological concept that refers to the set of shared beliefs, ideas, attitudes, customs, identities and knowledge commonly belonging to a social group or society. The Collective Mind forms our sense of belonging, identity and our behavior. Sociologist Émile Durkheim used this concept to illustrate how individuals are also bound together in deeper ways that reflect collective thought or behavior.[6]

For example, consider the world you were born into versus the world your parents were born into. Our collective consciousness had engineered this current reality. Think about the Industrial and technological revolutions and all the amazing revelations as well. Think of the global challenges we are all currently facing together. We chose this. Which means that if we can shift underlying systems of belief that have been handed from generation to the next, then we can change the future reality for us all. Consciously engineering a world that works for all, not just for some.

The Collective Unconscious is a concept originally defined by psychoanalyst Carl Jung and is sometimes called the objective psyche.[7] It refers to the idea that a segment of the deepest **unconscious** mind is inherited energetically or genetically from previous generations and is not shaped by personal experience.

For example, have you ever considered the accepted norms? That 9–5 job, the houses we live in and even how we live together as communities. Consciously and unconsciously we have directed our individual and collective efforts here. As captains of our own fate, we have played within the current rules and norms to end up here today. Choosing our global leaders and captains, giving our power to governments, people and others to captain the fate of spaceship earth. What if we appointed different captains? Imagine more women in positions of power. How would their underlying belief systems, guide and shape the world? What would happen if we chose more leaders—"captains"—that were working against the collective unified beliefs that we each hold as captains of our own lives and environments. Perhaps we need to address the collective unconsciousness, bring it to the surface and ensure that the captains we choose are leading our spaceship earth in the right direction. Not towards a 6th mass extinction or a world where health is not a basic human right available to all.

When left unchecked, the captain and crew may feel that they are forging their own path, when in fact they are simply following the routes of other captains and ships that have gone before them. Deep down it would be like wanting to go to Hawaii because that's where the captain, the crew and vessel are happiest. But finding that you continue to end up in the busy ports of Shanghai where no one is surprised to see you there—except you! You wonder why it keeps happening.

With realization you can course correct your ship by choosing your true north and calibrating your internal compass at any time.

What if you took a minute to pause, go inwards and allow your conscious captain to speak and align directly with the crew? Cast that new vision together, commit to weathering the storms and navigate the way to your new destination rather than the one you never really wanted to go.

Our conscious mind is still a big player in who we become. In the early 1900s E. Stanley Jones shared that, *"The conscious mind determines our actions and choices, the unconscious mind determines the reactions, and the reactions are just as important as the actions."*[8]

Perhaps it's the sum of how we act and react that shows the true character of our being. Not just how we think and consciously choose, but how we react in tough, painful and emotional situations that draw from our unconscious. Do we become a product of our choices and actions, or a product of our unconscious reactions based on past experience and perhaps emotional pain or trauma? Perhaps it is both.

Some people might be spending their life healing ancestral trauma, whilst others might have the breathing space to consciously engineer a whole new reality for us all. Some might not be thinking at all.

Regardless of how you view mind, the one thing that all neuroscientists, psychologists and philosophers agree on is that it's mighty powerful. The main thing to know is how to use it well. Yogachara-Chittamatra (an integration of quantum physics and Buddhist philosophy) have summed up "mind" saying that:

"The mind is the principle creator of everything because sentient beings accumulate predisposing potencies through their actions, and these actions are directed by mental motivation. These potencies are what create not only their lives, but also the physical world around them."[9]

This is a fancy way of saying that thoughts literally become things! This is a whole journey to explore on its own but mostly take from it that our mind is the most powerful generator of all! The karmic instigator!

THOUGHTS AS AN ENERGETIC FREQUENCY

"Turn on, tune in, drop out."
— *Timothy Leary* —

1. SCIENCE OF BRAIN FREQUENCIES

The human brain is filled with copious amounts of information, from your daily to-do list, to memories, to communicating with people and interacting with technology. Brain overwhelm and information overload are common expressions people use these days. So how can we know which thoughts to listen to, and when? Which ones serve us and which ones are unproductive and useless? When should we tune in or tune out?

Research published in *Nature*[10] by Laura Lee Colgin and her group from The Norwegian University of Science and Technology (NTNU) found that when brain cells want to connect and communicate with each other, they synchronize their activity and literally tune into each other's wavelength. Pretty cool, huh? Colgin and her team investigated how gamma brain waves were particularly instrumental in communicating across cell groups in the brain region of the hippocampus in rats. In summary, the lower frequencies are used to transmit memories or past experiences, whereas the higher frequencies are used in the present moment experience of what is happening here and now.

"The cells can rapidly switch their activity to tune in to the slow waves or the fast waves," Colgin says, "but it seems as though they cannot listen to both at the exact same time. This is like when you are listening to your radio and you tune in to a frequency that is midway between two stations—you can't understand anything—it's just noise."[11] This is similar to trying to be productive in the present moment, only to find we tune into the frequency of social media, news or others peoples thoughts and opinions.

2. TUNE IN

Imagine that you are in charge of tuning into your own "frequency" radio station each day.

If energy is a vibration with a specific frequency, which channel are you tuning into? A positive or negative frequency one? The high vibration channel or the low vibration channel? Each day we tune into different stations through all of our senses. We tune into auditory stations (a radio station, a podcast, audiobook), or what you see on visual stations (A TV station, YouTube, even social media platforms), and in reality (people, environments etc,).

Consider the stations, platforms, people or environments you energetically tune into. Are they positive and uplifting or negative and something that lowers your energetic vibration?

Every morning when you wake up, do you pick up your mobile device and tune into social platforms, or do you journal and write down what you are grateful for today? One is a comparison of a virtual reality, whereas the other is an embodied action in that present moment.

However, this might be changing as we speak. Open your phone and reflect on the type of people you follow on social platforms. Do they make you feel energetically inspired and empowered? Or do they make you feel insignificant and down in the dumps? Reflect on the type of audio books, radio stations and the type of music you listen to. Is it uplifting, or is the frequency and energy of the words quite negative?

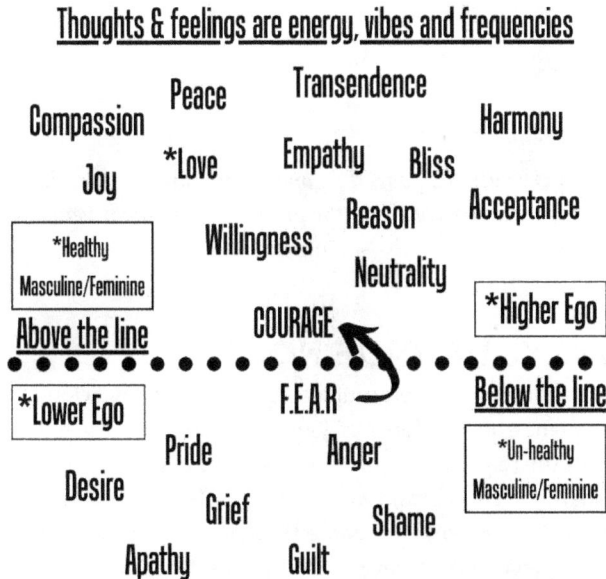

Thoughts & feelings are energy, vibes and frequencies

Transcendence

Peace

Compassion   Harmony

*Love   Empathy   Bliss

Joy

Reason   Acceptance

*Healthy Masculine/Feminine   Willingness

Neutrality

Above the line   COURAGE   *Higher Ego

*Lower Ego   F.E.A.R   Below the line

Pride   Anger

Desire   *Un-healthy Masculine/Feminine

Grief   Shame

Apathy   Guilt

3. EVERY THOUGHT HAS A FREQUENCY

In the book *Power vs. Force* by David R. Hawkins, there's a hierarchy of levels of human consciousness.[12] Although we can fluctuate to different levels during different times, there's usually a predominant "baseline" state where we commonly dwell.

Enlightenment	700-100
Peace	600
Joy	540
Love	500
Reason	400
Acceptance	350
Willingness	310
Neutrality	250
Courage	200
Pride	175
Anger	150
Desire	125
Fear	100
Grief	75
Apathy	50
Guilt	30
Shame	20

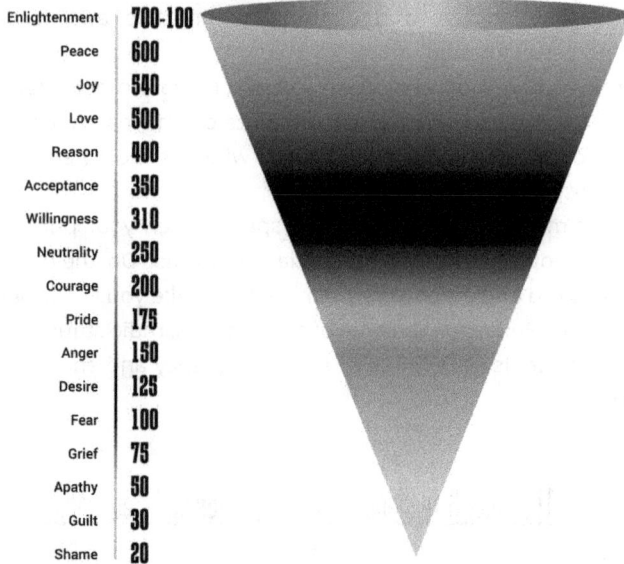

*"Don't cry over the past, it's gone. Don't stress about the future,
it hasn't arrived. Live in the present and make it beautiful."*
— Unknown —

ALIGNING YOUR TRUE NORTH

As the unconscious mind communicates with our conscious mind, it sends subconscious signals in the form of feelings, emotions, imagination, sensations, and dreams. It's the reason why you can't just tell someone to think better thoughts or convince them to live a certain way or make different choices.

They need to do the work and come to their own self-realizations in their own time. You can however, empower people to experience different events and ways of being. In the same way you could inspire and empower someone to travel with you to a place they have never been. They might borrow your courage and come for the ride!

This is a difficult change to make for anyone considering the strong cultural narratives and constructs of modern western society. How can we be happy, healthy, connected and abundant at the same time? Neuro-linguistic patterning shows us that we can change our own thoughts; we can reframe, restructure and rewire how we think. But, how do we achieve a cultural change; to change existing constructs that certain societies fundamentally accept as truth?

We need an inside-out approach, to go deep within and realign "our crew" with our "captain" and change our individual direction. Recalibrate our internal compass with a positive future vision that aligns with our "true north." To do this may require some emotional release and even healing ancestral trauma in our collective unconscious. The thoughts and emotions suppressed under the surface lead to "disconnect" between the conscious captain and the working crew. We need both alignment and synergy to find a sense of inner peace.

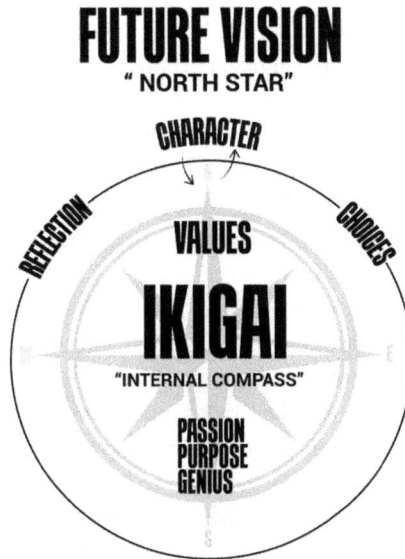

FUTURE VISION
" NORTH STAR"

CHARACTER

REFLECTION

VALUES

CHOICES

IKIGAI
"INTERNAL COMPASS"

PASSION
PURPOSE
GENIUS

Once we have made peace within, we can find ease and flow in our external environment. Easily navigating rough seas and avoiding storms with a tuned-in internal compass, that keeps realigning us with our true north, finding the path of least resistance towards our desired destination. Ensuring that the captain and crew get there together. Furthermore if anyone has connected with you and your path, it means you can accurately lead them through treacherous waters so that they too reach the desired destination with you.

It takes a decision to take ownership and go inwards first, so that you can individually make a decision to change the future narrative of your life and create a ripple effect of change that alters cultural narratives and inspires others t hat they can too.

Letting go of past narratives and reframing past experiences as lessons for future voyages requires work. Open your mind, open your heart and be prepared to feel more as you go deeper into the depths of your human vessel, before consciously engineering and manifesting your dreams in the external reality.

THE EVOLVING HUMAN BRAIN

How does our mind as a mechanism actually operate today? We have a modern biological brain that has to interact with both a natural world and a virtual consciousness all at the same time. To understand where our "mind" is going, we need to understand how it evolved.

Over time, the human brain tripled in size to become the largest most complex of the primate species alive today.[13] So what separated us from other animals? How did we become the self-proclaimed cleverest species to walk this earth? If it were brain size that separated us from other animals then elephants and whales would trump us for intelligence. Perhaps it was brain size relative to body size? Well actually shrews and mice do much better on that front too!

The truth is that we don't know. *"As it stands...it is not clear what it is about our brains that causes our minds to be special,"* admits Suddendorf, a University of Queensland researcher whose book *The Gap: The Science of what separates us from other animals* focuses on this unique separation between humans and other species.[14]

Although one could argue, how clever can we truly be considering we are, in fact one of the only species that destroys the natural environment that sustains them! The whales, naked mole rat and immortal jellyfish have a better understanding of long-term survival being both long-lived and ancient species. After all, our species of man has only been around for 200,000 or so years, just a small notch on the belt of time.

From an evolutionary perspective the human brain contains about 100 billion neurons, more than 100,000 km of interconnections, and has an estimated storage capacity of 1.25 × 1012 bytes (Hofman).[15] This would circumnavigate the world (40,075km) 2.5x over!

These impressive numbers have led to the idea that our cognitive capabilities are virtually without limit. However, every hypothesis looks for more mental constructs to reaffirm our own innate cognitive biases, that we are the smartest living species on this planet!

You may have heard that dolphins and bats use echolocation to determine the position of obstacles in their path. Humans had to use "bio-mimicry" to consciously engineer external technological devices to do this for us, which is cool but demonstrates that ultimately we are but vassals to nature's peak designs. We may actually never move in water like a dolphin does, or fly like a bat does at night, so effortlessly.

The hard truth for some is that we are not so special and we do not have unlimited capacity. *The Handbook of Intelligence* shows that the human brain has evolved from a set of underlying structures that constrain its size, and the amount of information it can store and process![16] So how then do we surpass this biological constraint?

The first clue is an organism's processing capacity and speed. The ability to *process* information about its environment is a driving force behind evolution, the more information a biological system such as the brain receives, and the *faster* it can process this information, the more successfully it will respond to environmental challenges thus increasing its chances of survival.

The second clue is an organism's functional capacity to use this processed information for actions and reactions. The limit to any intelligent system can be tested by its ability (or inability) to process and integrate big volumes of sensory information and compare them with memory and experiences in an extremely short amount of time. It suggests that the "functional capacity of a neuronal structure is inherently limited by its neural architecture and signal processing."[17]

So what was the secret that allowed us to bypass the functional capacity of our own brain? How did we begin to process more information and process it faster so we could survive and thrive within the context of any environment; from deserts to forests to icy regions?

It was our ability to consciously engineer, experiment and learn that helped us make the evolutionary leap to using and creating tools to manipulate our surroundings. It started with hammers to mold our physical environment, fire to utilize our chemical and elemental environment and continued to what we see today; spaceships, satellites, neural links, cities, smartphones, gene splicing technology and even wearable biofeedback devices.

Essentially we learnt how to use natural elements from our environment to create an external brain in the form of computers and smartphones. We also developed a way to create virtual consciousness, a "world wide web" and to share information at the click of a button. We then took it a step further and developed artificial intelligence to organize and connect information in a forward thinking way. In the same way a human mind problem solves in external environments.

The evolution of the human brain led to finding a way to bypass our biological constraints by creating a virtual mind, a virtual collective consciousness akin to an external hard drive for your biological mind with forward thinking artificial intelligence. Incredible!

The good news is that children in any corner of the world with a smartphone and internet access have the ability to access education from some of the world's greatest minds. Those teachers and mentors still alive as well as the pioneers of humanity who have come before us, leaving their wisdom "online" for others to tune into. Elon Musk and his team used their biological mind to consciously engineer rockets and satellites that may one day permit children in every corner of the globe to have access to the collective consciousness and virtual mind through global wifi, smartphones, online education platforms and anything in between, using Starlink and SpaceX.

This book will be that resource one day: a remnant of my own biological consciousness, a curation of collective consciousness and biological chemical reactions that resulted in these thoughts and connections. This *SelfCare* book becomes another framework for the collective and virtual consciousness. Something that future generations can build on or replace as the complex becomes simpler.

I AM VERSUS I FEEL

But it's not all about thought. How does the heavy mass of gray matter that is our brain give rise to the felt experience of sensations and thoughts? Thinking is only part of the puzzle. Our thoughts and our choices that shape our reality may be more emotional than they are conscious. In his 1994 book, *Descartes' Error*, neuroscientist Antonio Damasio reaffirms that, *"We are not thinking machines. We are feeling machines that think,"* suggesting, *"Emotion and its underlying neural machinery participate in decision making."*[18]

We are feeling beings that think, not the other way around.

Most marketing experts know that people largely choose and buy from emotion, not rational thought. We cannot simply learn to think better thoughts and make better choices; it's not how it works.

Descartes' Error, Damasio writes of brain-damaged patients like the famous Phineas Gage, who survived a steel pole penetrating completely through his skull and brain without losing any intellectual reasoning capabilities. Although this over-simplifying Gage's deeply complex and extraordinary story, his case baffled and even divided scientists—they never really came to an agreed and final conclusion. Damasio proposes that its emotion that guides our behavior and decision-making, and Descartes' error was in his emphasis of separating them in a dualistic way. He uses Gage's classic case in which to make his point of emotions being part of intelligence. He suggests that humans don't make decisions in a purely logical or cognitive way but instead there is an emotional governance at play. That the limbic system, amygdala and pre-frontal cortex are prime contributors. He says "Because the brain is the body's captive audience, feelings are winners among equals."[19]

To grossly simplify Damasio's theory, he suggests that our brains are stamped with a "somatic marker" so that every experience, every moment—emotion is branding our brains with "feeling markers." Let me explain.

The amygdala, that emotion center, is the ancient reptilian part of our brain that actually wires us for survival, to read and react to a situation quickly. It is extremely powerful in young people. It is thought that a maturing amygdala contributes to two behavioral effects. Firstly the tendency for adolescents to react explosively (fight or flight!) to situations rather than with more controlled responses.[20]

Imagine you are surfing in beautiful clear waters and you see a shadow move underneath you—you freeze; shark! Your fight or flight emotion center of the brain is on full alert, assessing the threat. Your reptilian brain kicks in as your heart and breathing increases.

Gradually, your limbic brain kicks in as you come to realize that it is not a shark, after all just a clump of seaweed moving with the ocean currents. That's your prefrontal cortex (ventromedial) kicking in to calm the amygdala's panic. The second limbic brain, stamps this moment with a "somatic marker" so that you don't respond in such a heightened way next time.

The second behavioral effect of a growing amygdala is the tendency for youth to misread people's neutral or inquisitive facial expressions as a sign of anger. Some people are more reactive than others or misread emotional and physical cues, the emotional center of their brain may not have had the stimulus or guidance needed to mature effectively.

We must be patient too, because the balm of calm within our brain—the prefrontal cortex—does not reach maturity until about 25 years of age. So until then, the amygdala is able to coerce the brain. In short, most teenagers see sharks (threats) even when it is clearly just seaweed.

Have you ever wondered why **emotional events are more memorable** than events that do not evoke any emotion? Emotion guides our decisions and allows us to remember events and experiences due to their emotional impact on us. A number of scientific experiments involving fMRI brain scans reveal the heightened activation of the amygdala (the emotion center) alongside the hippocampus (memory).[21]

Emotions turbo boost and strengthen the imprint of the memory.[22] It's the reason why creating an emotional experience for people is the best way to be memorable and create a somatic marker in their lifetime of experiences. You may not even have to experience the emotion yourself. A stranger's completely unrelated but emotional story can become a catalyst to making a task or experience more memorable![23] It is the reason why other people's emotional stories can help impact our future decisions. Their emotional story is embedded in your mind for future actions and reactions!

1 BAD EVENT : 5 GOOD EVENTS

THE 4 TYPES OF INTELLIGENCE: IQ, HQ, EQ, GQ

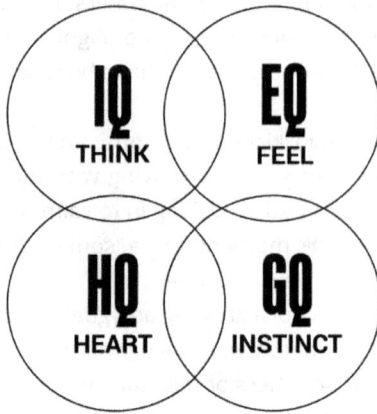

IQ is the intelligence quotient that often refers to our rational and conscious minds ability to think, recall information and solve challenges. However, like you I am curious about different quotients for intelligence. What about the heart, our emotions and even our gut? Do you wonder what that feeling, raised heart beat or butterflies in your stomach really tells you?

Howard Gardner proposed the model of multiple intelligences in his 1993 book, *Frames of mind: the theory of multiple intelligences* to help differentiate "human intelligence" into specific modalities, rather than just being dominated by one general ability.[24] As an example modern day schoolchildren are measured by their IQ (mind), more than their ability to think critically, feel and make good decisions in the ever-changing external environment.

Sir Ken Robinson's famous Tedx talk explains how modern schooling kills creativity, suppresses the feeling and reduces the need for critical thinking towards a solution.[25] Freeing young mind and hearts from old paradigms and systems of thought, is exactly what the modern world needs in order to move forward and thrive together in harmony with each other and nature.

Can we combine the intelligence of the mind (IQ), with the intelligence of the emotional (Emotional Q), with heart intelligence (Heart Q) and with the intelligence of our "gut instinct" (Gut Q)?

I see it as **IQ + HQ + EQ + GQ = True Intelligence**

According to Yogi Bhajan, *"Intelligence is when your senses (mind, heart, gut) and your consciousness calculate on the spot. Senses and 'feelings' will say one thing, consciousness and 'thoughts' will say something different. And when you can put it together, two and two, that is intelligence."*[26]

He suggests something important, that true intelligence goes beyond thinking. It is felt; it is intuitive based on life experiences. It explains why the best academics and scholars may be extremely knowledgeable (IQ), but lack the physical application and impact in the real world.[27]

Perhaps you can recall a time when "gut" overrode "mind." For me, it was as a young man when I had the opportunity to walk on by, unaffected, as my father lay homeless on the streets of our town. Or I could take a minute of my time to say hello, see if he was okay and recognize the existence of the man that gave me my first breath.

If I lacked compassion and empathy (EQ and HQ) then it would have been easy to walk on by, willfully and ignorantly disregarding his existence. I would have then spent the rest of my life rationalizing (IQ) why I chose not to say hello. My friends may have laughed at me, they may have judged me; it may have affected my sense of identity or social status.

However, deep down my gut instinct (GQ) kicked in, my emotional and feeling being was overwhelmed with a sense of compassion and my heart started beating harder as I stepped forward to acknowledge my father's existence. Listening to my gut first, before my heart, my emotions and then mind enabled me to make an uncomfortable decision in real time.

It was a decision that taught me my most valuable life lesson. It taught me empathy, compassion and ignited a feeling of faith within me that I will never forget. It also changed my rational mind. I no longer saw my dad as a homeless drunk. I saw him as my father, a man in need of support who was numbing his mind and emotional being with alcohol. He had been doing it for so long that each unguided decision led him to the point that he was surviving, not living, homeless on the streets where his son was born.

Every time we make decisions that ignore our gut, heart and our emotions, we disconnect from our internal compass and head down a path that takes us away from our true north. We then try to rationalize it with our mind (the captain), but find that there is a disconnect between our conscious mind, our deep unconscious mind and most importantly our internal feelings.

The disconnection between how we really feel, our unconscious mind and our conscious thoughts and actions can lead to disharmony between our internal and external world. Many human beings seek external mind-altering substances to numb the mind or seek out experiences that allow them to feel again.

If we lack compassion and empathy (EQ and HQ), then it's easy to rationalize (IQ) and make decisions at the expense of others or at the collateral damage of the environment and communities we live in.

Choosing different is emotional, not rational.

MIND OVER MEDICINE

Lissa Rankin, American M.D and author of *Mind Over Medicine* contends that mainstream medicine does not represent the universe of potentially valuable treatment protocols or modalities. Rankin was frustrated when Western medical treatments failed to help her own health challenges so she went looking for answers beyond the traditional guidelines.

She discovered incredible evidence to attest that; *"State of mind, emotion, human circumstance, human interaction and belief not only play a role, but have the ability to effectively turn on or off the body's innate ability to heal itself; they either keep disease and pain ever-present, or serve as a foundation for sustained recovery."*[28]

David Butler, world-renowned expert and author of *Explain Pain,* illuminates the true power of the mind. *"Pain is in the brain,"* and is more complex than just an input.[29] *"One of the most popular stories is the drug cabinet in the brain—the story of our own powerful and underused pharmacy and one which is hijacked by the pharmaceutical industry which prefers exogenous rather than endogenous medication. What is the most powerful pain reliever? Morphine? Oxycontin? Fentanyl? Oxymorphone? Think again..."*[30]

"The best relief for pain is distraction."

Yes, that's right; distraction is the most powerful pain reliever in the world! It means that pain relief does not need to come in the form of a synthetic medication. We can relieve or distract ourselves from pain by creating new experiences. Participating in hobbies, taking time to move in a meaningful way and spending time in nature.

Others partake in virtuous activities giving their time to volunteer in the service of others or the natural world. From dog shelters to planting trees, these virtuous activities, seem to evoke a sense of gratitude and contentment that distracts our mind from pain. Some people love new challenges and love to learn new things. With enough distraction, you too may find the road to recovery, or at least pain relief!

Understanding that pain is an output of the brain, not an input is the most powerful paradigm shift in modern medicine! It means we can influence and suppress it, creating space for more positive emotions.

We know the brain can change and heal itself. In his book, *The Brain's Way of Healing,* Norman Doidge shares that neuroplasticity is one of the most important discoveries of our modern time. He states that the brain's ability to change its own structure and function *"in response to mental experience—this is the phenomenon of neuroplasticity."*[31]

Doidge describes that, *"Neuroplastic techniques explain why we can see patients in whom years of chronic pain has been alleviated, and others who have recovered the ability not just to walk or talk but to live fully despite debilitating strokes, as well as cases of long-standing brain injuries cured or vastly improved.*"[32] This not only gives hope to the average person without disability, it gives hope to anyone who has experienced a debilitating injury. The brain can structurally change itself and change the way the body functions with the application of the right stimulus.

What should become increasingly clear is the power of your thoughts towards living your dream life, but also being able to heal and bounce forward from any situation you might find yourself in. Your amazing human vessel can heal and regenerate itself with the right stimulus over the desired amount of time. In the case of severe damage or irreversible disability, simply knowing that the human body is able to adapt and alter to accommodate its new able functions is a powerful point of hope for anyone!

I remember seeing my father days after he suffered a severe brain injury. He was comatose for close to a month without movement and supported by modern medical devices such as ventilators. After a month or so he squeezed my hand for the first time, before opening his eyes. This was his first sign of life, and a critical moment. I was not to know that the allied health team had been close to alluding that his life support be turned off.

What happened from there was a miracle of the human spirit. His return to life showed me how resilient this human body is. Even to self-inflicted harm. In his early recovery he could not speak or lift his arm, let alone throw a ball. Within 12 months however, he was painting again. He lacked the fine motor skills that he once had, but he could paint better than I could.

The amazing part of this story is that the brain damage impacted the part of the brain that housed his long-term memory. His injury actually freed him from the past emotional events that had led him to alcoholism as a way of numbing his painful thoughts. Within 24 months he was painting in a whole new way that I had never seen. Art became his therapy.

Incredibly his paintings were now colorful and bright, no longer dark and solitary. It matched the happiness and light heartedness that he had come out of hospital with. One could argue that he was happier after the brain injury than he was before. What an amazing human vessel we have! I hope this inspires hope in your life or in the life of someone you love.

MAKE PEACE AND MANIFEST

Remember anything is possible from here. Own it all. We each need to have the courage to accept, forgive and love to find inner peace and enlightenment in the context of any life. It means that you do not need to be the Dalai Lama to find inner peace in your own life; you can be anyone, anywhere, anytime.

Our collective purpose is to empower each other towards our own self-mastery. Mastering our internal reality will help us influence our external reality.

Feel more, think less, do better.

Realigning our collective thoughts will change the world. Our minds are consciously and unconsciously engineering our individual and collective realities into existence. If we can control our thoughts and keep them aligned with coherence and community and care, then we create that in our world. Control your thoughts; control your reality.

I would encourage you to make peace with your past; events that have already happened and are unchangeable. Each event has a lesson for us to take forward into a positive inspiring future vision. The future is yours to manifest and create.

MIND IS MEDICINE PRESCRIPTION

» Every day align your thoughts with your actions in order to head toward your True North.

» Make a list of past events you haven't made peace with. Write down the lessons you received from them and let them go.

» Create a positive and inspiring future vision board and put it up where you can see it every day.

» Take an inventory of the quality of your thoughts. Are the majority of your daily thoughts in a high frequency; love, forgiveness, acceptance, courage? (rather than lower frequency thoughts of blame, fear, victimization).

» Are you using all your intelligence? Are you developing the ability to feel first? (EQ). Do you listen to your gut instinct and heart? (GQ & HQ). Do you learn something new each day? (IQ).

To learn more about this medicine, or to contribute to this medicine, visit **selfcare.global/mind**. Here you will find blogs, videos and podcasts.

Selfcare.global/mind

NOTABLE EXPERTS IN THIS CHAPTER:

Dr David Hawkins, Bruce Lipton, James Justin, Russel Brand, Dr Joe Dispenza, Émile Durkheim, Carl Jung, E. Stanley Jones, Laura Lee Colgin, Thomas Suddendorf, Antonio Damasio, Howard Gardner, Sir Ken Robinson, Yogi Bhajan, Lissa Rankin, Dr David Butler, Dr Norman Doidge.

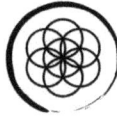

6

FOOD IS
MEDICINE

We don't have a food shortage, 40 percent of food produced is wasted every year.[1] Food journalist Mark Bittman told us that "1 billion people in the world are chronically hungry. 1 billion people are overweight."[2] We need sustainable and regenerative agriculture and effective distribution.

EVERY TIME YOU EAT, YOU'RE EITHER BUILDING IMMUNITY OR BUILDING DISEASE

Breaking News: Modern agriculture got it wrong! Farmers were quite excited when they used chemical fertilizers for the first time; it meant high yields, less work, more profits! But then they began to see the negative consequences on the ecology and health of the local environment; frogs, birds, bees and insects started to vanish. It turns out that these Endocrine Disrupting Chemicals (EDC) chemicals are not only poisonous for human consumption, but also poisonous for all other living organisms.

Over time these chemicals began to deplete the soil of nutrients, lowering the nutrient value in the crops they were designed to help—go figure! Short-term gains were taken at the expense of long-term consequences. For over a century we have known that continually consuming food from nutrient deficient soil results in us living in a state of energetic depletion.[3] Way back in 1910 American physician Dr Curtis Wood Jr aptly described the average North American as, "overfed but undernourished."[4] It just took us 100 years to understand what he meant!

So, before we get too deep into this food topic, let's state the obvious—

Food is a foundational building block for the growth and function of a healthy human body; it is not a complementary or alternative medicine, it is foundational.

Everything you eat has an effect. In fact, *"Every time you eat or drink, you are either feeding disease or fighting it."*[5] Nutrigenomics is the field of medicine that studies how the food we eat can ignite and activate our human potential *or* suppress our human function by promoting disease and dysfunction.[6]

What we eat shouldn't be complicated. Michael Pollan, a renowned lecturer on food, agriculture, health and the environment, sums it up nicely with seven simple words to live by, *"Eat food, not too much, mostly plants"*—the last word being the most important.[7]

How did we become so confused?

To understand Food as Medicine, we need to shift the conversation away from nutrition "isms," ideologies, fads, diets, superfoods, restriction based regimes (Ketogenic, Atkins etc) and quick fixes, and tackle the key question:

**How can everyone nourish their body every single day,
so that their body can regenerate itself naturally?**

It's starts by knowing what actually fuels and nourishes your body and why. What we consume each day; air, water and food empowers the body to regenerate fifty million cells every second—what clever engineering!

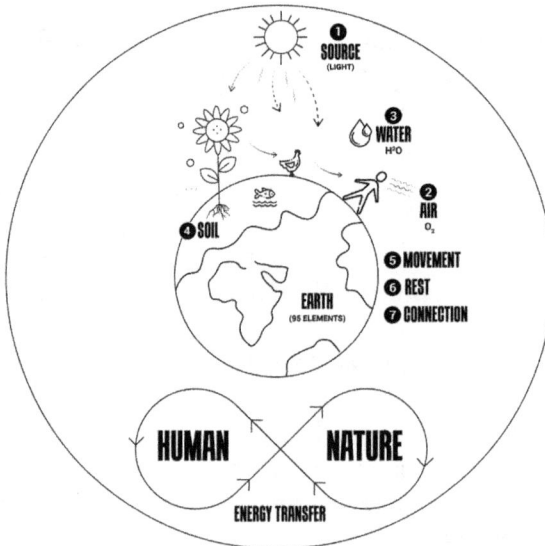

NOT ALL FOODS ARE CREATED EQUALLY

It must be understood that not all foods are created equally. Sad but true.

Nature's "food" has been overrun by packages of convenience and well-placed marketing on supermarket shelves. Farming practices, soil health and inefficient food chain systems also contribute to the nutrient and chemical values that reach our tables.

Understanding what *real food* is and its function will help you make better choices in relation to your self-care. It will connect you with the realistic needs of your unique body based on your lifestyle, level of activity and your environment. Athletes and office dwellers have vastly different needs. Learn to recognize your own fuel needs and how to find them naturally.

From here you can move away from consuming "food-like" products and return to foundational food to heal, transform and grow. Food from natural sources, grown in living biodynamic soil and healthy natural ecosystems, free of synthetic chemicals that is low on human interference. Just like our grandparents' day—simple! Lay down the building blocks now in order to reach the peak physical human body you'd like in 12 months time and beyond!

FOOD AS MEDICINE

The dichotomy of overweight yet undernourished has been slow to gain recognition. A Nutrition Canada National Survey back in 1975 found 50% of Canadian adults were overweight and of these 10% of males and 30% of females were obese![8] Yet these results did not get a lot of attention at the time despite their finding of a suboptimal nutritional status of the population. The researchers felt there was, "no evidence of clinically apparent malnutrition [and] it is difficult to judge the immediate health significance of this finding."[9] The "health significance" would be revealed with time.

For generations, our cultural constructs didn't associate obesity and increasing waistlines with malnutrition, it was considered the opposite. The governments of the day didn't see the impending cardiac and metabolic effects from the increasing lifestyle of excess. Indicatively the obesity prevalence rates nearly doubled in Canadian adults between 1978/79 and 2004, from 13.8% to 23.1%![10]

Unfortunately, what we now know from experience is that being overweight increases susceptibility to a number of diseases and consequently shortens one's life. A concept now commonly fostered as "increase one's waistline and shorten one's lifeline."

However the war isn't on obesity. Our waistline is the end result of a willfully ignorant and a consciously manipulated population whose lifestyle choices (yes personal choice, not blame) led to those pants not fitting. The war is about educating people on what food actually *is*. The war is within your own heart as you choose how to fuel your own body, your family's bodies, and consequently which circular economies you feed into and support.

Your local farmers market with biodynamic, organic, seasonal produce? Or the brightly colored processed bag in the supermarket isle with an "organic label" that didn't exist 100 years ago? This choice will unleash a new lifestyle that is conscious of the whole process of nutrients, from farm to your fork.

Nutrients as a concept, have been recognized since the early 19th century, when the English doctor and chemist William Prout identified what came to be called the "macronutrients": protein, fat and carbohydrates. They were thought to make up the bulk of food's qualities until doctors began to notice that even with an adequate supply of the big three, people were not necessarily nourished.[11]

This mystery became apparent in the 19th century when British doctors were puzzled that while their Chinese laborers in the Malay states were dying of a disease called beriberi, the disease did not seem to affect the Tamils or the native Malays. Finally it was realized that the Chinese ate "polished" or white rice that is mechanically milled. The others ate non-milled rice. A few years later, the essential nutrient (vitamin B-1) was discovered in rice husks of unpolished rice that protected against beriberi, this was one of the first vitamins or micronutrients discovered.[12]

Each Day Human Beings Need to source 25–27 of the 118+ currently known universal elements from the natural environment to maintain life and growth.[13] We call these elemental molecules—**Nutrients.** The overarching elements we need each day are sunlight, air and water, which we'll look at in more detail shortly.

Second to these we need to source big "macro" nutrients of proteins, fats and carbohydrates, which are ultimately just different, compound arrangements of carbon, hydrogen and oxygen. We also need small "micro" nutrients and some elements in their trace form. These remaining elements need to be present in the organisms we eat, based on the soil they are grown in.

If the soil is missing these key building blocks, as in often the case in modern agriculture, then the plants are deficient and the element cannot reach our bodies. Arguably, all nutrients are equally important for our optimal health. I'm sure we've all had a heart palpitation or a muscle cramp. The simple deficiency of one trace element can stop our bodies from performing, in the same way dysfunctional spark plugs in a car's engine will stop even the most expensive machine from starting.

Carbon, hydrogen, nitrogen, oxygen, phosphorous and sulfur (CHNOPS) are the 6 key elements making up most of the biological molecules on Earth.[14] The first four are also known as the **"Big 4"** accounting as they do, for 96.2% of what humans need to consume daily.[15] The small remaining ratio is made up of micro and trace elements found in different natural foods.

To get you thinking in new healthful holistic terms, let's take a look at what you need and why.

Big 4 Essential elements that make up (96.2% of daily needs)[16]
1. Oxygen (O) (65%)—The air we breathe and water we drink
2. Carbon (C) (18%)—*From carbohydrates and proteins in the plants and animals we eat
3. Hydrogen (H) (10%)—A key element found in water, H+ Ions are responsible for the pH of water.
4. Nitrogen (N) (~3%)—*From proteins in the plants and animals we eat.

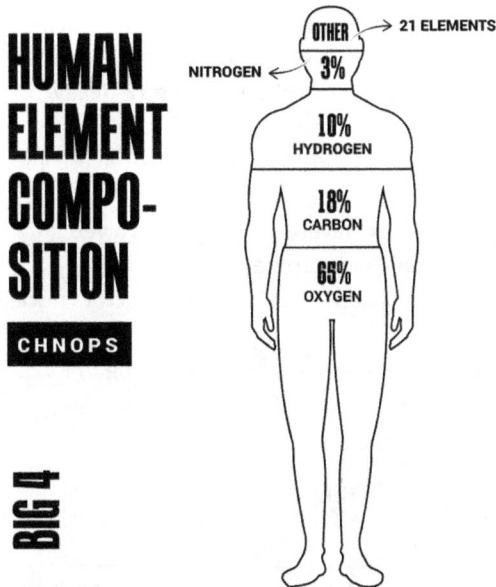

HUMAN ELEMENT COMPO- SITION

CHNOPS

BIG 4

OTHER → 21 ELEMENTS

NITROGEN ← 3%

10% HYDROGEN

18% CARBON

65% OXYGEN

7 major elements for the human vessel (~3.5% of daily needs)[17]
1. **Calcium (1.5%)**—Bone development, regulation of muscle contraction and myocardium activity, blood clotting, nerve impulses transmission, regulation of cell permeability.[18]
2. **Phosphorus (P) (1.0%)**—Protein synthesis, ATP synthesis and transport of energy in biological systems.
3. **Potassium (0.35%)**—Muscles and myocardium activities, neuromuscular excitability, acid-base balance, water retention and osmotic pressure.
4. **Sulfur (S) (0.25%)**—Essential amino acids, cartilage, hair and nails formation, enzyme activity in redox processes and cellular respiration, intestinal peristalsis.
5. **Sodium (0.15%)**—Fundamental regulation of cell permeability and body fluids; deficiency is rare, but an excessive intake may be associated with high blood pressure.
6. **Magnesium (0.05%)**—Bone formation, nervous and muscular activities, lipid metabolism and protein synthesis, CVD protection.

7. **Chlorine (<0.05%)**—Hydrochloric acid formation (digestive juices for digestion process).

13–15 minor trace minerals and micronutrients for the human vessel (0.70% and trace amounts of daily needs)
8. **Copper**—Functionality of several enzymes in blood and muscles.
9. **Zinc**—Helps the body's defensive (immune) system and plays a role in cell division, cell growth, wound healing, and the breakdown of carbohydrates.
10. **Selenium**—Protection of the muscle membrane integrity, antioxidant.
11. **Molybdenum**—Production of enzymes associated to uric acid.
12. **Fluorine**—Protection and prevention of tooth decay, bone development; diseases related to excess.
13. **Iodine**—Essential for the synthesis of hormones that are involved in the growth process and body development.
14. **Manganese**—Synthesis of several enzymes involved in the metabolism of proteins and sugars, bone development.
15. **Cobalt**—Constituent of vitamin B12: growth factor, nucleic acid synthesis, hematopoiesis.
16. **Iron**—Blood and muscle tissues: hemoglobin, myoglobin.

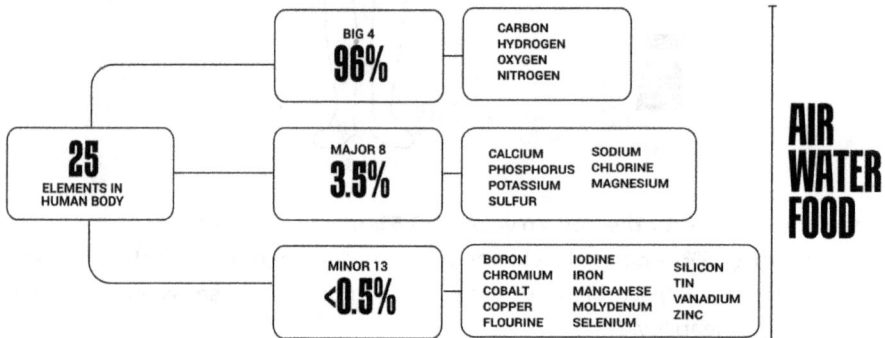

We also require traces of Lithium, Strontium, Aluminum, Silicon, Lead, Vanadium, and even Arsenic and Bromine. Defining these nutrients in more detail, allows you to cross-reference anything you consume. Note that there are synthetic, inorganic and man-made versions of these required elements however they are not the same. These versions can all be expected to negatively disrupt normal cell function.[19]

In addition to all this, the human body has actually been found to contain traces of up to 60 elements! Remember we only require between 25–27 for normal human function. All other elements can be disruptive or even toxic—"carcinogenic."

Where do they come from and how do they get into our human body? Well simply take a look around at the industrialized environment that you live in; every breath, every sip of water, every bit of food consumed and even the absorption through your largest organ (the skin).

How much do we need of each element to function for survival and healthy performance?

High performing people obviously need to consume more for their energy output than sedentary people, with minimal movement and energy output each day. For the average person the essential elements can be divided into macronutrients and micronutrients. The human body composition by nutrient density at rest looks a little like this;

Body composition by nutrient molecules	To Build (% elemental composition)	To function (% total calories)	Recommendations for normal human function (metric)
Sun (light energy)	* Source of all energy	0%	10–30+ minutes of midday sunlight
Oxygen	*65% of Elemental composition	0%	11,000 liters of air per day (more with exercise) to provide approximately 550L of oxygen per day
Water (H2O)	55–65% wet weight	0 %	3.7L of H2O a day for men 2.7L of H2O a day for women
Carbohydrates	1%	45% to 65% percent of your total daily calories	225–325 grams of carbohydrates a day.
Protein	16% *45–55% of dry weight)	15% to 25% of total daily calories.	0.8–2.0g per kg of body weight
Fat	16%	20% to 35% of daily calories Saturated fat: 10% or less of daily calories	44–78 gram per day Less than 22 grams of saturated fat
Vitamins & Minerals	6%	0%	See selfcare.global/food

HUMAN MOLECULAR COMPO- SITION

CARBOHYDRATES (CHO)

1%

VITAMINS + MINERALS
(Ca, Na, P, Mg, Fe etc)

6%

16%
FAT
(CHO)

16%
PROTEIN
(CHO)

62%
WATER
(H2O)

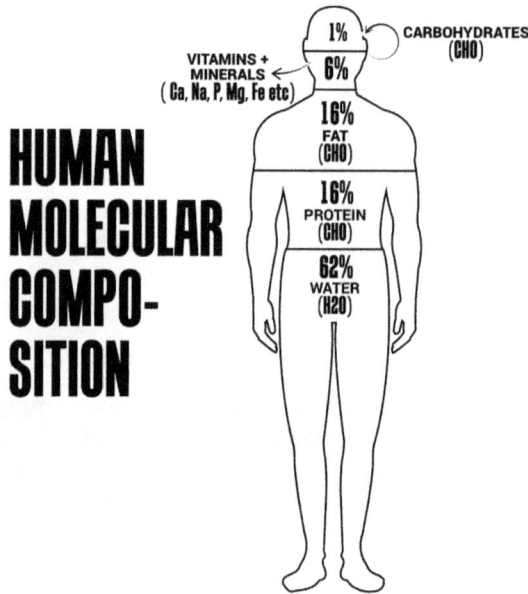

So how does all that information translate to the ultimate meal?
The universal meal for humans is CHNOPS plus our spark plugs!

Hunger and thirst are the first elements of self discipline; if you can control what you consume, eat, drink and breathe, then you can control everything else.

1. **Oxygen**
   » 10 deep breaths (550 Liters+ over day). Examples; The 4-7-8 breathing technique, also known as "relaxing breath," involves breathing in for 4 seconds, holding the breath for 7 seconds, and exhaling for 8 seconds. The Wim Hof method and even moving in nature to take in "prana's" life force!

2. **Water**
   » 2 glasses of natural spring water (2.7–3.7 liters daily). Example: eat more plants (mostly water), carry a 1 liter refillable water bottle and fill it 3x over the day!

3. **Food**
   » Soil and food package: vitamins, minerals and trace minerals will be present in the above food sources as part of the whole "food package" providing they are sourced from no compromise sources and biodynamic soil.

» 45–65% Carbohydrates (225–325g): Fruits, vegetables, tubers, seeds, nuts and whole grains.

» 20–35% Fats (44–78g): Seeds, nuts, coconut oils, avocados, cacao nibs

» 15–25% Protein (0.8–2.0 g per/kg of body weight): From incomplete protein sources in plant form (yellow split pea protein, brown rice, hemp and pumpkin seeds). If you are a compassionate omnivore consume complete proteins from animals like fish and wild game.

Overall simply remember the sage advice from Michael Pollan at the beginning of this chapter, "eat mostly plants," from non-compromised (free of toxic chemicals) and natural sources.

WHAT SHOULD HUMANS EAT?

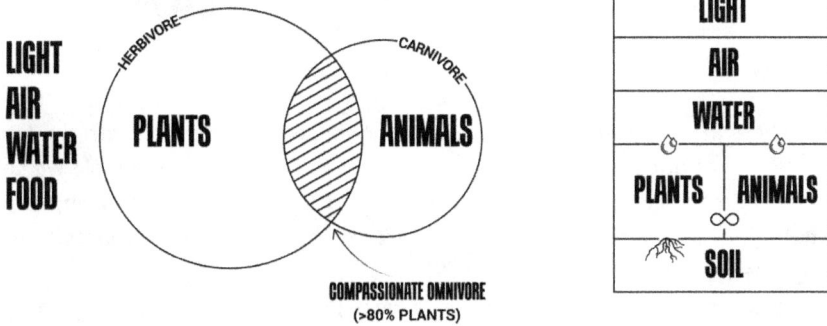

COMPASSIONATE OMNIVORE
(>80% PLANTS)

THE NAME GAME

SATURATE DAILY CONSUMP- TION

16	**MINERALS** (MAJOR >TRACE9)	MICROS
13	**VITAMINS** (FAT SOL WATER SOL)	
2	**FATS** (SATURATED UNSATURATED	MACROS
3	**CARBS** SIMPLE COMPLEX FIBER	
20	**PROTEIN** AMINI ACIDS	

THE 35%

3L	**WATER** H20	
550L	**AIR** 02	
∞	**LIGHT** SUN	

THE 65%

Somewhere in our recent history, we lost our sense of connection with the land, the integrity of our produce and the impact it was having on the people we sold it too. Food marketing took off in the 1980s and "real food" began disappearing from the supermarket shelves, gradually replaced by "advertised nutrients," which are not the same thing.

Staples like fruit, vegetables and eggs were pushed aside for brightly-colored packaging, clever marketing "icons," processed and packaged breakfast cereals and canned goods which boldly stated new terms like "fiber" and "cholesterol" and "saturated fat."

There were rather crafty economic and political motivations behind the calculated introduction of these new words into our lexicon. Carefully chosen in place of the more candid yet provocative, "eat less meat or diary" for example. What cattle rancher or dairy farmer wants to hear those words from an official government dietary pronouncement? Historically, the food industry in America has responded with powerful political and economic voices that created new cultural habits for the Western diet.

We were unconsciously and even willfully educated *towards* convenient food-like substances that we created, not nature. More recently "organic," "natural" and "superfood" have come into the marketing realm as old strategies stopped working.

All **food from nature is super, that's all we need to know.**

In an integrated natural future, fake and food-like products should need to pay for the certification to be classified as "safe for human consumption," thus increasing their supermarket price, whilst natural and organic food becomes cheaper and accessible to every family. Not just those who can afford it.

BIODYNAMIC ORGANIC IS "NORMAL"

Organic, biodynamic and ecological agriculture looks to address the deficiencies of a century and should be the baseline for global techniques. Our food should not contain toxic or harmful impurities, which sounds common sense, but most of the food we consume today is unfortunately compromised.

Bhutan is a living example of this principle in this modern reality. They are the closest country to supply between 70–100% of the food for their people from organic and biodynamic sources. The next closest is Denmark at 15%! Let's develop agricultural systems like Bhutan and monitor the burden of chronic preventable disease over the coming decades. My gut feeling is that the prevalence would decrease drastically for the next generation.

All food was once organic and should still be. Our ancestors would be baffled at the need to define "organic food!" Organic food production has existed for thousands of years (since the beginning of agriculture) and will continue indefinitely, provided that we collectively come to understand that nature supports us, not the other way around.[20]

It sounds fancy but biodynamic farming is simply a holistic systems approach to food production. It operates according to the interconnected relationship between humans, nature and all that is living and non-living. Relying on crop rotation, cover crops, seasonal phases, animal and plant manures, biological pest control to balance host/predator relationships, manual weed control, and returning organic residues back to the soil.

These agricultural systems recognize the biodynamic and living nature of the soil, ensuring vital minerals and nutrients are available in the soil to be absorbed by the crops and subsequently by us. No chemicals, nothing synthetic, no nasties. Grown from soil and returned to the soil, a complete circular economy.

This elemental information is not currently part of the labeling process. If we consider the definition of "organic food" from DEFRA in the UK, it states that *"Organic food is the product of a farming system which avoids the use of man-made fertilisers, pesticides; growth regulators and livestock feed additives.[21] Irradiation and the use of genetically modified organisms (GMOs) or products produced from or by GMOs are generally prohibited by organic legislation."[22]*

These standards are basically saying that organic food is natural (from nature), and it is low in human interference in that it hasn't been modified or synthetically human-made.

However, you might notice that this definition is missing something vital. It is more about what's *not* put on our growing food versus what we really need to know: the nutritional density of the food and the quality of the soil it was grown in! I would be more mindful of the soil quality and biodynamic farming methods than the organic labels, especially when clever marketing has realized that you will pay more for an organic certification.

We need self-governance of organic standards as a community expectation. When the Soil Association in England published the first organic standards in 1967, farmers were invited to register their farms with the Soil Association and sign a declaration that they would abide by these guidelines; a self-certification. It was self-governed and the farmers maintained this natural standard. Each farmer took pride in their own produce and sold it to families and restaurants knowing that this level of care translated to better taste, texture and nutrition for their long-term wellbeing.

TO HEAL, FIRST—DO NO HARM

While this healthcare principle is usually associated with modern interventional medicine, my aim is to change conventional thinking and apply it more directly to the lifestyle choices that we make each day. The balance between natural healing mechanisms and external intervention is akin to the balance of opposing forces. For the majority of lifestyle related dysfunctions and diseases, "first, do no harm" could help us better evaluate our food and activity choices, preventing much of the harm to ourselves in the first place!

Smoking, drinking alcohol, consuming fake food and added stress are examples of significant yet subtle choices we make. If one day you were in an accident (God forbid!), the "harm" has already occurred and you'd need acute and urgent help from specialists. For lifestyle related dysfunctions and disease, the challenge for modern medicine is to intervene from the foundation of the body's natural healing mechanisms.

Remember what we consume each day either fights disease and abnormal function or promotes it. It disables natural healing pathways or it enables them. There is a balance and internal harmony that is powered by our choices. If we make consistently better choices, dietary and lifestyle choices, our human vessels will respond accordingly, in good health, vibrancy and resilience for all future events.

However we cannot fully achieve good health and wellbeing if the interface between the outside and internal world is not functioning optimally, if it is not in balance. An alarming amount of people in the 21st century report some form of digestive dysfunction: irritable bowel syndrome (IBS), intestinal permeability (leaky gut) or a range of chronic inflammatory conditions like diverticulitis or even Crohn's disease. Digestive dysfunction is very closely correlated with chronic preventable disease.

It is extremely hard to promote nutrient saturation if our digestive health is in a state of dysfunction. For the most part our digestive system is inflamed because of our lifestyle choices in what we consume; unconsciously causing self-harm.

The gut-brain axis and impact of stress is also well documented and needs to be addressed. Are you familiar with any of these feelings; a history of digestive issues and tiredness, foggy brain, regular illness or even "hangry?" Are you sometimes tired and super reactive? Even with the people you love? Have you ever been in a stressful situation and felt butterflies in your stomach or felt like you wanted to be sick?

Hidden in the walls of the digestive system is your second "brain" in your gut. It's revolutionizing modern medicine's understanding of the links between digestive, emotional, and even mental health. Knowing that our digestive system is our second brain, the powerhouse of our immune system and that its internal harmony is closely linked with our mental, emotional and physical health might help us make better lifestyle choices each week!

Avoid those situations that expose you to prolonged stress (work, social, personal), avoid excess soda and alcohol consumption and walk past fake food-likes substances in the supermarkets that just leave you feeling bloated and lethargic anyway!

Science has found evidence that;
1. People with mental health issues often have a comorbid digestive issue such as Irritable bowel syndrome (IBS), or leaky bowel syndrome as a naturopathic doctor might call it. An Ayurveda doctor might refer to it as disharmony between different elements of the body.[23]
2. People who lack energy to get through their day commonly have digestive issues too. A prior systematic review also revealed that IBS is common in patients with chronic fatigue syndrome.[24]
3. People who live in stressful environments commonly develop "functional gastrointestinal disorders" which according to a Harvard health study affects 35% to 70% of people at some point in life, women more often than men.[25] These disorders have no apparent physical cause—such as infection or cancer—yet result in pain, bloating, and other discomfort. It also means that your gastrointestinal tract is sensitive to emotion; anger, anxiety, sadness, elation—all of these feelings (and others) can trigger symptoms in the gut! And vice versa.

The simplicity of the challenge is that Dysbiosis and inflammation of the gut, *"have been linked to causing several mental illnesses including anxiety and depression, which are prevalent in society today."*[26]

The simplicity of the *solution* is that healthy gut function has been linked to normal central nervous system (CNS) function.[27]

And vice versa. Our external daily lifestyle choices influence our internal harmony. Our internal harmony determines our ability to externally function optimally in the context of any external environment. From here the process continues indefinitely!

A HEALTHY DIGESTIVE SYSTEM =
Healthy Immune System, Healthy Endocrine System (Hormones),
Healthy Cognitive System (Thoughts), Better Emotional Health,
Improved Clarity Of Thought, More Energy And Thus
Better Physical Health.

The implications are massive. A healthy digestive system is linked to an improved quality of life and even length of life!

If you aren't "feeling" good, if your mental health isn't great, if you're getting sick all the time, if you feel inflamed, if your energy is low and you are finding it hard to get moving...then flip your approach from outside-in...to inside-out! Less shelf help books, less cognitive therapy, less willpower based movement sessions, less emotional release techniques and more daily habits and rituals that promote internal harmony.

The choices are many; eating mostly plants from natural and organic sources, intermittent fasting, avoiding self-harm, rebalancing the gut micro-biome with pre and pro-biotics, healing the walls of the digestive system with the ancient wisdom of powerful plants and not forgetting "drink more water; get more sunlight" are two of the easiest most effective treatments for a myriad of human dysfunctions!

If you want to FEEL better then: manage external stress, make lifestyle choices that minimize harm internally and promote internal harmony. Your digestive system and integrated internal systems will do the rest. Your integrated systems led by the bi-directional gut-brain axis will give you the resilience of immunity to weather any storm.

It will increase your energy for any physical performance needs. It will enable clarity of thought and a balanced hormonal system that will enable you to act and react in a way that promotes external harmony and tunes you into the abundance of the world. Rather than feeling like it continues to break down and requires maintenance, every time you are just about to get going!

Avoid certain carbohydrates: FODMAPS are short-chain carbs that are resistant to digestion. Imagine you are eating a big bowl of highly processed wheat based pasta or any other "high-carb" society meal and later that night you notice bloating, discomfort and even some pain. To know why, you need to understand FODMAPS.

Monash University defines FODMAPs as a, "group of simple carbohydrates (sugars) that are not completely digested or absorbed in our intestines."[28] These carbohydrates are very different to ancient grains like quinoa or that pasta your Italian Nonna handmade for you from a non-compromised source.

When FODMAPs reach the small intestine, they move slowly (or block the bowel) attracting water (like making glue with water, flour and heat). When they pass into the large intestine, FODMAPs are fermented by gut bacteria, producing gas as a result. The extra gas and water cause the intestinal wall to stretch and expand. Because people with IBS have a highly sensitive gut, "stretching" the intestinal wall causes exaggerated sensations of pain and discomfort.

Common FODMAPs include "de-natured" versions of:
- **Fructose:** a simple sugar found in many fruits and vegetables, it also makes up the structure of table sugar and most added sugars.
- **Lactose:** a carbohydrate found in dairy products like milk.
- **Fructans:** found in many modified foods including grains like wheat, spelt, rye and barley.
- **Galactans:** found in large amounts in legumes.
- **Polyols:** sugar alcohols like xylitol, sorbitol, maltitol and mannitol. They are found in some fruits and vegetables and often used as sweeteners.

Let's be frank, to reduce sensitivities and intolerances, stop consuming fake, denatured food-like products that do not adhere to "no compromise" standards! Your body is very sensitive (possibly even allergic) to things that do not serve your internal health and wellbeing for a reason.

If you'd like more information about "What to Eliminate" see **selfcare.global/food** for more tools and resources.

QUALITY OVER QUANTITY—LESS CAN BE MORE

Let's return to the most vital nutrients of all sun, air and water. The source of all energy starts with the sun. There are well known reasons to be wary of too much sun exposure; heat stroke, heat rash, sunburn and skin damage however for many of us, the pendulum has swung too far and we do not get enough!

Spending your days cooped up inside an office often means you're not getting enough vital vitamin D. Carey Bligard, MD says like many other things, sunshine should be enjoyed in moderation in relation to your environment and individual conditions, however there is no doubt it is one of the most effective mood lifters of them all! Sunlight also impacts your melatonin levels, which tell your body when to sleep, so a good dose of sunlight will help you sleep well that night.[29] Who doesn't want that? Ask yourself; can I take that call outside? Can I read that report in the sun? Make time for it!

AIR, OXYGEN = LIFE FORCE!

It goes by many names but remains the most vital building block for life. Breathing saturates your body with oxygen (O2) and exhales carbon dioxide. The oxygen floods our amazing lungs and is then sent via red blood cells to the whole body to be used to produce energy. When we focus on our breath through meditation we are attracting life force "prana," reaching every cell of our body. There are many benefits to being aware of and also heightening our oxygen levels such as relieving stress and maximizing energy.

How then do we factor in the modern scourge of air pollution on our health? Air pollution is the result of invisible gasses like ozone and carbon monoxide mixing with tiny solid or liquid particles.[30] Ozone pollution comes from gasses like exhaust from tailpipes and smoke from factory chimneys. Particle pollution is mostly created by traffic, manufacturing, power plants and farming. These high concentrations of chemicals and gasses moving around our environment for us to inhale can result in all manors of health affects from headaches and irritation to asthma and lung diseases and many more.

This is particularly relevant as I pen these words in the "lockdown" period of 2020.

Air pollution associated with the long-reigning industrialized era compounded the impact of a virus that apparently targeted the respiratory system. The temporary isolation of masses of people that no longer transported themselves around in a billion or so smog-making machines, allowed something unexpected to happen. Air quality improved globally, Indians could see the Himalayan Mountains clearly for the first time in decades. Even the atmospheric ozone layer started to heal.[31] The Earth took a breath to heal and regenerate, which will hopefully allow us to do the same.

Since the Clean Air Act[32] was passed more than 45 years ago, air quality has improved, even in the face of climate change. Standing in 2020, I see the next 45 years becoming a world where clean air is a human right, not just an action plan. Something we all stand up for and fight for as we realize the enterprises that pollute our air, are polluting the health of the people we care about most and even future generations.

THE CITIES WITH THE CLEANEST AIR IN THE WORLD

If you want to live in environments with clean air here are the top five major cities with the cleanest air in the world:[33]

- Honolulu, Hawaii
- Halifax, Canada
- Anchorage, Alaska
- Auckland, New Zealand
- Brisbane, Australia

Wherever in the world they're located, the cleanest cities have certain things in common. They all promote walking and cycling and the use of electric cars instead of motor-based transportation, they have great public transportation systems and feature car-free zones in their city centers. They also rely on solar or wind power to generate electricity.

THE POWER OF PURE WATER

Not all water is not the same. The most pure water on earth is widely accepted to be natural spring water, as long as it's been sourced naturally and not exposed to factors such as pumps, pipes, faucets or BPA-laden bottles. Spring water is formed over thousands of years or more, when surface water sinks through multiple layers of organic matter such as sand, gravel and rock, finishing up in underground aquifers. This process is an incredible form of natural filtration, thoroughly cleaning the water of impurities. Finally, a spring bubbles back up to the surface as the pressure builds from the aquifer.[34]

You may hear other fancy concepts such as reverse osmosis, distilled or alkaline water. Reverse osmosis works by pushing water through a semi-permeable layer that removes chemical contaminants and pesticides. The downside of reverse osmosis is that all the minerals are removed from the water at the same time as the contaminants.[35]

Distilled water is made by collecting the condensed steam from boiling water, this removes all chemicals, contaminants, and minerals from the water like reverse osmosis.

Alkaline water has a higher pH than regular tap water, which is why many claim that it can neutralize acid in the body and also provide more hydration.[36] However there's very little proof that it does either of these things. "Alkaline water filters are, in my mind and in the opinion of most of my colleagues, a complete scam for its price point," says Dr Stillman. "Especially when natural spring water is found free in nature."[37]

We do know that internally amongst all 12 integrated systems of our body and our blood, we like to keep the body in the healthy alkaline corridor. An internal environment that is too acidic promotes dysfunctional cellular processes. Fake foods and chemicals in everything we consume sends the body towards acidic disharmony, where as, more plants and vegetables from biodynamic organic sources rebalance the body back towards the alkaline corridor. We are over 65% water, so it makes sense that natural spring water is a vital part of our longevity.

BE A COMPASSIONATE OMNIVORE

"It is easier to change a man's religion than to change his diet."
— *Margaret Mead* —

Dr. David L. Katz concedes that, "Yes—from an evolutionary standpoint, eating some meat, preferably from lean, well-fed, well-exercised, and kindly tended animals is assuredly consistent with human health."[38]

But the health of modern humans and the planet argue consistently for Michael Pollan's concise and pithy advice, creating a win for all, not just some, "Eat food, not too much, mostly plants."[39] I can't say it enough.

Catherine Friend, author of *The Compassionate Carnivore*, put it this way; "Most of us have distanced ourselves from our meat, protecting ourselves from the truth that we are eating animals. Yet we don't need to protect ourselves. Ignorance is not bliss. Being a carnivore asleep at the wheel means someone else is driving. Being a carnivore who wakes up, looks around and engages means you're in charge. Being in charge is good."[40]

Finally, what we eat more of has implications for what we eat less of. Eating more meat means eating a lower proportion of calories from plants, vegetables, fruits, nuts, seeds, beans, lentils, whole grains, which are decisively associated with better health.

The impact of nutrition on our genes—nutrigenomics—can't be underestimated. If we think back to the chapter "Genes is Medicine," our genes load the gun, but our lifestyle and food choices pull the trigger. Which means that our fork is so powerful it not only transports food to our mouth, it can be used as a genetic on and off switch to alter our weight, blood pressure, blood cholesterol, cancer growth, and even our chances of healthy aging.

RAISE OUR STANDARDS

By now it's clear that all foods are not created equally. We need to raise our individual and collective standards, and become non-compromising in our choices because the right foods are a powerhouse of valuable nutrients that can influence our cellular biology and our epigenetic expression in profound ways! No compromise means that we are in tune with the natural environment, the nutrient density in the soil and therefore the plants that we consume or the animals we consume that eat the plants. These nutritional building blocks transfer into our cells for our optimal daily function.

I ask you to raise your standards to energetically change your life.

Here are a few ways to ensure you are eating "no compromise" food. The choice is yours. Choose your way of life. Choose the quality of your building blocks.

Choose how your human vessel will express itself. With the knowledge of self-care you can choose wisely. You don't have to force it on others. Inspire them through your actions, not your words. Others will begin to model your way of being.

🌸 FOOD IS MEDICINE PRESCRIPTION

» **Eat more plants!** Reach for a juice or smoothie instead of an artificial drink.

» **Be a compassionate omnivore!** If you eat animal products, do your best to source it from compassionate and regenerative sources

» **Check your soil.** Is your food from living, nutrient dense, biodynamic soil that is not compromised with impurities? Could you visit the farm and see abundant ecology if need be? No compromise is the quality of anything you consume!

» **Check local first.** Can you source more food locally and buy organic? Do you have a local farmers market?

» **Water.** Can you source clean, fresh water free from impurities and other nasties? Natural spring water? Carry a reusable 1 liter water canister. See if you can fill it 3 times in a day!

» **Grow and recirculate.** Reuse, recycle, redistribute. Don't forget your green thumb. Start a vegetable patch, plant a fruit tree or at least some herbs. Compost and return any organic matter back to the soil to continue the process in your home or local community.

» **Sun, water and oxygen.** Are you making time to breathe fresh air, get quality water and get some Vitamin D from sunshine? The most essential nutrients of all!

To learn more about this medicine, or to contribute to this medicine, visit **selfcare.global/food**. Here you will find blogs, videos and podcasts.

Selfcare.global/food

NOTABLE EXPERTS IN THIS CHAPTER:

Dr Curtis Wood Jr, Michael Pollan, Dr William Prout, David Wolfe, Monash University, Dr Carey Bligard, Clean Air Act, Dr Leyland Stillman, Dr David L Katz, Catherine Friend.

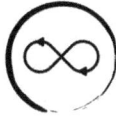

7

MOVEMENT IS MEDICINE

*"Movement is a medicine for creating change in a person's
physical, emotional, and mental states."*
— *Carol Welch* —

Look at your hand. Look closely at your fingers. Slowly bend and straighten your fingers, notice the muscles and tendons slide and glide in harmony. Notice how your mind thinks about moving your fingers and your hand responds accordingly. What a miracle movement is: so many layers, so many integrated systems. All of it resulting in something most of us take for granted each day. How would you cope if one day this miracle movement stopped? Imagine losing movement in a limb or the limb itself. No arms to wrap around someone, no hands to experience touch or to hold another hand.

Now meet Bethany Hamilton. As a young rising surf star, at the age of only 13 Bethany lost her left arm to a tiger shark attack. People thought this would end her dream career. One month after the attack, Bethany returned to surfing. Unbelievable! Within a couple of years she won her first national surfing title. Bethany's foundation of faith has been her backbone; her source of truth, hope, and strength.[1] At 17 years old, her dream of surfing professionally came true and she continues to be an active surf competitor to this day.

Next imagine (if you can) being born with no arms and no legs—then radiating the attitude; "No arms, no legs, no worries!" Nick Vujicic has inspired millions by doing just that. He was born in Melbourne, Australia in 1982 and without any medical warning, Nick was born without arms or legs: a rare condition called tetra-amelia syndrome.

While still young, Nick experienced many obstacles as well as fear and hopelessness for his future, but a turning point came when he decided to embrace his situation. With persistance he was able to do more tasks on his own, actions that most people can only do by using their limbs, such as playing sports, brushing hair, typing on a computer, swimming, and much more. Nick believes that persistence can help fulfill your biggest dreams but not without choosing to embrace failure as a learning experience.

Nick is a highly successful motivational speaker, author, CEO and advocate for social and emotional education in schools, teaching students to make positive changes in their lives and their communities. Nick is a shining example that the only physical disabilities we face are those in our mind. *No legs, no arms, no worries.* Nick is married to his wife Kanae and they have four beautiful children. He continues to inspire people globally, even as you read his story now.[2]

MOTION IS LOTION

Our bodies love to move. For the entire human system. It promotes the healing, maintenance and regeneration of all the integrated human systems. We were born to move, but our environments and technology are reducing our need to do so. Our modern lifestyles are deprived of nourishing movements. There is a reason our spines, hips and knees are stiff and restricted!

While reading this chapter, I hope that you are inspired to put this book down— to stop thinking about it—and get up and simply move. Move in a way that feels good, as you remember the variability of movement you had as a child swinging from monkey bars, dancing and playing in nature. Movement needs to be part of our lifestyles and integrated into our daily rituals.

As you put this book down you may be called to look around at the sedentary lifestyle you have accepted for yourself. Driving the car to work instead of catching public transport, too many hours on the couch, avoiding a morning walk in favor of a coffee, thinking caffeine will give you the energy and clarity you need for the busy day.

Movement in its essence is very complex but don't worry, nature has already figured it all out for you. All you need to know is that motion is lotion for every cell in your body, from your blood, to your brain, to your muscles and even down to your genetic blueprint.

Every movement creates an amazing healing stimulus for all of the 12 integrated systems that make up our amazing dynamic human body. In the same way a bird doesn't need a flight manual, we don't need a rulebook, expensive methods, workout gurus or strict regulations and philosophies in order to move.

In the 21st century we simply need to put our technology down, look around at the natural environment and remind ourselves to embrace movement as a way of life, not as a chore. Movement is meant to be fun so it should integrate naturally into your daily lifestyle. Dance, bushwalk, swim, surf, jump, stretch, trapeze!

MEANINGFUL MOVEMENT GOALS

Plan a movement goal for 12 months time, big or small; run a marathon, master a handstand, walk pain free, increase your PB—what will it be?

Write down some small movement goals to get you started. It could be to garden more, to walk to the end of the street every day, to walk the dog, to stretch before bed. Whatever it is, just start somewhere.

Write them down here.

My first small movement goals:

....

....

....

....

....

I wish for you to find the answer to achieve that functional end goal within these pages, so that you can live life dynamically and without restriction.

And for those of you who wish to push the limits of your human potential, mastering movement in any of nature's elements; amongst water, on land and even in the air, you will have access to the methods and strategies to do so. All you have to do is find the right community and mentor and be internally driven to apply the stimulus needed to one day function in the way your mind envisions.

From ultra marathons to freediving one hundred meters underwater on one breath, feel and know that anything is possible. The rest is up to you. Just keep moving!

MOVEMENT AS MEDICINE

"Normal movement or activity may be considered to be a skill acquired through learning for the purpose of achieving the most efficient and economical movement or performance of a given task and is specific to the individual."[3]

Remember how much you loved to move? Think back to running and jumping in your childhood and the mindless joy it created. Before we look at how to regain and retain much of that freedom of movement even as we age, let's examine movement and what it takes to excel at it! The four basic elements to movement are:

- joint mobility
- balance (static and dynamic)
- coordination and control
- alignment and posture
- strength and functional capacity to master our external environments

A person feels pain and restriction when dysfunction occurs within these areas. Technically movement can be described as the interaction of the individual, the task and the environment.[4] From the individual comes the controlled movement to meet the demands of the task, which is constrained by the environment.[5] The individual's ability to meet the interacting task and environmental demands determines that person's functional capability—we know this as being "good at it" or not so good at it, perhaps even terrible at it.

A person's level of ability develops from the specific interaction of their individual;

- Perception (integration of sensory information)
- Action (motor output to muscles)
- Mind and cognitive systems (including attention, motivation and emotional aspects of motor control).

These interactions are different for everyone. Our mind also affects both perception and action systems at many different levels.

BENEFITS OF MOVEMENT—SHOW ME THE EVIDENCE!

When did moving become such a chore? When we created sedentary jobs? Or created gyms and the overwhelming concept of going there for deliberate exercise? Finding the movement that ignites joy for you will mean you'll start to look forward to it every day!

Here are just a few more examples of the benefits of simply moving.

- **Movement and food/medication**

"There is no medication or nutritional supplement that even comes close to having all of the effects exercise does," says David C. Nieman, PhD, "It's truly the best medicine we know of."[6]

- **Movement and your sex life**

A 2003 study published in the *Annals of Internal Medicine* found that men over 50 who were physically active had a 30% lower risk of erectile dysfunction compared with those who were sedentary.[7]

- **Movement distracts the mind, allowing you to be more present**

Distraction is one of the best methods for pain relief. Pain is in the brain. When we move it forces us to shift our attention. Hence why we can feel better mentally, physically and emotionally after movement or exercise.

- **Movement and immunity**

"People who exercise regularly have reduced risk of getting the common cold," says Dr Nieman, who points to studies that indicate people who are physically fit report 60 to 90% fewer colds than those who are sedentary.[8]

- **Movement and a healthy heart**

Cardiovascular exercise is not just important for weight control and general fitness. It can significantly lower the risk of death from heart disease (and cancer), according to a 20-year study published in the *International Journal of Obesity* in August 2005—even for individuals with a body mass index in the obese range.[9]

Let's look at some movement recommendations.
- At least 150 minutes of moderate aerobic exercise per week (brisk walk, swim, mowing the lawn).
- Or 75 minutes of vigorous aerobic activity per week (running, dancing, surfing)
- Spreading this out over the week into daily movement has increased health benefits
- Mobility equals longevity
- Master and control your body weight in multiple planes of movement before aiming for strength and power. You want to build on a functional foundation, like you see in mixed martial arts—precision can trump power.
- Aim for strength training exercises at least twice per week. Train functional movements not the individual muscles. Use a weight or resistance level heavy enough to fatigue your muscles and the movement within 8 or more repetitions. For example, when doing a chin-up see if you can lift yourself over the bar.

- This may not seem like much, however the average person struggles to prioritize adequate movement into their daily rituals.

IMPACT SCALE OF MOVEMENT?

Not all movement is ideal for where you are right now. If you are deconditioned and haven't moved for a while, then anything in the water, walking, restorative yoga, clinical Pilates, a daily beach walk or riding to work might be a nice way to pace yourself into it.

Don't be concerned if things feel a bit stiff and sore initially, especially if it feels like your human vessel has been hidden away inside, gaining dust and some mild "rust." Your body is amazing and it will adapt and loosen as you continue to lubricate the physical body with motion as lotion.

As the body conditions itself to movement and starts to beat gravity again, it will permit you to run, jump and get the variety of movement that you had when you were younger. We can beat gravity each day but for many people it's a struggle to get through the day without pain, let alone do Crossfit, intensive workouts or explosive sports. So ease yourself back into it.

Impact x Relative to body weight	
10x + Very High impact	Gymnastics, parkour
6–10x High Impact	Running, jumping, contact sports
3–6x—Medium impact	Jogging, skiing, snowboarding
1–3x—Mild impact	Walking, riding
0–1x—Low impact	Tai Chi, Yoga, Pilates, surfing
-1–0—Anti-gravity No impact	Water and air-based activities

MASTER MOVEMENT AWARENESS

Even with disease and dysfunction, our goal is to master normal movement patterns with efficiently and flow. I want to share some examples of how this is possible for you, too. Like children, we need variability. There's no single form of movement that gives us everything we need in terms of muscular control, strength, cardiovascular fitness, coordination, balance, and range of motion. Here are some therapies that can help you regain normal movement.

MOVEMENT CONTROL

You may have heard of Pilates? Founder, Joseph Pilates (1883–1967) originallly called his exercise method Contrology. Now it is famously known as Pilates. In his book, *Return to Life,* he claims that "Contrology develops the body uniformly, corrects wrong postures, restores physical vitality, invigorates the mind, and elevates the spirit."[10]

The principles of Pilates are breath, whole-body health and whole-body commitment; with the whole-body encompassing mind, body and spirit. It is in the honoring of the Pilates Principles that the depth of the work is achieved.[11]

These Principles are traditionally cited as:
- Breath
- Concentration
- Centring
- Control
- Precision
- Flow

A final word from Joseph Pilates shares that, "It is only through Contrology that this unique trinity of a balanced body, mind, and spirit can ever be obtained." However, this is simply one approach. The concept of control and developing the right foundational "normal" movement patterns, before loading the body up, is the key point. Train the movement, not the muscles and progress to functional movement patterns relative to your desired skill level as soon as you can. There is no point training on the mat for years, if your daily tasks or performance skills all involve standing.

MASTERING STRENGTH

The launch of his company CrossFit in 2000, was the culmination of an idea that started during founder Greg Glassman's teenage years as a gymnast. He discovered that by using dumbbells and a barbell he became stronger than other gymnasts using only bodyweights. As his training continued to strengthen his talent, Greg was interested to find that he could out-lift his gymnast buddies and out-tumble his cycling friends. His curiosity was roused that he could find people that could beat him in one area but not all. [12]

And so Crossfit's "Jack of all Trades, Master of None" strategy came to be. CrossFit's goal is not to achieve specialized abilities but is general physical preparedness. Training enhances 10 key physical qualities: cardiovascular/ respiratory endurance, stamina, strength, flexibility, power, speed, coordination, agility, balance and accuracy.

These skills are built by incorporating movements from a variety of disciplines: gymnastics, weightlifting and sprinting or high-intensity work in various forms. In addition, CrossFit also emphasizes set, measurable outcomes. Specific weights, distances and movements are repeated to allow for a clear measurement of performance.

MOVEMENT MASTERY

So what makes us good at some things and terrible at others? Have you ever wondered how ballet dancers, gymnasts and surfers for example appear to move with such ease, flow and grace? These movements have been targeted and honed for many years. If we examine such highly efficient movement we see three qualities emerge;

- goal achievement
- minimum energy expenditure
- minimum movement time.[13]

This level of movement mastery requires an advanced level of neuro-muscular control.

**Movement control occurs because of physiologic processes
that happen at cellular, tissue, and organ levels.[14]**

They have developed a mind-body connection that is subconscious. It can't all be conscious and awareness based. It is inherent and reflexive too. Consider that a baby giraffe knows how to walk only minutes after birth, where as a human child can take a year or longer!

Our physiological processes are designed for timely and efficient movement, even with the unexpected. Imagine if you trip and fall suddenly, *"What good does it do if you extend an outstretched arm after having fallen down? Extending your arm in a protective response has to be quick enough to be useful, that is, to break the fall."*[15] This ability ebbs and flows from infancy to illness and old age, but its always there waiting to be reactivated depending on our alignment with movement as medicine.

We can in fact train ourselves to move and fall in safer ways. Take the training technique, "parkour" as an example, where people run, climb, swing, roll, vault or jump over obstacles, sometimes from heights of three meters or more, without injuring themselves.

Movement mastery requires nourishing and stimulating your inbuilt human potential for the functional demands and capacity in which you hope to perform. An elite surfer, mixed marital artist, marathon runner, cross country skier, snowboarder, free diver and calisthenics gymnast have all activated their human potential relative to the context of the environment in which they wish to perform. Their body has adapted accordingly to the repetition of stimulus.

Imagine mastering movement in all environments. On land an ability to master gravity, in water; an ability to master movement in the flow of a natural environment, under water: an ability to adapt to a pressurized environment, in the air and even in space where gravity no longer exists as it does on land. Would that be the ultimate movement mastery, mastering all the elements with ease and natural flow?

Movement control comes with practice.

I remember the first time that I tried surfing, I felt like a baby giraffe trying to walk for the first time. The movement control required to surf is challenging: to master dynamic balance on a piece of foam in an external environment that is unpredictable and changing is something to be admired.

When I started it required an in tune mind; knowing the functional capacity of my ability, minus the ego. As I paddled out to surf that first time, subconsciously I was integrating sensory information from my environment. How big are the waves? Are the conditions right and is my board big enough? Is the person guiding me someone that I should listen to? Am I in the right spot? What's the worst case scenario? Are there sharks? How do I not drown?!

All of that "information" from the external environment (and my conditioned beliefs and fears) was processed by my central nervous system (brain and spinal cord), resulting in my first attempt at a controlled movement through coordinated muscle activity as I tried to stand for the first time on a wave. As I stood up there was an unfamiliar feeling of dynamic joint stability from my feet, to my knees, hips, trunks and flailing arms. Not to mention activating postural control of my trunk that provided a stable base. All this would one day result in precise and finely coordinated muscle activity throughout the movement, without having to think about it.[16]

I didn't succeed in my first attempt. I actually started on the wrong board and in the wrong environment. I had the wrong mentor and guide. So I retreated for a while and listened to an old friend that had been surfing for 40 years. He advised me to start with a longer, wider and more stable longboard. He took me out in a more predictable environment and boom! I was surfing. It didn't look good at first, but as the years went on, it has become more effortless and skilled. I even moved on to shorter boards and everything in between, depending on the external conditions. Today, I am still not a master but I have enough skill to enjoy it.

For me, "surfing is medicine" just as Dorian Paskowitz, a doctor and surfer that lived the endless summer, famously wrote. He didn't care about being a great doctor or rich or famous, he just wanted to be a good husband and a good father, and thus a good man. I admire his philosophy greatly.

THE SUCCESS CLUES

Anthony Robbins has repeatedly told those who want to succeed that "success leaves clues." If someone is wealthy and healthy year after year, then perhaps it's not luck that got them there. Maybe they are doing something worth noticing. If someone is a successful artist or entrepreneur, perhaps they learned a thing or two about business and marketing. Maybe they have a winning strategy that they practiced along the way. Maybe that strategy or formula is worth knowing about, right? Maybe it will save you years of learning the hard way.

Learning new skills can be defined as the experience and practice of processes, which create a relatively permanent improvement in a person's capability for responding to a specific task and environment.[17] If we apply Malcolm Gladwell's somewhat controversial 10,000-hour rule to this concept of practicing a specific task then anyone can achieve physical success.

Gladwell's theory suggests that takes 10,000 hours to master any skill or task. This can be accomplished with 20 hours of work a week for 10 years.[18] We each have 8736 hours in a year. Which is why many of these athletes below were able to master their skills and win championships, most before their 18th birthday by applying their drive to skill mastery in a single desired activity.

Shaun White, became a professional snowboarder at 13 years of age. He started skateboarding around five years of age and began snowboarding soon after. By 13 he turned professional and began competing in big events and amassing multiple awards and victories. He now holds 3 Winter Olympic gold medals and 15 X Games gold medals.

Soccer royalty, Pelé, was only 16 years old when gained a spot in the Brazil national team. At 17 years old he made his international debut and won his first World Cup; a Guinness World Record.

Angela Lee is one of the most influential MMA fighters in the world. She was just 19 when she won the One Championship Atomweight title, which made her the youngest World Title Champion in any major fight promotion. Currently 23, Lee continues her fighting reputation with a 10–2–0 record!

The point is that if you find an activity you love doing, put the time in, seek the support and mentorship to master the skill, and practice and apply that learning in the context of any environment, then it is likely you will master at least one skill in your lifetime. Find the ease and flow of movement in your life.

HOW TO MASTER ANY MOVEMENT

"Anyone who has learned how to play a musical instrument knows that translating notes on a sheet into finger movements is effortful at first, but gradually becomes more automatic over time." The well-known psychologists Fitts and Posner first described this widely appreciated feature of motor learning in 1967.[19] In their book *Human Performance*, they also proposed three stages of learning motor skills: a cognitive phase, an associative phase, and an autonomous phase.[20]

3 STAGES OF MOVEMENT MASTERY

Stage 1—movements are slow, inconsistent, and inefficient, and large parts of the movement are controlled consciously.

Stage 2—movements become more fluid, reliable, and efficient, and some parts of the movement are controlled automatically.

Stage 3—movements are accurate, consistent, and efficient, and movement is largely controlled automatically. However, it has not been clear exactly how the different stages of motor learning map onto neural systems in the brain.[21]

The ability to maintain and change posture and movement is the result of a complex set of neurologic and mechanical processes. Those processes include motor (move), cognitive (mind), and perceptual (senses) development.

"The development of motor control begins with the control of self movements, and proceeds to the control of movements in relationship to changing external environment conditions." [22]

As the nervous and muscular systems mature, movement emerges.[23] Motor control allows the nervous system to direct what muscles should be used, in what order, and how quickly, to solve a movement problem. If you want to hack your movement mastery, find a movement master in your skill of choice and be a student of life!

MOVEMENT MASTERY

Improvisation	An ability to adapt and move with balance and flow as the external environment around us changes.	Autonomous performance, minimal energy expenditure and maximal efficiency.
MOVEMENT MASTERY "10,000 HOURS"		
Functional Adaptation	Challenging the movement pattern from many different movement strategies or sports	Snowboarding, skating
Functional performance	Ability to adapt movement pattern into the sport or activity they are participating in.	Optimizing squat technique for jumping.
Power	Ability to perform movement quickly whilst beating gravity or imposed load.	Box Jump squats, double and single leg.
Strength	Ability to repeat movement under load.	Squat with load. Progressively load until the technique is lost. 5 x 10 repetitions.
Endurance	Ability to repeat movement. Aerobic.	Running, swimming, repeating body weight movements like a squat through range 100 times with body weight or low resistance/load
Control	"Contrology" Pilates, motor control training, patterning, mastering body weight	Breaking down the movement. Lower back and pelvic dissociation, knee and foot position. Practice movement with good control
Mind—Body	Visualization, observation, learning, modeling	Watching the techniques of the people with the best movement mastery. Visualizing doing it your mind
GET THE FOUNDATION RIGHT		
Principle 4—Motion is lotion, increase your variability of movement		
Principle 3—Make movement an active lifestyle, not a chore		
Principle 2—SAIDS—Specific Adaptation to Imposed Demands		
Principle 1—Train the movement, not the muscle		

Fit to functional: set functional goals with an emotional driver that will get you out of bed each day. E.g. a 5 mile run for cancer might drive you if someone you care about died from cancer versus, just going for a run.

INTEGRATED MOVEMENT MASTERY

What is the common element between the different examples of success we have cited so far? They are all *movers*. Ido Portal is a man who defines himself as a movement teacher. He has begun a "movement culture." He learned from yogis, dancers, fighters and circus performers and slowly started developing his own perspective of movement, which he named the "Ido Portal Method."[24]

Ultimately, all of Ido's teachings aim for you to become the master of your own body. Here are some tips from Ido you can integrate into your daily movement philosophy.[25]

- Always look for a teacher
- You're gonna get what you practice
- You have more excuses than a pregnant nun
- Range of Motion equals anti-aging
- Get strong based on normal and functional movement patterns

Just as we should aim to eat organically we should aim to move organically too—move your spine! In China they say, *"You're as old as your spine."* Move your body and make it part of your lifestyle. Imagine if we could beat gravity on every plane to achieve any desired outcome from our movement capabilities. That is true strength and movement efficiency, conquering so much physical pain and dysfunction in our human vessels.

THE MOVEMENT PARADOX

The last piece of the integrated SelfCare puzzle is that not all physical pains, restrictions and ailments are, well...physical!

From stress, emotion, your workplace of choice (or necessity), the relationships you choose to connect with and the environments you choose to live in. All of these factors and more can lead to "physical pain," where movement alone or treating the physical body might not be the missing piece of your puzzle. Either way movement helps, but it pays to know the underlying drivers too.

Imagine that your work choice, your work environment and how that impacts you socially (finances, relationships and so on) could be the driving force behind your physical pain. Recent studies have found that musculoskeletal pain in the low back and upper extremities has also been linked to stress, especially job stress, exacerbated by technology, computers and sedentary work places.[26]

What if your physical pain didn't require a physical therapist, but an emotional release therapy instead? We have found that physical treatments and movement-based therapies might help maintain health through other pathways, but if the stress remains, the physical signals and symptoms are likely to continue irrespective of movement therapies and physical treatment. Basically, the physical treatment becomes a "band aid approach" to the underlying challenge, longstanding micro-stress.

Did you know that with sudden onset of **acute stress** or anxiety our muscles can tense up all at once, and then release their tension when the stress passes? Which means that stress presents itself as a physical signal or symptom. Chronic stress can even cause the muscles in the body to be in a more or less constant state of guardedness. It can also increase our pain sensitivity as a whole.[27] Remember that pain is an output of the brain, not an input.

When muscles are tense and tight for prolonged periods of time, this can trigger other reactions of the body and even induce more stress-related issues. A common example is those "tension" based headaches that seem to come out of nowhere. If acute, some physical treatment might help. If longstanding and chronic, the physical treatment might not do all that much.

The key point to understand is that when physical symptoms are caused by injury, bacteria, or an allergen for instance, medical and physical treatments can work. However, when physical ailments are caused or exacerbated by emotional stressors, often the approach within traditional western medicine is limited. A placebo effect may offer some relief; yet many times the frustration caused by unsuccessful medical interventions can worsen our emotionally-induced issues and symptoms..

No one is immune to the physical reactions caused by emotional stress!

Which means that we are all vulnerable to suffering from unexplained physical symptoms when emotions overwhelm us. Emotional factors, such as losing a loved one, or internally suppressed feelings can elicit a whole range of physical symptoms.

"Emotional centers in the brain link with many important structures of the body, including our large voluntary muscles (anything you can flex) and our involuntary muscles, such as the gastrointestinal system."[28]

**When you treat the physical body, you need to treat
the environment in which you spend the most
time, and take care of your mind and emotions.**

Now that you know the science and holistic benefits of movement, find something you love doing and do it for at least 30 minutes a day! And commit to not missing 2 days in a row! The only limitation is in your mind, your human body will find a way. Movement nourishes the entire body. Get variable, swim, do yoga, tai chi, bush walk. Do it with friends!

∞ MOVEMENT IS MEDICINE PRESCRIPTION

» Move more—at least 30 minutes day.

» Avoid sitting for more than 50% of your day.

» Make movement part of your lifestyle, not a chore.

» Design variable movement opportunities into your day and week.

» Do you have ONE movement activity or skill that you enjoy doing each week and would like to master?

» Who is a movement mentor that you learn from?

» Are there any healthy tribes you can join?

To learn more about this medicine, or to contribute to this medicine, visit **selfcare.global/move**. Here you will find blogs, videos and podcasts.

Selfcare.global/move

NOTABLE EXPERTS IN THIS CHAPTER:
Ido Portal, Bethany Hamilton, Nick Vujicic, Carol Welsh, Anne Shumway-Cook, Marjorie Hines Woollacott, Kathleen Haywood, Nancy Getchell, Dr David C. Nieman, Joseph Pilates, Greg Glassman, Dorian Paskowitz, Anthony Robbins, Malcolm Gladwell, Angela Lee Lee, Shuan White, Fitts and Posner, Donna Cech, Suzanne Tink Martin.

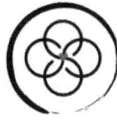

8

WORK IS MEDICINE

*"Work to live, don't live to work. If you wake up every day to do
something you love, you will never work a day in your life."*
— *Unknown* —

WORK TO LIVE, LOVE, CONNECT AND CONTRIBUTE TO THE WORLD

Before she was twelve years old, Hanalei Swan started her own business as a fashion designer. Sketching designs since she was only three years old, she had incredible talent, passion and importantly supportive environments in her parents and positive lifestyle.

Hanalei recalls that instead of asking her what she wanted to be when she grew up, her parents had asked her what she wanted to be *now*; it was a definitive moment she'll never forget. Hanalei draws on her experience living within different cultures around the world to influence her designs and create sustainable, simple and stylish collections that support local people working for her studio and her suppliers in Bali.

Her fashion label stands for "slow fashion," using sustainable fabrics and conscientious processes. Hanalei believes in the slogan, "Don't invest in fashion, invest in the world," helping to spread the knowledge that your consumer choices have a huge impact on the prosperity of local communities, economies and ecosystems.[1]

Hanalei is a world traveler, speaker, model for her fashions and even an author. She is a global inspiration, showing us that age is no barrier to achieving integrated success from passion and belief in doing something you love that the world needs right now.

KNOW YOUR VALUE AND WORTH

Traditionally we trade our time for the money that buys our needs and wants. Day after day we spend our time earning that money. In essence you could say when we buy something, we actually buy it with our time spent earning the money in the first place. Your time is your most valuable, irreplaceable commodity.

With this value in mind I ask you, does your current work still seem worth your time? Or does this existence seem limited and scarce? Would you prefer to spend your time doing something that you love every day? Something you are passionate about, something that benefits the world, something of high value that people will pay you for? Something you would never want to retire from doing?

These questions portray your "ikigai," a Japanese word for finding meaning and fulfillment each day. Embracing this concept in your life can free you from old constraints; free your time and your location in order to truly live, giving you freedom to choose. By tuning into your individual reason for being, or "ikigai," frees you from cultural and social constructs dictating what success should be for you.

To consider the value of your time, let's consider the story of Picasso selling a drawing on a napkin. Author Mark H. McCormick[2] retold a famous anecdote about the great painter Pablo Picasso. The story (whether true or not) shines a light on the relative value we perceive in life. The value we hold for ourselves and for others.

It's been said that a diner approached Picasso in a restaurant and asked for a sketch on a napkin.

"Fine," Picasso said and took some charcoal from his pocket to make a quick sketch of a goat. His sketch required only a few strokes, but it was without doubt— an original Picasso.

The diner reached for the napkin, but Picasso did not hand it over.

Picasso said, "You owe me $100,000."

The diner recoiled in shock. " $100,000? Are you serious? It didn't take you any longer than 30 seconds to sketch it!"

Picasso thrust the napkin into his pocket. "You are wrong," he said. "It took me my entire lifetime."

The question remains; considering we may be lucky enough to have 6 million hours in the average human lifespan. What's five minutes of your time actually worth? The question remains; considering we may be lucky enough to have 600,000 to 1 million hours in the average human lifespan, what's your time actually worth? Where could it be spent better?

PATH TO FIND YOUR "IKIGAI"

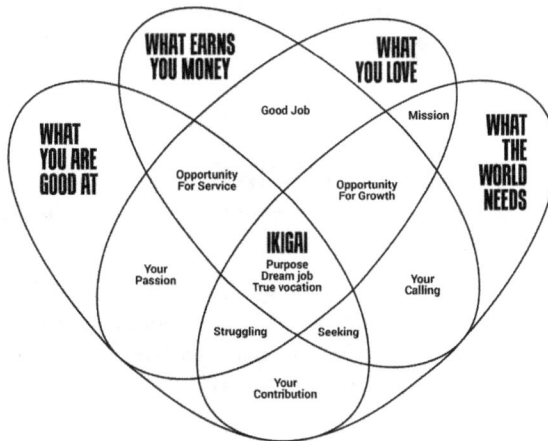

Some of us want a simple life, others like Elon Musk want to live and leave a legacy of discovery; ultimately you get to choose. Even though he was touted as the richest man on the planet recently, he still takes his kids to school every day, spends time with family on Sundays and has been almost bankrupt multiple times. He understands what it means to submerse yourself in the end feeling of what your ideal life would be—free from time and money constraints. Make decisions in your life toward that end goal, that "emotional feeling of success" without comparison or fear of judgment. Ten X your vision or live simply!

This chapter aims to inspire you to integrate working and living into the same ideology of fulfillment, that there is no separation. This chapter will enforce the key values of working to live, love, connect and contribute positively to the world by showing you;

- The value of your time, your most valuable resource
- That money is just "energy," a mental construct we created to exchange material value
- How to align your internal compass to your values
- How to create a future vision relative to your version of success or to living

your ideal day every day in a meaningful way
- How to work smart, leveraging your value in order to free your time
- The future of shared and circular economies that are a win for all
- Investing and utilizing in positively-geared and decentralized financial systems.

When you find your "ikigai," you can serve from overflow, redistributing energy and resources to areas of the world that need it most through shared and circular economies. You will want to "work" until your final days, leaving this world with no regrets and living a legacy of positive impact. Even if it only impacts your family and local proximity of friends and community: that will be enough.

DEFINE WORK AS MEDICINE

For thousands of years, individuals within societies have worked to achieve their purpose; hunting, gathering, worshiping, healing, honoring, protecting, creating, preserving, providing, constructing and inventing plus so many more callings that created human history. As societies connected we bartered with one another, exchanging items we deemed "valuable," from shiny metals to coins and then lighter, more effectual notes. These items gave us a sense of tangible value and security for survival.

Most of our "value exchange" now occurs online—in fact, *"92% of the world's currency is digital in 2020. This means that most of the money you earn, transact with, use to buy goods/services and so on exists only on computers and hard drives. Only an estimated 8% of currency globally is physical money."*[3]

Today our concept of money is just mental energy and it doesn't actually exist. It has become a mental construct for the agreed value of the work we do that appears as numbers on a screen. Money exists in virtual reality more than it does in our physical reality. It is healthy to understand this disconnection so you don't give it more thought than it deserves.

Having said that, this virtual "construct" to connect and share information can be used to the advantage of our health and well being. Technology can now help us free our time and location to work in a way that suits our ideal lifestyle. An accountant can do their work sitting on a beach in Bali, or sitting in an office minutes away from their place of birth.

This knowledge can free people from their modern western working lives that are often simply presumed to be a means to an end; they continue to choose to live to work; to work to survive and ultimately to build someone else's dream that is not aligned with theirs.

I want you to reconsider your work and the value of your irreplaceable time. Are you working like a dog for a large salary and a stomach full of stress? Are you working for a pittance and can't get ahead in your dreams? Are your dreams aligned with your inner self or are they society's "dreams" and "expectations" on the material ladder?

Work as Medicine highlights the value in finding meaning in your work of choice weighing up everything you've learned thus far in this book. Consider your work and how it relates to your inner values and ideals and direction in life. Do you believe in the work you do or in your employers' mission and principles? Ask yourself how can you get where you want to go and importantly how do you want to feel along the way?

There are opportunities nowadays for people to learn to work smarter not necessarily harder, while still exchanging value, solving problems on big and small scales, and freeing up more of their time.

Irrespective of working hard or working smart, contemplate exactly what it is you're working towards. Is it;

- To cover your basic human needs?
- To cover all your personal debts and basic needs?
- To live debt free and in personal abundance?
- To live with an abundance of resources and an ability to meet the needs of your family?
- To live simply, with just enough to have the breathing space to truly live a life of choice?
- To live in a meaningful way with enough resources to self fund your own passion project and have a positive impact on the world?
- To live with enough resources to buy all the "wants" that you feel you need to live the lifestyle of your dreams (houses, cars, boats)?
- Value yourself in a way that you can attract more, earn more, receive more and have the ability to share and circulate more.
- Just don't do it at the expense of others, your health, or what truly matters to you

For those that follow leading entrepreneur Robert Kiyosaki, he suggests there is a "cash flow quadrant" to how we work.

Quadrant 1:

Employee: You have a job. 90-95% trade their time for money, trying to follow strategies like that of Scott Pape, The Barefoot Investor. Having a job means using employee wages to get ahead in 20 years' time. Often working a "job" that we don't enjoy or find fulfillment with.

Quadrant 2:

Self Employed: you are your business. Thanks to technology, Peter Diamandis suggests that there will be over 1 billion people freelancing, consulting and working for themselves. If you do it well, you may even be able to live the 4-hour work week like Tim Ferris suggests.

Quadrant 3:

Business owner: People work for you, and hopefully you can pay yourself. However the hard reality is that 95% of businesses fail in 10 years due to a lack of cash flow, poor financial management or an inability to sustain growth. Business owners who don't automate their business or learn to delegate, end up creating expensive hobbies that rob their time, lifestyle and even their wellbeing.

Quadrant 4:

Investment: Passive and residual income. This is nice in theory, but the harsh reality as mentioned previously is that 80% of people live on less than $10 a day, with not much left over to meet their basic needs, let alone, invest. We are also taught strategies like debt reduction and negatively gearing properties, where ultimately the banks win with the compound interest you pay. We need to shift to positively geared systems like decentralized finances; utilizing compound interest, force multipliers and Metcalf's law in our favor. Investing at the right time. Timing is everything.

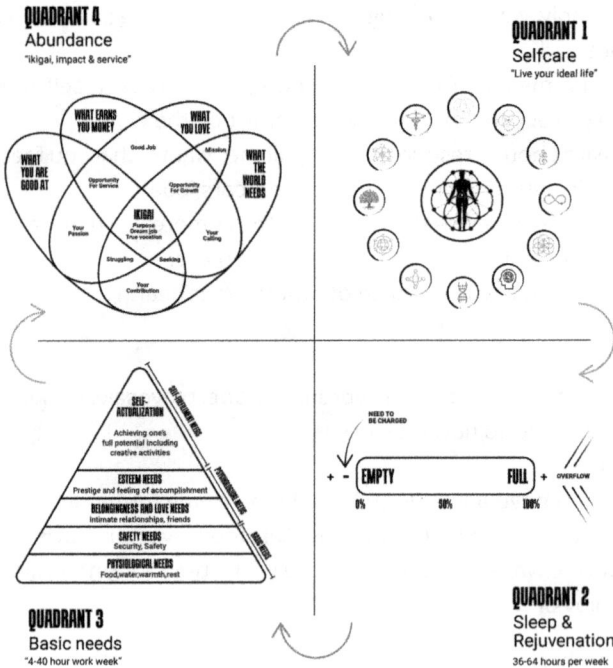

QUADRANT 4
Abundance
"ikigai, impact & service"

QUADRANT 1
Selfcare
"Live your ideal life"

QUADRANT 3
Basic needs
"4-40 hour work week"

QUADRANT 2
Sleep & Rejuvenation
36-64 hours per week

We suggest a new WORK TO LIVE quadrant.

Quadrant 1:

Selfcare, lifestyle medicine and living your ideal day. Working to live, rather than living to work. Enjoying the journey, rather than leaving it on your vision board for some future day. Live it now, even in small steps!

Quadrant 2:

Sleep, rest and rejuvenation. Learn to rest well and slow down so that you can speed up when needed.

Quadrant 3:

Having enough cash flow to meet your 7 basic human needs. Notice if you can work to cover your basic living expenses in 1 hour or 80 hours. We all need to find a strategy to ensure that our basic needs to thrive are met. Otherwise we will always live in scarcity. This number will differ depending on where you live and how you live. On $250 per week, most people can live a great lifestyle in places like South East Asia. In Europe, that may not even cover your weekly food bill.

Quadrant 4:

Abundance. Imagine having a bank account that automatically fills each week with enough money to cover your basic human needs for you and your family, with some left over.

Whatever you are working toward, know that there is a strategy and pathway to get you there. There is someone like you, with similar values (internal compass) and a similar true north (vision) that needs someone who is hungry and coachable to help them get there. Seek, find and surround yourself with more people like that and with a consistent work ethic, you can create the life of your dreams. Once you start on this path, you'll find it opens up doors and possibilities that you had never imagined.

The empowerment you feel from working in a meaningful way, doing something you love flows onto your whole human experience. Filling your own needs this way allows you to share from abundance with your local community and beyond.

Work to live and serve from an abundant
overflow of time, money and resources.

CAN MONEY BUY HAPPINESS?

A wealthy investor once asked me if I was a slave. He said "If you were to balance all the money you earn each week and the debt you owe personally, how much would you have left over?" Would you be in abundance (GREEN) or living in scarcity (RED)? This includes mortgages, student loans, credit cards and anything else. Also consider how free your time is to spend it in areas that truly matter (e.g. with family).

Overall, would you say that you are:
RED (living in debt) ◄————————————► GREEN (living in in abundance)

Don't feel bad if you are living in debt. In the USA nearly 300 out of 320 million people are too. Yes—most people do not own those fancy cars, big houses or expensive suits they buy. The Survey of Consumer Finances, which the Federal Reserve releases every three years showed that;

- Under 35s were living with ~$65,000 of personal debt,
- 35–54 year olds were living with close to $134,000 of personal debt and
- Those who were 75 and over were living with an average personal debt of $35,000.[4]

When you add that all together, household debt in the USA totalled 13.2 trillion dollars in 2018. If you had to write that check it would read $13,210,000,000,000!

This isn't just applicable to the USA either; world debt is close to 60 trillion dollars. Yet despite this large number only 19.41% of people globally (out of 141 countries assessed) actually have access to "credit" cards and thus debt.[5] This means that the other 80% of people who are living on $10 a day, or less without access to any form of credit are simply living within their means.

The paradox and the good news is that this 80% of the world is not living in personal debt, which suggests that they are in fact living in a better financial position than the 300 million Americans and the rest of the developed world who are living beyond their basic needs. What a contrary thought! The so-called "less developed" world is financially in a better position than the "more" developed countries. It might also explain why that Balinese rice farmer may give you a smile and a wave as you drive by. He or she is living in abundance, meeting their basic needs, plus the needs of their family. Without debt and credit cards with heightened interest rates.

Furthermore, a report in the *Wall Street Journal* summarized their findings as to whether money can buy happiness; "*It turns out there is a specific dollar number, or income plateau, after which more money has no measurable effect on day-to-day contentment.*"[6] The study, which analyzed Gallup surveys of 450,000 Americans in 2008 and 2009, suggested that there were two forms of happiness:

1. Day-to-day contentment (emotional well-being)

2. Overall "life assessment," which means broader satisfaction with one's progress in life.

While a higher income didn't have much impact on day-to-day contentment, it did boost people's "life assessment." The magic income in Australia was found to be roughly AUD$75,000 a year, meaning day-to-day happiness was found to rise as you earned more money, until you hit $75,000. After that, it is just "more stuff" with no gain in happiness.

If money did represent happiness, then 80% of the world would be considered unhappy yet for anyone that has traveled, you might have noticed more smiling faces in developing countries than in the developed ones, reinforcing that connection is the best medicine and money can't buy happiness after all.

Imagine if we took the "western wage" and moved it to a developing country? How would that $75,000 per year fare? I'm sure even $20,000 would surpass meeting our basic human needs for health and happiness as well as excess to live in abundance.

Besides happiness, there are a few other things that money can't buy. Roy T. Bennett author of *The Light in the Heart*, sums up the transient value of money by sharing the top 15 things money can't buy;

> **"Time. Happiness. Inner Peace. Integrity. Love.**
> **Character. Manners. Health. Respect. Morals. Trust.**
> **Patience. Class. Common sense. Dignity."**[7]

Living by these virtues would fill anyone's soul with satisfaction and gratitude. Remember what money truly represents nowadays; the energy of exchanging value for our labor. We use this energy to meet our basic human needs, to be at "enough" and potentially have excess to serve from overflow. Spending money that we don't have is likely to create stress. Link that stress to everything else we have already spoken of and you can connect the dots between your work habits, spending habits and the health of your human vessel. We each get to define success in our own terms and measure what really matters.

7 WAYS TO ALIGN YOUR INTERNAL COMPASS

Including our conditioning, we are also the unconscious products of our education. The modern education system is only 200 years old. Formal education used to be reserved for the elite but industrialization changed the way we worked, and created a need for universal schooling. Western culture has been teaching within the principles of adherence to the system for two centuries; you can choose to deviate from this path.

Rather than looking to be part of the 95% of people that work as employee's to build someone else's dream, I would love to explore what makes you tick, what you actually love doing and think about most. Outside of social and cultural constructs, who do you really want to be in this world? Not everyone knows their answer immediately; here are some questions to get you started;

- What do you love doing? (akin to flow state feeling)
- What are you good at? (every one has a unique genius)
- What can you be paid for? (exchange value, think outside the box)
- What does the world need? (does it have a positive impact?)

#1: CREATE YOUR FUTURE VISION

As your answers grow, they will help create your future vision for your ideal day, what does it look like? Script or make a vision board!

Explore all these tools and templates @ selfcare.global/tools

Take a minute and imagine what it would be like to live that day in reality, forgoing time, money constraints, external constraints and internal beliefs of what you think might be possible for you right now. Dream with me for a minute.

- What would it actually feel like?
- Where would you wake up?
- Who would you wake up with?
- What would you do in the morning?
- How would you spend your time?
- How would you finish your day?

When we hold this end vision clear in our mind, we start to realign some things internally. When we feel aligned, energy flows and we attract everything that we are meant to be. In real time, we then get to use our values to guide our day-to-day decision-making. If you don't know whether to go left or right, to say yes or no, then stop, take a breath and ask yourself;

1. Does this feel in alignment? With your true north?
2. Does this take me towards or away from my vision?
3. Does it work against my integrity, character and core values?
4. Does this add stress to my life or relieve it?
5. Does this add value to my life? or just take it?
6. Will this free my time in the future, or is it just a time expenditure?

Alignment is a choice. The alternative is choosing to continue to bounce between extreme experiences of pain and pleasure, hope and disappointment. Change isn't easy otherwise everyone would do it. Our primitive nature often leans towards safety and comfort but now we have the resources to achieve our potential like never before; potential for a peaceful lifestyle or a busy professional one, potential to know our passions and how they can benefit the world; the potential to live in true and meaningful abundance. Potential to free our time or to keep giving it away. Imagine waking up one day with all the resources and networks you need to truly live with all of your time available.

Imagine for example, a young man who decided to stop chasing other people's version of "success" and cast his own vision of success and created his own ideal day. It involved having the time to travel, to explore, to surf and spend more time in nature surrounded by good people. He realized that this lifestyle did not require 90 hours a week working in a busy law firm. He realigned his real needs and values and applied his skills to earn enough money working from his laptop, doing what he loved as he traveled and lived life according to his version of success. He was wholly content.

Imagine a busy single mother who, out of necessity was forced to work a 9-5 job that covered the basic needs of her young family. One weekend, she was inspired to cast a new vision for her future. She wanted to live a life where her kids did not need to go to daycare all week. She wanted to make more memories with them. This was the whole reason she wanted to be a mother in the first place, but she had become so out of alignment she found herself doing the exact opposite.

She decided this was her new vision for her life and for her family and thought back to her writing skills she hadn't used for a while. She got up the courage to look and ask around for opportunities and to her surprise, there they were! She was able to work from home and create more abundance for herself and her children. She halved the time her children were in daycare meaning their time together doubled! She was living her ideal lifestyle with opportunity to keep increasing her abundance!

No doubt there is someone out there who has already walked the path towards the ideal lifestyle that you are currently painting in your mind. Cast a vision and make decisions towards that "true north," that ideal lifestyle in the coming months and years. With some work and open minded seeking, you too are likely to see opportunities in many areas you had not previously noticed. Hustle to attract and find the flow, often the universe manifests and creates from what we put out into it.

It often requires finding someone that already knows how to "fly that plane" or "walk that path," someone who can show you how to improve your chances of parachuting into the right opportunity. Cast a vision, seek and lean into each opportunity as it presents itself. Once you have found it, transfer that energy and flow to where it needs to go and keep it circulating. Don't build a moat with it. Remember abundance is found in "we," more than just "me" and no one is happy going this journey alone.

#2: DEVELOP AND EMBODY YOUR TRUE CHARACTER

Jim Rohn's outlines the traits he believes people with strength of character embody.[8] We might already have them or aspire to them;

- **Integrity:** The origin of the word integrity means "whole" or "undivided." Integrity is about being congruent, displaying congruence with your words, actions and values.
- **Honesty:** As the old adage says—honesty is the best policy. And "the truth shall set you free."
- **Vulnerability:** This is our ultimate power; to own our strengths and our shadows. However, be mindful of false vulnerability, where people overshare for attention and not for connection, or play victim to a sad narrative to manipulate you.
- **Loyalty:** Everybody fails at some stage in their life. A loyal person stays with their friends even during tough times. A loyal person stays true to themselves. Notice who shows up when the times are good, but most importantly, who shows up when times are challenging.
- **Self-Sacrifice:** Self-sacrifice is what a leader does. A leader can sacrifice for the good of the whole and inspire others to contribute to the greater good. As Simon Sinek says, great leaders eat last.
- **Accountability:** We all have blindspots and need other people to be accountable to so we can be self-responsible and head down the road of success. Surround yourself with the right mentors and people who keep you accountable to being your best self. Even if it requires critical conversations and honesty at inconvenient times. Welcome people who challenge you, not just validate you.
- **Self Control and Discipline:** The ability to remain poised, disciplined and in control helps one make good decisions. Good decisions lead to good actions and good actions lead to good character.

Which of the 7 do you have to help you align with your internal compass? Do you naturally possess some and never noticed?

#3: LIVE YOUR PURPOSE

Do you believe that everything has a purpose? Aristotle, the ancient Greek father of western philosophy thought so, and he called that purpose, "telos." Meaning the ultimate reason for each thing being the way it is, whether created that way by human beings or nature. I want you to apply that concept to yourself and ask yourself these questions:

- Why do you get out of bed each day?
- Why should anybody care?
- Do you do what you say you will?

These questions can require some soul searching but perhaps when you surrender to finding your purpose it will come to you. Author and Speaker Charles Eisenstein explains it this way, *"Some of us may have experienced it when we find ourselves cooperating naturally and effortlessly instruments of a purpose greater than ourselves that, paradoxically, makes us individual more and not less when we abandon ourselves to it. It is what musicians are referring to when they say 'The music played the band'."*[9]

If you were to guess, what is your purpose, your personal why? What would it be?

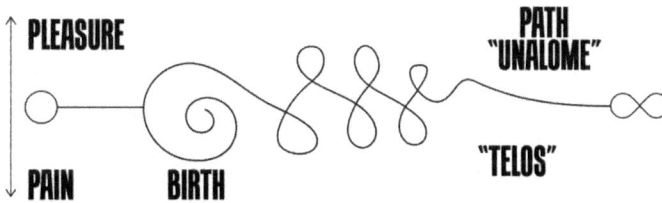

#4: IGNITE YOUR PASSION EVERY DAY

I define passion as your heart and soul's work. It is more than enthusiasm, it is a driving energy to reach the outer limits of creation. Passion is also synonymous with action and can only be proven by doing such. I love passion particularly because it gets you off the couch and into experiences. Without passion, you would not be reading this book! An example of passion is when I wrote the first version of this book nearly 6 years ago, 5 weeks of my life disappeared. Time stood still.

In March of 2016, I entered my room whilst living in the south west of Australia as the download came and my mind started connecting every piece of information, experience and curious question at once. It felt like my brain exploded and every synapse fired at once—5 weeks of 16 hour days, late nights and even hearing the birds as the sun rose, realizing that a whole day and night had passed in the blink of an eye.

I walked out of that room in April 2016, feeling like it was still March. Notice the things that make time stand still and ignite every cell in your body. Over the next 6 years, that same passion drove me to stay aligned with my true north. Even during a global pandemic.

Name **one** thing you are passionate about. When does time stand still for you?

#5: DISCOVER YOUR OWN STYLE OF GENIUS

*"Everybody is a genius. But if you judge a fish by its ability to climb
a tree, it will live its whole life believing that it is stupid."*
— Albert Einstein —

To be a genius, be a fish in water or be a monkey in a tree. If you feel like you are in an environment surrounded by people who do not see your magnificence or unique gifts, then seek to find your tribe. Go where you are loved, appreciated and valued for your unique skills and passions. Never settle for less.

Roger James Hamilton drives the modern entrepreneur movement. He helps people find their unique genius, their flow and collective business opportunities. The question I have for you at this point of our journey together is, *"What is your genius?"* What is your unique skill or talent that you can give to the world, exchange value for and is something that the world needs?

Genius comes without comparison or judgment. Who is to say the mothers or teachers of the world are any less valuable than the investors and entrepreneurs of the world? Imagine if we all worked from our zone of genius and shared our skills with each other, collaboration, co-creation and common-unity towards a world that works for all of us, not just some of us.

#6: KNOW YOUR VALUES

People place value on an array of different things; money, possessions, travel, creating experiences, creating memories or supporting their families needs. What do you **value**? This is an important question to ask when discovering why we do what we do. Why we live in personal debt, why we live beyond our needs for "wants" that we never really wanted and often regret buying.

What if you don't actually value that expensive house or car? You thought you wanted it, but perhaps the stress associated with buying it reduces your ability to live a life that you truly value; a fleeting, emotive purchase decision that changed everything. Imagine buying that cheap car that still gets you from A to B and paying it off in a year, versus that expensive car that you are still paying off 10 years later.

Dr John Demartini is a leading behavior specialist. He describes why we value these "unconscious voids" (wants disguised as needs) and that what we perceive as most missing (void) in our life therefore becomes what we perceive as most important (value).[10]

Consciously you might not want or need that expensive car, but unconsciously your society or culture may determine you as being successful based on the car you drive, they don't care if it sends you into a large amount of personal debt and stress.

If deep down we didn't care what others thought, or didn't buy into this cultural narrative as more people are doing, then perhaps we would be happy riding a bike or catching public transport. Both strategies solve the problem of getting to work on time and create far less stress.

> **The hierarchy of our voids (what we feel is most missing in our life) determines the hierarchy of our values.**

If we are taught unconsciously that we need money to be happy, then we will spend our whole life chasing this "void" in the search of happiness. Only to realize that when we get enough money, it may have taken us away from what we truly value; time with friends, family and memorable experiences.

The more important a value is, the higher it will be on your hierarchy of values and the more discipline and order you will have associated with it. As an example you can say you value your health and wellbeing, but your waistline says otherwise. You may in fact spend more time at work, which takes you away from living a healthy life. Yet, you consciously rationalize that you are doing it for your family. Even though you spend no time at home with them. I have learned to self-reflect on my own patterns of behavior, not just my words or good intentions. It's what we do that matters. The same applies for others too. I often work with people based on the way they treat people who have less. People who treat the janitor the same way they address the CEO. If you learn to trust patterns of behaviors, not just words, then clarity will unfold.

Our highest values will always show up in how we act each day, **not just what we say we value.** This is the harsh reality and mirror moment we must all face at some stage in our life. The less important a value is—the lower it will be on your hierarchy of values and the less discipline and more disorder you have associated with it.

As an example, if you value your family more than you health, you will be happy to serve from an empty cup each day, as long as they are okay. However, you may one day realize that you cannot truly serve and support them, if one day you can no longer support yourself. All of a sudden your health and wellbeing is linked to your highest value of family and things can change in an instant.

When it comes to seeing the value systems of others, patterns of behavior are the only measuring stick, not words. If someone's loyalty can change overnight, due to money or circumstance, then the harsh reality is that their patterns of behavior have already shown you what they value. Unfortunately it wasn't you, and that's okay, because you deserve better. If you value yourself, then how others value you will never matter. If someone can be there by your side at your best, but not in your depths, then it's all you need to know. Ask yourself, would this person be there if I lost my health (mental, physical, emotional), had an accident, went bankrupt or found myself in a challenging situation that I couldn't have prevented? If you can't confidently say yes, then, perhaps your gut and heart already knows. As Jay Z eloquently shares too "I never ask for nothing I don't demand of myself. Honesty, loyalty, friends and then wealth." Don't expect things of others that you are not willing to give yourself.

I'm sure you can relate in your own unique way. Dr John De Martini's value assessment has been a great tool to remind me of my own internal compass. It helped me know when to go left or right even when stepping into the unknown. I hope it can do the same for you.

#7: LIVE IN ABUNDANCE

Consider the contrast between scarcity and abundance mindsets. The scarcity mindset believes, "There is **not** enough for everyone." I first learned about the scarcity mindset from Stephen Covey's book *The 7 Habits of Highly Effective People*. Here's what it said about the scarcity mindset:

"Most people are deeply scripted in what I call the Scarcity Mentality. They see life as having only so much, as though there were only one pie out there. And if someone were to get a big piece of the pie, it would mean less for everybody else."[11]

This mindset limits people to thinking that there is only one scarcity pie to be distributed amongst all 7.2 billion of us. It restricts people from seeing that there is an endless amount of pies available or that we can expand the pie to create more abundance for us all to share and circulate. Where the most valuable ones are the ones you create or co-create with others. What if you knew that we could all bake our own abundance pie and share it!

On the other hand is the abundance mindset that believes, "There is **more** than enough for everyone." Here's how Covey describes it:

"The Abundance Mentality, flows out of a deep inner sense of personal worth and security. It is the paradigm that there is plenty out there and enough to spare for everybody. It results in sharing of prestige, of recognition, of profits, of decision making. It opens possibilities, options, alternatives, and creativity."[12]

As an example the scarcity mindset would focus on the fact that nearly 1 billion people will go to bed tonight hungry. Whereas the abundance mindset would recognize that today we grow enough food to feed 10 billion people and that over 40% of it is wasted! If we focused on sustainable agriculture, renewable food sources and effective distribution, we could solve this problem in our generation. Imagine if every community or household had its own permaculture garden.

As inventor and futurist Buckminster Fuller suggested last century, we do not have an issue of scarcity, we have an issue with distribution. We have enough food to feed 1.5 times the global population, yet 1 in 8 people still go to bed hungry in 2020. The scarcity mindset would suggest that this is just the way it is.

The abundance mindset would start looking towards a solution. How can we share, distribute and ensure that the abundance of food gets to where it needs to go. By solving a challenge that impacts 1 in 8 people globally, it is likely that they would find abundance in the context of their own life too. What is your default?

- **Scarcity**—There is only one pie to be shared and distributed amongst everyone
- **Abundance**—There are more than enough pies for everyone, and if there is not enough we can just bake another one. Or better yet, what if we simply increased the size of the pie by 1% or 10%? The math wizards can do a quick calculation: Volume of circular pie = $\pi r2$ calculation to see the difference. What if rather than being a 2D pie, we make it a 3D sphere? All of a sudden abundance is everywhere and everyone gets some pie! However, it is important to note and see who is selling the narrative that the size of the pie is limited and even decreasing. Some people use scarcity to gain money, power, control and feed their own greed to build higher fences at the expense of others. One mindset is apathetic and designed to win at the expense of others. Let's all win together!

Living in Bali, I see people with seemingly "nothing," living on less than $10 a day but living in gratitude and happiness for what they do have, sharing, circulating and giving with ease and flow. For me, I choose to base myself in this "environment" because this culture understands abundance, even though they might be seen to be living in the western version of scarcity. One could argue however that a culture living with less personal debt and more happiness, understands abundance more than most.

**Abundance is knowing your time is your
most valuable resource, not money.**

Time freedom is being able to do the things we love with the people we love exploring every inch of this human experience. We all get 168 hours in a week. What if we could work smart and find a way to cover our basic needs and even have enough money and resources to live our ideal life by working just four hours a week! This leaves 164 hours to explore this human experience, free to truly choose.

Tim Ferriss challenges us to forget the old concept of retirement and putting off our dream lifestyle. His book sat on my desk for years until I had had enough of the daily grind and knew there must be more to life! *The 4-Hour Workweek* shows you how to maximize your niche skills and reach your ultimate end goal whether it be to escape the rat race, achieve high-end world travel, or earn a big income with minimum management.[13] It inspired hope that I too could one day live the life of my dreams, working in a way that freed my time, my most valuable resource; much more valuable than money and material possessions that I was taught to value by society and pervading cultural values. Some successful entrepreneurs like Jack Ma and rapper 50 Cent share valuable insights. They both said that they never went to Harvard University, but Harvard graduates now work for them. Even Jeff Bezos, founder of Amazon shared—"If your team requires more than one table (two pizzas) at a restaurant. It's too big." We can leverage a distributed web of talented freelancers, co-creating and collectively build each other's dreams. Abundance is about leveraging and co-creating teams with a common vision.

You too can leverage technology and systems available to all of us, that can free your time and location to work from anywhere in the world at any time. As I write this book, I sit in Bali on a Sunday night curating this consciousness to share with you. Anyone can free their time and location. Now it's your turn.

THE FUTURE ECONOMIES WILL BE SHARED AND CIRCULAR

Everyone is familiar with linear economies; having such a long history in the western world. Imagine you support a linear economy and buy one of the two billion books printed in the US each year, these require thirty-two million trees to be cut down in order to fulfill that production. A linear economy would finish there. Perhaps we could create a book depository to share these books around but ultimately over time, more books would be printed requiring more trees to be cut down.

Eventually this creates a degradation issue such as the one we have in the Amazon Rainforest. The Amazon biome lost an average of 1.4 million hectares of rainforest per year between 2001 and 2012![14] If the rate of deforestation exceeds the rate of regeneration due to our consumer "demands" (not just books!) then the earth biome will change too, an act of "human induced" climate change— whether we like it or not. What we do in the bookshop clearly affects rainforests like the Amazon.

A circular economy understands the full cycle of production. It's model is built on economic, natural, and social capital. It is based on the three RRR principles:
- Reduce: Design out waste and pollution
- Reuse & Redistribute: Keep products and materials in use
- Regenerate natural systems

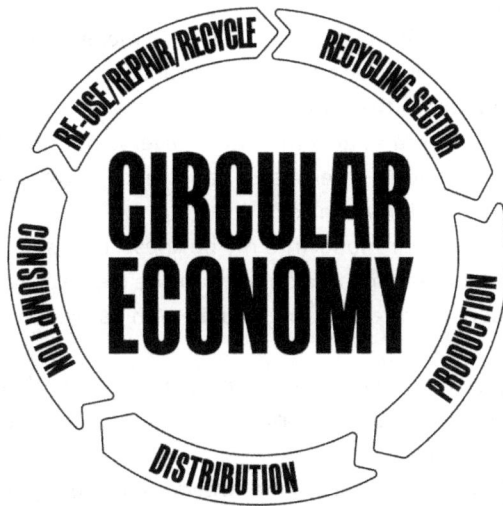

For example, a single book requires 0.016 trees worth of resources to be produced. Knowing this, imagine for every book bought, one tree is planted or one hectare of ancient rainforest is protected as part of the production and exchange process. All of a sudden, a linear economy becomes a circular one, where the rate of regeneration exceeds the rate of destruction. In 50 years time, with this approach we may all be living in abundance.

You might point out that we could all choose electronic "ebooks" instead, meaning no trees would directly need to be cut down. However this technology requires mining and natural elements in its production too, creating other environmental affects. The production process of so many modern consumer "wonders," has a huge impact on the natural world.

The ecological footprint of passenger planes is another hard truth. The amount of fossil fuels burnt and the amount of mining needed from production to commercial use and maintenance is extremely inefficient. It is the reason that Greta Thunberg sailed in a yacht to the UN climate talks.[15] She understood the incongruence of standing up for the environment at the UN Climate Action Summit in New York while flying in a plane to get there!

It might seem impossible at the moment to travel overseas without flying. However, bullet trains in Asia and Europe are becoming a more efficient and even faster way of traveling long distances. The challenge is to apply that idea to traveling "across" or "under" our oceans. In the mean time imagine if we planted ten trees for every plane trip we went on or ten trees for every online conference meeting that prevented the need for us to fly anywhere! We could offset one behavior with multiple positive outcomes. Providing that we all did it— the challenge is finding a way that we each personally offset our own behaviors.

Richard Branson, founder and CEO of the Virgin group agrees with the circular economy, "It seems entirely straightforward to me that we should take from the planet and give back," he says. "For me, it's a choice to do that, of course, but more than that, it feels a real responsibility."

Paul Dunn (who wrote the foreword in this book) and Masami Sato from B1G1.com have set up a platform where every day consumers like you and me, plus our conscious enterprises, can create a giving impact for every conscious consumer decision we make.

I have implemented their model into my business. (See **selfcare.global**). Every time you engage, comment, or share our content we create a giving impact in your honor. The same applies for everything you do with us. We hope to lead through example.

Zero waste might not be possible, but circular and abundant economies that connect humans with the natural world and each other are very much possible right now and in this moment.

The future of work will value time freedom more than money. Helping every individual meet their basic human needs by collectively solving issues of distribution in an abundant world. The future of business will be shared and circular. We will no longer accept handing over a world to future generations that is scarcer than when we arrived. It is our individual and collective duty to ensure that this is the true north for all of us.

In a circular economy, everyone benefits from the economic activity that builds and rebuilds overall system health. It recognizes the importance of the economy needing to work effectively at all levels; large and small businesses, organizations and individuals, local and global ecosystems. How can you optimize your passion and time within your local circular economy?

> *"There's a myth that time is money. In fact, time is more*
> *precious than money. It's a non-renewable resource.*
> *Once you've spent it, and if you've spent it*
> *badly, it's gone forever."*
> **— Neil A. Fiore —**

Whatever you choose to do in life, do something you love. To make an prosperous business, ensure that it's more about others than you. Be customer centric, build a movement, leverage each other and cast a vision that people can all get behind and support! Don't limit yourself by asking "What can I alone do?" Ask better questions like: "Who do I know?" and "Who do you know?" and "What could we do together?" Free your time, have an empty calendar one day, whilst having all your basic needs met. Then live truly and freely by choice! And decide what you believe in. The abundance pie, or the scarcity one! Ultimately, what you believe to be true will shape your reality and even mine. The future is abundant for us all. I believe that.

✸ WORK IS MEDICINE PRESCRIPTION

» Find your reason for being. Take the internal compass tests online (**selfcare.global/assess**).

» Do what you love and you will never "work" a day in your life.

» Create your future Work Is Medicine vision. Write it down every 12 months and review.

» In the essence of Elon Musk, "Stop it or swap it."
  - Replace Netflix marathons with sleep
  - Replace fake influencers with inspiring creators
  - Replace toxic low vibration people with high-vibing mentors and friends
  - Replace low vibration thoughts (fear and victimization) with high frequency thoughts like courage and gratitude.
  - Replace scarcity with abundance
  - Replace alcohol with water
  - Replace suppressed emotions with vulnerability and radical honesty
  - Replace overthinking with aligned action, one small step at a time.
  - Replace processed food with high energy natural food from uncompromised sources.

» Value your time and energy.

» Learn to leverage each other. Ask, "what can we do?" versus "what can I alone do?"

» Answer this: ONE HOUR OF MY TIME is worth

....

....

» Start thinking "circular" instead of "linear." A circular economy is shared and conscious. How can you contribute to a shared economy? How can we make a bigger pie so that everyone can enjoy some?

» How do we build longer tables, not just higher fences?

To learn more about this medicine, or to contribute to this medicine, visit **selfcare.global/work**. Here you will find blogs, videos and podcasts.

Selfcare.global/work

NOTABLE EXPERTS IN THIS CHAPTER:

Hanalei Swan, Tim Ferris, Elon Musk, Roy T. Bennett, Jim Rohn, Aristotle, Albert Einstein, Roger James Hamilton, Dr John Demartini, Stephen Covey, Buckminster Fuller, Greta Thunberg, Richard Branson, Masami Sato, Paul Dunn, Neil A. Fiore.

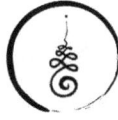

9

LIFESTYLE IS MEDICINE

"The biggest adventure you can take is to live the life
of your dreams, in real time."
— Oprah Winfrey —

Popular travel vloggers, Ryker Gamble and Alexey Lyakh led a movement for young people to explore the world and be "High On Life."[1] They lived and embodied their message with an irresistible desire to wander and travel, searching for the whole human experience. I was lucky enough to meet them in 2018 as we were both traveling around Bali. Little did I know that it would be the last time I saw them.

Later in 2018, they were living their best lives while capturing the beauty of Shannon Falls, near Squamish, British Columbia. Ryker and Alexey, along with Megan, Alexey's long-time partner trekked up to a higher tier to enjoy the views when Megan slipped and fell off the 100-foot waterfall into the fast flowing system of granite pools. Without thinking, Alexey jumped in to help her. Ryker then jumped in after his best friend Alexey.

None survived. Megan was 29; Alexey and Ryker were 30-years-old. Ryker posted frequently on his social media platforms about his belief in fully experiencing each moment free from any weight of the past or any anticipation of the future. Free to realize that only you can control how you feel, about anything. Free to see things for what they are and free your time, have an empty calendar one day, whilst having all your basic needs met. Then you can live truly and freely by choice! This is a tribute and reminder to live your best life, just as their lives symbolized the joy of being present in the here and now.

For me, meeting them was a brief spontaneous connection in the presence of people truly high on life, not trying to escape it with drugs, alcohol or mind-numbing jobs. These amazing humans and others inspire me every day to know that life can be done differently.

They inspired many to love life and live it fully! They weren't without controversy of course, but living greatly often inspires naysayers. If not for their tragic accident, I'm sure they would still be sharing the same message of being high on life. And though, sadly, they aren't here to say it themselves— their message still lives on today, inspiring and encouraging people to live with passion and zest.

The world is vast and full of possibilities. Follow your bliss. Stop looking for reasons why you can't and look for reasons why you can. Tomorrow is not guaranteed for any of us. I dare you to wake up tomorrow and choose to be high on life; choose to live your ideal day, your ideal life.

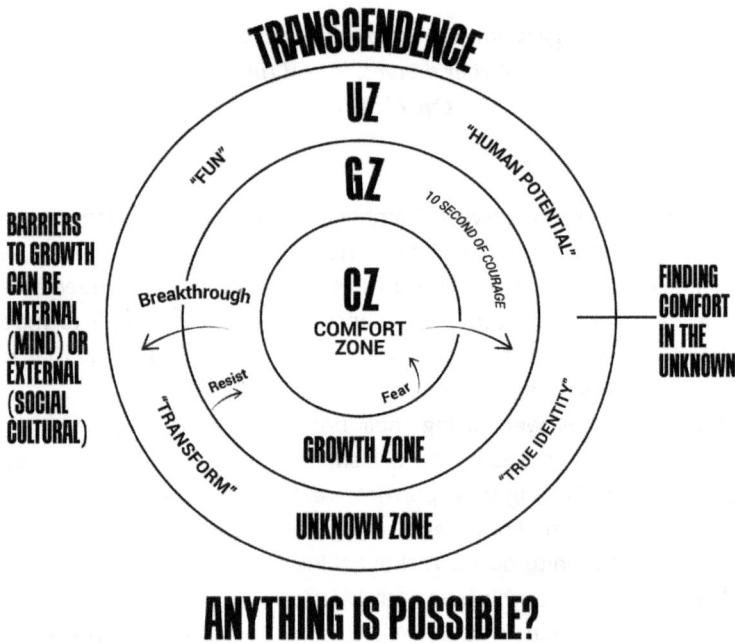

Image: Extension of David TS Wood's work https://thekickasslife.com/about

LIVE YOUR OWN ADVENTURE

During my 20s, I was fortunate enough to be mentored by speaker, author and founder of Amplified Living (amplifiedliving.com) David TS Wood. He once shared with me that, "a comfort zone is a beautiful place, but nothing ever grows there."

Over the years he gave myself and others permission to "play full out." In fact, he dared us to live beyond our comfort zone. It was a taste of new freedom.

Imagine what your life would look like if you didn't rationalize every action with a thought process that came place of comparison and self-judgment of "what will they think?" or "I don't want to embarrass myself" or "I don't want to risk rejection." David dared us to think beyond our insecurities. He kept reminding us that all the fun happens outside our comfort zone. However, he also understood that living in the unknown zone takes a special type of person. Many of us seek safety and security, which isn't a bad thing either. Perhaps we need periods of both?!

So, I'd like you to take a moment and think about your own comfort zone and life expression on a scale of 0–10.

0: Comfort zone

5: Uncomfort zone

10: Unknown zone

I invite you to play in the full human experience. From 0–10. All it takes is 10 seconds of courage to step outside of your comfort zone. In the movie *Yes Man* with Jim Carrey, he starts saying yes to everything. An amazing journey unfolds as he leaned into each new human experiences. I feel that this outlook (with some healthy boundaries) may be a good default operating place.

But that's me. What about you?

What is your default?

Where do you choose to operate from?

You could remain reserved, listening, observing and being a passenger of life (0–5), or you could continue to show up and live in your highest vibrancy, unapologetically. (5–10) leaning into the unknown with every choice and action. For example:

0–5: would be to continue doing the same thing you are doing right now. Safe, secure and engrained in your daily rituals.

5–10: would be buying a one way ticket to that place that you have always dreamed of going. Listening to your heart as it gives you that 10 seconds of courage to DO something that you have always wanted to. What happens from there? Who knows, but I'm sure it will be something that you never regret. Take a chance. You can always return to the comfort of your current experience.

- Imagine if you simply danced like no one was watching.
- Imagine if without thinking you connected with that good looking or high vibing person that you had been thinking about all along.
- Imagine if you said yes, more than you said no.
- Imagine if you invited new experiences into your life.
- Imagine if you learnt a new skill or tried new things every year.
- Imagined if you traveled to a new environment and destination each year enriching your human experience with connections and cultures that you never even knew existed.

SOMETIMES YOU MUST DARE GREATLY

I often remind myself that it can sometimes take only 10 seconds of courage to overcome F.E.A.R (false experiences appearing real). This thought empowers me to step outside my comfort zone. If I am ever unsure, I ask myself—*Would I regret not doing it?* It can also mean letting fear win, "forget everything and run," or letting courage win "face everything and rise." Whether you operate from fear (below the line) or courage (above the line) is completely up to you.

At a conference in Brisbane I got a choice to play in my version of 10! I got to dance on stage in drag clothes, something completely outside of my comfort zone. I was singing a song that I had only just learned hours before and wasn't sure if I would remember the words and be able to walk in heels. Now, I could have played small and live by the "play-it-safe" rules. To this date is one of my fondest memories and it certainly expanded my life experiences from which it could never return.

Now, it may be energetically draining for some to live in so boldly all the time. However, next time you meet someone living in their highest expression, please celebrate their courage and applaud their ability to play in the unknown. Whilst many people live a double life, wearing multiple masks and showing up in a way that other people expect of them, others show up exactly as they are. Happy in their own sense of being. That's a beautiful thing.

If we are lucky, we each experience a catalyst in our lives that inspires us to stop living a life that doesn't fill us up each day; I hope this book is your catalyst! Why waste a minute living a life that leaves you feeling unhappy, unhealthy and misaligned? Time is quicksand, and seems to flow faster as you grow older; it is your most precious resource.

Casting an incredible future vision and choosing your "true north" is a beautiful and positive start. Vision boards and consciously engineered scripts and gratitude journals are great, but there comes a point where you will need to be courageous enough to embrace action and go for it!

In this chapter, I remind you that having a healthy human body is also a wonderful starting point. It's what permits you to go on every adventure.

Grace Hopper, a 20th century Rear Admiral in the US navy, saw life in a similar way, "a ship in port is safe, but that is not what ships are built for, sail out to sea and do new things."[2] Imagine our human vessel as a beautiful ship, built to sail the seas and explore the furthest corners of the globe, resilient enough to weather any of life's storms.

Lifestyle is Medicine explores how happiness is at hand for all of us and aligns wholeheartedly with many of the previous medicines to springboard you into action.

- What type of human vessel would you need for the journey?
- Do you have an allied health team to support you in your self-care, using a human and nature centric approach?
- What are your own standards for living and being? Live fast and die young or live towards longevity? Or a mixture of both?
- Write a bucket-list or a f*ck it list and live a life with no regrets.

Create a bucket list and vision board that you courageously lean into each day. Take each breath with compassion, empathy and a grateful heart, savor each movement and shared embrace. Living in your ultimate alignment creates a living legacy, to serve, to contribute and to pass on to future generations, meaning you will die with no regrets, the finest aspiration of all.

> *"Life should not be a journey to the grave with the intention of arriving safely in a pretty and well preserved body, but rather to skid in broadside in a cloud of smoke, thoroughly used up, totally worn out, and loudly proclaiming 'Wow! What a Ride!'"[3]*
> *— Hunter S. Thompson —*

DEFINE LIFESTYLE AS MEDICINE

Lifestyle as Medicine has been the most powerful in my life. It is the ambition to work to live your ideal day every day. The awareness of this medicine aligns your daily habits and rituals with the resilience of the human vessel that you require to live this lifestyle you're creating.

Our human bodies are designed to adapt to all of life's stimuli. You are the captain of your ship and the master of your own fate. Whatever your ideal; trekking in the deepest part of nature, bouldering and climbing amazing rock faces, surfing waves with no one around or sharing the kick of a football with a loved one, we all need a human vessel that can go the distance. Maintaining our human body is the first step on any journey that our mind can conjure up and that our heart drives us toward.

Fortunately as human beings, if an environment is no longer nourishing our journey, we can choose to live in more nourishing environments. Shift your mind from seeing life's challenges to seeing opportunities for growth and a life well lived. Stay grounded in your values, the foundations of your character and the integrity of your decisions even if they do not match society's conventions; they are your truth!

> **Lifestyle as Medicine is about courage, leaning in and taking a step towards living a life of your dreams.**

For me, **Lifestyle Is Medicine** is the embodiment of all the other medicines, aligning our thinking with dynamic action. We become the sum total of how we choose to think, consume, move, work, connect and which environments we choose to spend the most time in. Thus we each need to choose wisely, act wisely and find flow in the unknown. We need to solidify our vision, taking moments to pause, ground ourselves and then to go deeper as we get ready for the next stage of growth in our lives.

Now it's your turn.

CREATE YOUR IDEAL LIFESTYLE VISION

Pause. Breathe. Write it down. Make your vision tangible.

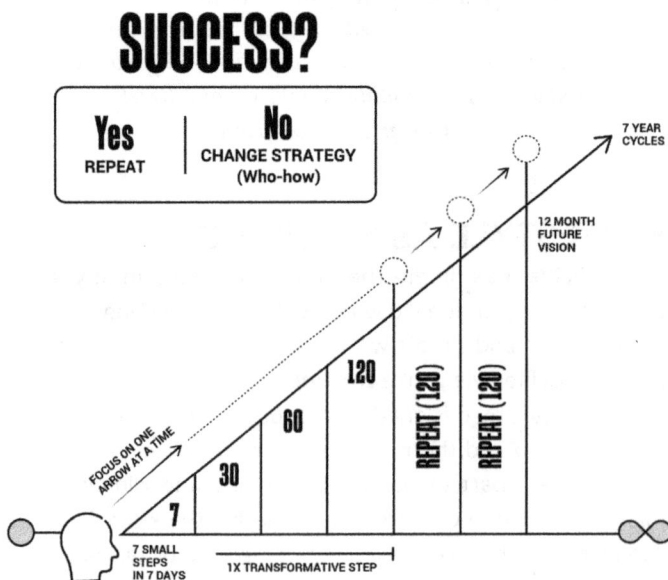

Look at the little character above. Let's call him Freddie. Freddie is walking towards time or infinity in a straight unchanging line of his life.

Above him, is a choice to cast a vision arrowing upward towards a 12-month goal. Over the long term, it is interesting to remember that human life works in 7 year cycles, both physically and mentally as we move between birth and 7 years; 7–14 years and so on. Each stage represents the maturing of our rational mind and emotions, our sexuality and sense of responsibility to ourselves and to humanity, heading ultimately toward the "Source" and what we might call our "rebirth."[4]

Let's assume Freddie will live for 70 years and so he has 10 "chapters" of his life to write and rewrite as he travels along. One day he is compelled to reflect on the pain and dissatisfaction of past experiences and he decides to step away from repeating the process, to rise above life's negative distractions, projections, addictions and requests from others and script a new future for himself.

He looks internally to recalibrate his "true north," tuning into his values, purpose, passion, abundance, self-care and external impact he wants to make.

Taking the first step can be hard, so he breaks it down into 7 small steps he can take in the first week. Perhaps he focuses on the living less stressed and focuses on his breathing for the first time, to feel oxygen's life-force reenergize his output for the first time in years. Perhaps he knocks on his neighbor's door simply to ask if he or she needs anything. Perhaps he reconnects with nature or plucks up the courage to go to visit old friends, something he'd never made time for before.

Gradually these small steps grow month-by-month and he moves up toward his future vision of who he wants to be and how he wants to feel. Too often we fail to articulate our strategy for ourselves, fail to write it down, to make it a real plan with a blueprint to follow. The beauty of structuring your future this way is that it is solid and therefore more likely to manifest and importantly you can review and restructure every 12 months!

What do your next seven years look like?
Your next 14?

To download your own FREE "Lifestyle Vision Template" find it, below and if you have the courage, want accountability or wish to inspire someone else.

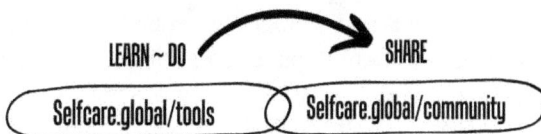

LEARN ~ DO → SHARE

Selfcare.global/tools   Selfcare.global/community

And get started planning your wildest and best life today!

HAPPINESS AS A LIFESTYLE

Before you aim for happiness, you might be wondering where to aim your arrow. Is happiness found by a direct hit or an accumulation of the experience? Can you even "make" it happen? Is it a feeling? Or is it the end result of wisdom and rational thoughts? Is our happiness at the mercy of things that happen *to* us? Or is it a quality that can surpass the events in our lives?

Though I have mentioned happiness at the beginning of the book, I have included again here because many people don't make the link at happiness as a lifestyle, they instead believe it's something that happens due to "external forces." And though many events and circumstances can alter our feelings, they aren't the cause of our lifelong relationship with happiness.

The pursuit of happiness is as old as civilisation, contemplated for thousands of years by Hindu religions, Buddhists, ancient Romans, and Greek philosophers like Plato and Aristotle. The ancient Greeks defined happiness as a phenomenon using the word "eudaimonia." The literal translation of "eudaimonia" is "good spirit," however it's more widely accepted to encompass the notion of "human flourishing," fulfilling your universal potential as a human being. Aristotle likened it to an acorn becoming the magnificent oak tree it was meant to be and nothing else.

According to Plato's definition, happiness was not achievable by the vast majority of people; it took understanding, discipline and hard work in many subjects in the pursuit of understanding what goodness is and fulfilling your potential.[5] Aristotle deviated in this philosophy by extolling virtues of "good actions" as being central to a well-lived life; that happiness is the end result of virtuous actions.

This differs quite a bit from the **modern concept of happiness**. We are inclined to see happiness as an emotional state, where we hope for the highs of achievements and wins, or achieve sanctuary from the suffering of the world. We think of those perfect moments that are exciting and euphoric, yet also momentary.

Aristotle explained happiness as a virtue by actively fulfilling one's purpose in line with one's values.[6] We have touched on this previously as finding your "ikigai" or reason for being. Is yours to live simply? Or is it to live and leave a legacy? How do different purposes and pathways all lead to the same end feeling of happiness?

Aristotle believed it was firstly through the embodiment of good thoughts, by appreciating what is good; friendships, virtue, honor, what brings pleasure and abundance as a whole to your life, remembering we are each limited to our own view point of what makes a "whole life."[7]

He also believed in the *experience* of applying these principles to the context of everyday situations and life's events, evaluating which course of action is best supported by reasons. This can be the most challenging; we cannot acquire wisdom solely through learning general rules. To embody the wisdom we need to create an experience of our own to learn from. If the result of our actions and reactions is positive and feels good; keep going. If the result does not feel good and is termed negative; it still becomes an opportunity for a learning experience to choose a different action or reaction next time.

Aristotle broke down the sum of happiness as, "being acquired, through practice, daily rituals, those deliberative, emotional, and social skills that enable us to put our general understanding of well-being into daily practice in ways that are suitable to each occasion."[8]

So what does this ancient wise one have to do with our modern times? He simply shows that our pursuit for happiness has not changed and we can apply our understanding of happiness to every situation!

> Imagine living in such a state of good health and well-being, whilst living a good life, with a good spirit that you live in a perpetual state of "eudaimonia!" Feeling the full depth of the human experience and emotion, and choosing to act and react in a higher vibration—transcendence!

Aristotle's version of happiness promotes firstly the "learning" dynamic of participating in rational activity and thoughts that lead to happiness through our daily actions. It is the reason why self-help books can be considered "shelf help," because while the teachings are great, if they are never actioned into your human experience, then what's the point? Again, to know and to not yet do, is to still not yet to "know." This book aims to be the hand pulling you off your chair, out of the office and into your life!

Which leads us to the most important part of Aristotle's definition, the "embodiment" of those thought's as you experience life and how you then choose to live, act and react within the realms of those thoughts; with honesty, justice, courage, and the virtues of what really matters. Happiness is the end result of good thoughts and actions.

Happiness therefore may well not be about emotion at all. In fact, someone can go through intense hardship and still be happy based on their actions, reactions and thought processes during that time. As an example a death can be a celebration of one's life; or a mourning of their death; or both. "Eudaimonia" is about living a good life with "good spirit" as a human, regardless of life's context or circumstances, whilst allowing for the full depth of our human and emotional experience. Grief is "okay," happiness is "okay": all feelings are "okay" and even necessary.

Mike Dooley, author of *Notes from the Universe* has a similar modern principle that happiness cannot be found in looking back at the past, but is more likely to be found in the pursuit of everyday moments. We should, *"chase happiness, forget the details and dreaded how to's."*[9]

In this high-tech world it can be hard to break down and rationalize a feeling. But think about those moments of looking into a loved-ones' eyes, the euphoric rush of hugging someone you haven't seen for a long time, even seeing your favorite animal each morning when you wake; you can encapsulate the gratifying feeling and thought of all these moments together to become a state of being.

To have happiness in our life, we simply need to align our internal thoughts with our external actions and reactions, to find inner peace, harmony and bliss in the context of any situation and environment. Whether you are a parent lovingly bathing your infant in New York City or in a run-down building on the Gaza Strip during a civil war, human beings have shown that we can feel happiness in any context, whether connecting with others, with nature or with your "ikagai."

When have you felt a *bliss* moment? Bliss is that intense feeling of inner peace and pure presence that empowers you to feel full of love and gratitude for that moment.
- Where were you?
- What were you doing?
- Who were you with?
- What were you thinking?
- Why did you choose to be there?

These questions might help you find and preserve that feeling of happiness. Good thoughts become good things. Learning to find a grateful heart in every situation will go a long way to the incarnation of the happiness within us all.

MAKE FLOW STATE A LIFESTYLE HABIT

Do you often lose track of time? Perhaps you've been entrenched in a puzzle, an intriguing work problem, a good book, a painting you're working on, tinkering in your shed, surfing, gardening or anything where you've been completely focused on the task at hand. Eventually you look up to find hours and hours have passed in what feels like no time at all! It's fair to say you've been in the "zone," but what does this actually mean?

Dr Mihaly Csikszentmihalyi, Ph.D. is known for his work on creativity, but is best known as the man behind the idea of "flow state" or "getting in the zone." He is the author of over 120 articles and books about what it takes to be fully immersed in whatever you are doing. The "flow state" is often described as the most productive and creative state of mind for us to be in.

Dr. Csikszentmihalyi would argue that achieving the flow state regularly is a key element of our happiness. In other words, when we learn how to enter the flow state, we increase our productivity, creativity, and happiness all at the same time. He shares four ways to "get in the Flow Zone."

1. **FREEDOM:** *"It is when we act freely, for the sake of the action itself rather than for ulterior motives, that we learn to become more than what we were."*[10] Ulterior motives can lead you down a negative path in life, which is something that Mihaly agrees on. Selflessness is important.

2. **SUCCESS:** *"Success, like happiness, cannot be pursued; it must ensue...as the unintended side-effect of one's personal dedication to a course greater than oneself."*[11]

3. **INACTION:** *"Few things are sadder than encountering a person who knows exactly what he should do, yet cannot muster enough energy to do it."*[12]

4. **GOING OUT OF THE COMFORT ZONE:** *"Most enjoyable activities are not natural; they demand an effort that initially one is reluctant to make. But once the interaction starts to provide feedback to the person's skills, it usually begins to be intrinsically rewarding."*[13]

The more time we spend here in this state the happier we will be. Achieving the flow state can also be looked at as an experience of mindfulness. It is that heightened sense of awareness that an athlete experiences during a game or what an artist feels in their most creative state. The good news is that you don't need to be either of these to be in the flow state. All it takes is the choice to increase mindfulness by taking the following steps.

Once you are in the Flow Zone, here are 6 ways to stay in a Flow State.
1. **Intensely focused attention:** Producing flow requires long periods of uninterrupted concentration, deep focus. This means multi-tasking is out. Only concentrate on one thing at a time.
2. **Clear vision and goals:** If you set some clear goals, your mind can stick to them rather than wandering off on another tangent.
3. **The challenge/skills ratio:** If the task is too dull, attention can wander, and you will not be focused on what you are doing.
4. **High consequences:** When there is danger lurking in the environment, we don't need to concentrate very hard. Adrenaline gets us into the zone.
5. **Creativity:** If you look under the hood of creativity, what you see is pattern recognition. This is the brain's ability to link new ideas together and create focus. Risk taking gives you the courage to bring those new ideas into the world.

6. **Equal participation and skill level:** Flow is most likely to happen in a group setting when all participants have an equal role in the project. If amateur rugby players compete against professionals, the amateurs soon feel out of their depth, and the professionals get bored.

Being in flow not only increases happiness, but can also encourage more positive emotions. Due to those positive emotions, you'll find that you're better able to cope when things take a downturn, or negative thoughts try to creep in. It's also been shown that people in the flow state achieve a higher level of performance in their work and daily habits. Pursue a lifestyle where you experience moments of flow often, whether it's in your work, hobbies, or passions.

HEALTHY LIFESTYLE MODERATION REDUCES RISK BY 80%

I want to remind you how can we maximize our physical potential for our lifestyle journey. Dr Michael Greger, founder of NutritionFacts.org[14] suggests that it might be simpler than you think to make way for healthy moderation and believes it's something that anyone can achieve!

Greger reminds us that, "...for most of the leading causes of death, our genes account for at most 10 to 20% of risk."[15] He suggests perhaps it's time we stop blaming our genes, "knowing that at least 70% of strokes and colon cancer are avoidable, as are over 80% of coronary heart disease and over 90% of type 2 diabetes." He also asserts, "We can focus on the 70%+ that is under our control. That may be the real solution to the healthcare crisis."[16] My sentiments exactly.

Rates of heart disease and cancers differ immensely between various populations too, and interestingly it is found that, "when people migrate from low- to high-risk countries, their disease rates almost always change to those of the new environment."[17] Once again we see that **Environment is Medicine** more so than genes and place of birth! Yet another inducement for us to co-create future environments that promote good health and wellbeing in the context of any lifestyle.

Dr Greger campaigns adopting four simple lifestyle choices to dramatically cut our risk of developing chronic disease; not smoking; not being obese, exercising half an hour a day and eating healthier. Voila!

Statistics show that these simple behavior changes can reduce the risk of type 2 diabetes by 95% and reduce the risk of heart attacks by 80%.[18] Imagine reducing the risk of stroke by 50% and reducing cancer rates by a third simply by integrating these behaviors into your daily lifestyle!

An important study by the Centers for Disease Control and Prevention in the USA followed about 8,000 adults for six years. Their results concurred with Greger's key pillars of not smoking; consuming a healthy diet; and engaging in sufficient physical activities in order to reduce the risk of early death.[19]

So what does this mean in terms of living longer? Dr Greger draws upon a study[20] that also measured the level of vitamin C in participant's blood, a biomarker for plant food intake, and these results showed a drop in mortality rates equivalent to being 14 years younger! How impressive is that!

If you are not yet listening, this is especially applicable to any of the 4–7 billion people living in the red and orange zones on the integrated health and wellbeing spectrum. If you can't stop it, then try to swap it or at least moderate the level of self-harm you impose on those cells of yours.

By "not smoking" they just mean not currently smoking. Remember that those beautiful lungs of yours regenerate every five or so years. Even if you smoked a pack a day in your 20s, you can still regenerate healthy lung cells in your 40s and beyond.

By "healthy diet" they simply mean complying with rather simplistic dietary guidelines set by governing bodies in each country. Eat more plants; get your 2 fruits and 5 vegetables each day. Drink plenty of water; avoid harmful processed "franken-foods" full of sugar and low on the nutritional density you need to build healthy cells.

By "physically active" they simply refer to at least 21 minutes out the 1440 minutes that we all have access to each day. You can move in a way that doesn't feel like a chore, just get the heart rate up to a moderate level where it's difficult to hold a conversation and you will be in the zone that creates a positive change in your body.

Dr Greger shares that those who simply, "managed at least one of the three behaviors had a 40% lower risk of dying"[21] prematurely. Those that integrated, "2 out of the 3 behaviors, cut their risk of dying in half!" While those that integrated, "all 3 behaviors cut their chances of dying by 82%!"[22]

By knowing how not to die, how to minimize self-harm and how to integrate the basic foundational behaviors into our lifestyles, we can now focus on living towards longevity and optimizing our human experience with a human vessel that is resilient enough to withstand any adventure you choose.

Actively follow your chosen lifestyle; and providing you don't get hit by a bus or eaten by a shark, you can choose what type of old person you become!

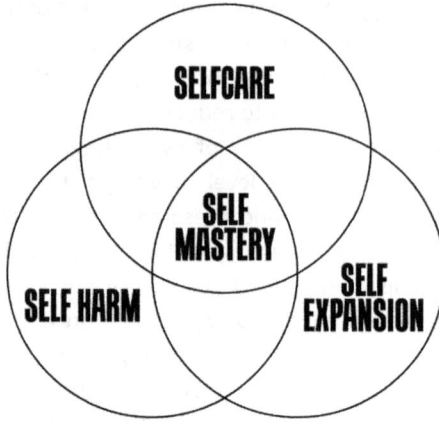

PREVENTION IS THE LIFESTYLE CURE

I am confident by now that you have embraced the life-changing impetus of this book that simply adopting a holistically healthy lifestyle can prevent 80% of chronic diseases. This truth is slowly pervading modern society however according to Yale-Griffin PRC Director David Katz, MD, overall the general public lacks clear and consistent advice about the role of lifestyle medicine in promoting health. He says too many competing voices, capitalist driven motives, and conflicting messages in the media have left many people confused about how best to improve their health.[23]

To overcome this confusion and educate the public about lifestyle medicine, Dr Katz assembled a global coalition called the "True Health Initiative." It consists of over 300 leading experts and influential leaders from the paradigms of the 12 Medicines; Nature, Environment, Connection, Food, Modern medicine, Lifestyle, and many more.

These health experts collated their knowledge about lifestyle as medicine and agreed on 6 core principles of healthy living that could add years to lives, and life to years:

Minimizing Self-harm
(1) Consuming minimally processed, low human interference mostly plant-based foods;
(2) Avoiding toxins such as tobacco and excess alcohol;

Move more and rest well
(3) Adopting a physically active lifestyle;
(4) Getting plenty of sleep;

Find harmony in your work and lifestyle

(5) Reducing psychological stress;

And finally;

(6) Cultivating supportive relationships and social bonds.

In other words connection, connection, connection! A message I reference, over and over again. Focus on just one of these actions to get started and your results will give you the energy to embrace them all!

LIFESTYLE MEDICINE IS THE FUTURE

The future of modern medicine is lifestyle-based medicine; integrating ancient wisdom into our modern world and shared human experience. The True Health Initiative has a vision where, "all people live long and healthy lives, free of preventable chronic disease."[24]

This too is my vision. There is growing understanding that we need to build healthy environments to enable every global citizen to live in a state of good health, free of chronic preventable disease. A world that gives everyone access to modern healthcare facilities for intervention as needed, using evidence based truths, on a foundation of our body's innate natural healing mechanisms.

We can refer to an official definition of lifestyle medicine as, "the application of environmental, behavioral, medical and motivating principles towards the management of lifestyle related health challenges in a clinical setting."[25] However, when we consider lifestyle medicine beyond the clinical healthcare setting it becomes so much more.

It becomes an empowered way of living and being, connected as communities living in tune with the natural world that nourishes and supports us all. It also creates space for the personalization of one's path by asking, "what would your ideal lifestyle be," without the need for comparison or judgment.

The modern "rediscovery" of lifestyle-based medicine and holistic practitioners is integral right now. Not just in the management of the current burden of chronic and preventable disease but in turning the tide toward prevention, and ultimately one day the absence of this burden that is plaguing our modern human experience.

Our modern approach to chronic and preventable disease is predominantly interventional in the form of "pharmaco-medical" treatments. We can all agree that while necessary in some cases, they should not be considered as the complete solution to the problem.

As it stands, "the global market for pharmaceuticals reached $1.2 trillion in 2018, up $100 billion from 2017, according to the Global Use of Medicines report from the IQVIA Institute for Human Data Science."[26] If money is energy, then we are channeling more and more vital energy into managing this burden of disease yet the number of people living a restricted life with a chronic preventable disease has increased to 1 in 2! This tells me if money into pharmaceuticals was the solution, then we would not be facing an increasing burden!

A new approach is needed right now. A human centric approach founded in nature and supported by communities that enable daily self-care within the context of any geographical setting. The challenge with changing this modern day approach is that it is so profitable. IQVIA Institute suggests that, "Going forward, the global market will grow by 4–5% CAGR, reaching $1.5 trillion."[27]

Imagine if instead, we invested this money in co-creating environments that enabled self-care on a daily basis, supported by nourishing communities that learn to empower self–regulation and self-government: real global blue zone communities, thriving together.

THE 4 PRINCIPLES TO LIFESTYLE MEDICINE

As explained previously chronic and preventable diseases have many known risk factors and markers, which are often the sole focus of clinical intervention.

However, these factors and markers have deeper roots and causes that can be above, below, internal and even external to the signal or symptomatic "marker" itself. Which means that like the principles of Ayurveda and other ancient medicines, we need to consider the whole person within the context of their current environment. We can think of this new perspective as involving "lifestyle interventions" towards the management of chronic disease.

These principles focus on taking radical self-responsibility. What we can individually do. But it also addresses how we can leverage each other and co-create enabling environments and communities that make our daily lifestyle choices a little easier.

Here they are.

PRINCIPLE #1: SELFCARE; ACTIVE RATHER THAN PASSIVE CARE.

The requirement for modern day practitioners, coaches and healers to be able to help guide, mentor and support individuals up the health and wellbeing spectrum, must be founded on the person seeking a health and wellbeing solution to be more active, rather than passive in their own care.

It is done with a process that should ultimately enable people to continue sustaining healthy lifestyle habits into their future. Seeking guidance when they get off track, or when they are inspired to take their health and wellbeing to a whole new level. A side note is that modern day practitioners, coaches and healers must also be walking their talk and I naturally include myself in this expectation. After all how can we guide patients to a place where we have never been?

PRINCIPLE #2: MODERN AND MEDICAL INTERVENTION IS SECONDARY TO OUR NATURAL AND INNATE MECHANISMS.

This may seem contradictory but it needs to be. Individual diets, psychologies, connections with nature and community should not be considered alternative or complementary medicine; they should be primary. Modern and medical intervention should be secondary to our body's innate wisdom and the nourishment that is available in all of the 12 medicines.

In an article for the *Medical Journal of Australia*, Egger, Binns and Rossner explain that, "Medication, in the lifestyle-medicine paradigm, is seen more as an adjunct than an end treatment in care, and side effects are recognized as part of the outcome."[28]

For example, erectile dysfunction from antidepressant medication in middle-aged men; "can potentially exacerbate depression. Not to mention not being able to be intimate might create an emotional disconnection with his partner in times of passion. Hence this effect should be weighed against the possible benefits of a lifestyle-change option such as exercise, for which a strong evidence base in managing depression and promoting healthy blood flow down stairs already exists."[29]

PRINCIPLE #3: WORK AS AN ALLIED AND INTEGRATED TEAM.

In the same way it takes a village to raise a child, it takes a community to help heal the sick. It also takes a community to thrive together in the blue zone towards longevity. As an allied team of health and wellness practitioners, coaches and healers we must actively work together for the benefit of the individual person (not just a patient), to ensure that they are being actively empowered to live in a state of good health and wellbeing.

Which means that at some stage, we as "health care providers" should make ourselves redundant, in that the person no longer needs an allied team to stay healthy in the context of their own life. Knowing however, that we are there to support them if they ever find themselves falling into the orange or green zone of the health and wellbeing spectrum.

Having a human and nature centric approach to good health and wellbeing means that we are all part of this team. Those influencing the natural world we live in, the communities and environments we grow with and the sense of connection we have as individuals, cultures and communities, these things are arguably all just as important as the accredited allied health professionals we seek for wisdom and tools to move up the health and wellbeing spectrum at our own pace. Which means the farmer who produces the food we all eat, is arguably a more important doctor than those administering the synthetic medication.

PRINCIPLE #4: 3 PILLARS TO WIN YOUR MORNING, WIN YOUR DAY.

We need to take radical self-responsibility in order to master our own morning rituals, especially before trying to help anyone else. We can't be part of the problem while trying to give others solutions.

There are 3 simple pillars we can all master each day.

Pillar 1. Mind is medicine

Pillar 2. Movement is medicine

Pillar 3. Food is medicine

It can be as simple as listening to an empowering podcast as you take the dogs for the walk in the morning, or having a plant-based smoothie bowl after a morning jog.

See if you can achieve all 3 pillars in a day. Then see if you can get two or three days in a row. Then seven. If you can get to 21 days, you start to develop a sticky habit. After 16 weeks, it starts to become a lifestyle change.

Your 3 pillar morning is personalized and unique to your life.

LIVE SIMPLY AND LIVE A LIFE WITH NO REGRETS

Good health and wellbeing must be a way of living and being. SelfCare will be the foundation for allied healthcare, promoting active empowerment rather than passive care. We should want to feel good each day, have energy to burn whilst looking after our cells for today and tomorrow. The only challenge is making better lifestyle choices. Create that vision for your ideal day, living in your ideal environments; a life truly of your own design.

Ask yourself what may be the underlying cause of your dysfunction and unhappiness. You may possibly trace the source back to the misalignment of your values or your truth that you haven't been listening to. Many years ago, I asked myself just such a question and the answer set me on a whole new path of natural truths and possibilities. I have benefitted from this state of being every single day since. In fact, I have built my entire lifestyle around it.

Start living your new choices and watch your health and wellbeing improve within 12 months. Most of us are stuck, choosing lifestyles that have never served us. Just because you were born into that societal or cultural construct for how you should live your life, doesn't mean that you have to keep living that way. Take time to measure what truly matters, take steps to feel good every day and serve from overflow. Cast that new vision, step outside your comfort zone and start really living. You are one courageous choice away from doing something your future self will thank you for.

⚕ LIFESTYLE IS MEDICINE PRESCRIPTION

» Download Your Lifestyle Vision Template and start charting your best life today. What does your seven year cycle look like?

» Go to **selfcare.global** and connect on social media with our like-minded SelfCare warriors who are all supporting one another in their lifestyle changes.

» Create your own 3 pillar morning routine
  - Mind: podcast, journal, meditation
  - Movement: walk, run, surf, gym
  - Food: water, breathwork, eat more plants

To learn more about this medicine, or to contribute to this medicine, visit **selfcare.global/lifestyle**. Here you will find blogs, videos and podcasts.

Selfcare.global/lifestyle

NOTABLE EXPERTS IN THIS CHAPTER:
David TS Wood, Hunter S. Thompson, Grace Hopper, Plato, Mike Dooley, Dr Mihaly Csikszentmihalyi, Dr Michael Greger, Dr David Katz.

1 HOUR MORNING MASTERY

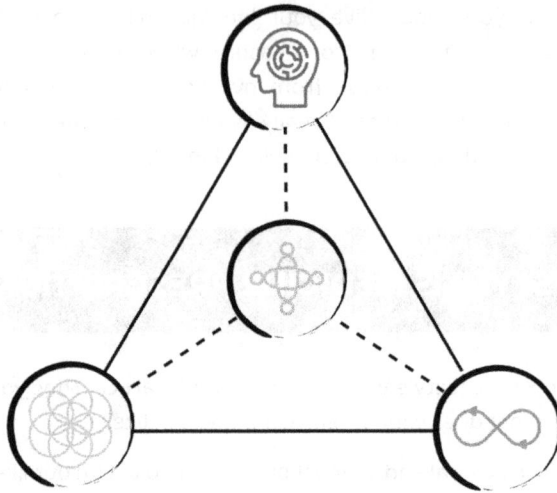

HOW TO MASTER YOUR MORNING IN 1 HOUR

MIND   20" Mindfullness Practice

FOOD   Hydrate, Breathe, Saturate

MOVE   30" Motion is Lotion

CONNECTION

Together is better, find your tribe

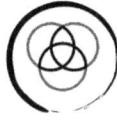

10

SPIRIT IS MEDICINE

*"Our spirituality is a oneness and an interconnectedness
with all that lives and breathes, even with all that
does not live or breathe."*
— *Voltaire* —

ZERO, ONE AND INFINITY

Spirit is often called many other names, and its significance (or lack thereof to some) is different for everyone. God, Source, Spirit, Allah, Brahman, Jehovah, Tao, Infinite, Nothing, Supreme Being, Wankan Tanka, The Great Mystery, Yahweh, the list goes on.

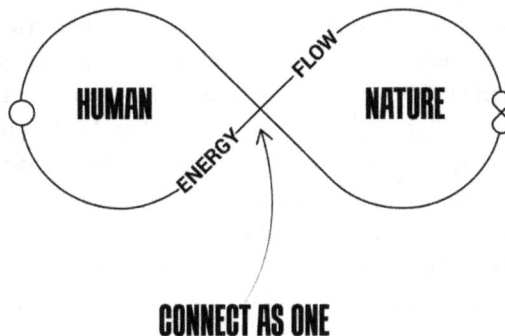

I have indulged my creative reflections with a little fictional story about the way we all see and experience our definition of Spirit differently. I have used three popular and different spiritual leaders to explore this; after all, "Spirit" is in fact a deep and personal exploration. It doesn't come with a set of rules or ways to live. It all stems down to your own personal relationship with your own soul.

That's the crux of any spiritual journey, an intimate and often unnameable exploration into the Infinite.

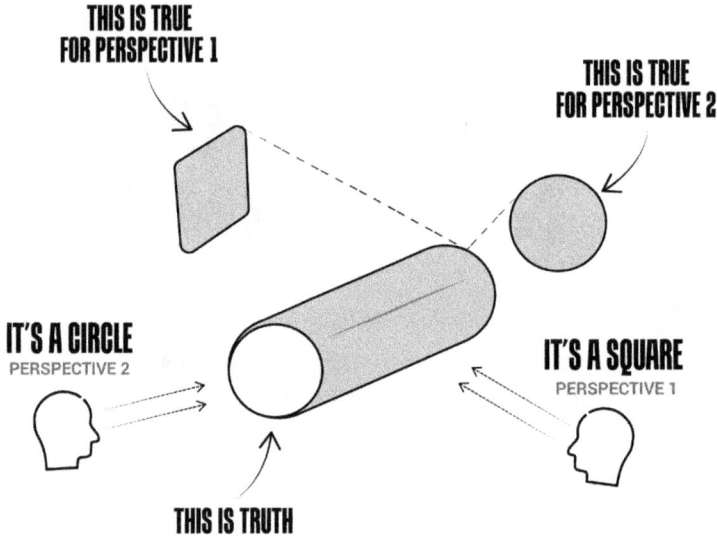

THE DAY THREE LEADERS FED THE DUCKS

In 2020, as the world paused to reassess its direction together, Michio Kaku, Deepak Chopra and the Dalai Lama sat down by a pond to discuss the universe, love and everything in between. They sprinkled breadcrumbs for the ducks to eat as their conversation unfolded. The ducks swam, pecked and quacked happily.

The Dalai Lama asked Deepak Chopra how he would describe Michio Kaku. Deepak pondered and eloquently shared that Michio is a modern-day superhero of the incomprehensible. He stretches his mind to 11 dimensions, understands what Einstein failed to grasp, and is a pioneer for expanded consciousness and other like-minded physicists and scientists like him.

Michio Kaku was flattered by the description and joked that they had forgotten to include his induction into the New York's 100 smartest people, but since Madonna was in there too, he wasn't sure how valid and reliable it was.

Not to be in the spotlight on his own, Michio Kaku deflected the attention and asked Deepak how he would describe the Dalai Lama.

Deepak looked at The Dalai Lama (currently Tenzin Gyatso) and shared that he believed the name "Dalai Lama" is also believed to mean Ocean of Wisdom and that he belongs to the Gelugpa tradition of Tibetan Buddhism, the largest and most influential tradition in Tibet. He said that the institution of the Dalai Lama is a relatively recent one; in our short human history, there have been only 14 Dalai Lamas and that he is a very sacred and important person for humanity and in our unity between East and West.

Deepak shifted his gaze to Michio Kaku and shared that the institution of modern science was equally young. He shared that the difference was only in that science primarily uses the mind to form testable explanations and about the universe within the context of our limited senses. He felt that science was a curious explanation of the universe and a reflection of human beings' requirement to "know before they do." Whereas Buddhism looked to connect, tune in and spread thoughts and feelings of peace, love and unity.

Deepak went on to share that according to Buddhist belief, The Dalai Lama is a reincarnation of a past Lama who decided to be reborn again to continue his important work. Buddhists also believe that a person who decides to be continually reborn is known as tulku. The first tulku was Gedun Drub, who lived from 1391–1474 and the current Dalai Lama in 2020 is this great soul, Tenzin Gyatso, sitting right here now.

The Dalai Lama bowed in reverence and clasped his hands in a gesture of thanks. He was rather impressed with Deepak's knowledge. With a big smile the Dalai Lama asked Deepak Chopra; "And how would we describe *you*?"

Deepak Chopra chuckled and said, "you or anyone else can describe me as you see and sense how you feel, or think I am in the context of your own thoughts and mental constructs."

They all nodded. The ducks kept paddling and ducking up and down in the water.

Michio spoke up and shared that Deepak is the author of many books on alternative and integrative medicine starting his study at the All India Institute for medical science, before moving to Boston, where he started his career as a Doctor. Whilst practicing within the scope of Western Medicine, Deepak became very disgruntled with the approach and the results. He reflected back on his roots and the principles of Ayurvedic medicine that treated the whole person within the context of their life and the environments they lived in. As a result, he founded the Chopra center for wellbeing in Carlsbad, California in hope to bridge the gap between ancient wisdom and the modern world. Michio shared he also founded the Chopra Foundation as a way of building a happy, healthy and sustainable future together.

The Dalai Lama smiled. Deepak acknowledged that his background, life experiences and beliefs had been different to that of Michio and The Dalai

Lama, however, he believed that ultimately, they were all on earth for a united mission. They were essentially talking about the same thing in different ways.

As they sat there, Deepak noticed a bee. Out of curiosity he asked Michio and the Dalai Lama what they thought a bee would sense, see and feel about the universe. The Dalai Lama and Michio said they weren't sure how a bee would perceive their own reality, let alone the sky or stars above.

Deepak went on to explain that a honeybee experiences the world through ultraviolet radiation which is invisible to the human senses. Whereas snakes experience their reality through infrared radiation at the other end of the spectrum. If you were to observe a human being, a bee and snake in the same physical context, they are all energetically experiencing the exact same physical reality, but from the context of their own senses, their worlds would look and feel completely different, even though they are sharing the same physical space. Perhaps the only difference between human beings and other living organisms is that we have developed the ability to communicate and explain it to each other.

Deepak concluded that humans would never truly understand what a bee sees and senses. It is beyond our human sensual perception. However, when a honeybee sees a flower, it doesn't see a flower in the way humans see it, it senses the flower from a distance and tunes into its attractive abundant energy as it completes its daily activities, bouncing from one flower to the next.

If you were to describe the importance of bees it would be easy to comprehend that if humans ceased to exist, the natural world would flourish. However, if the bees ceased to exist human beings may only have four or so years left on the planet. Even the humble bee is connected to our very existence.

They all went on to discuss how bats, dolphins and even chameleons might experience the world. Bats and dolphins using ultrasound, chameleons using two eyeballs to swivel on two different axes to see. It's all beyond human comprehension yet every living being is existing in the same physical reality. hey agreed that much of reality is a mental construct of our individual conscious projection, limited and created by our human senses.

Michio Kaku's mind began to wander and he shared with his friends a childhood story directly related to this experience. He shared that when he was a child, he would sit in the Japanese Tea Gardens in San Francisco and spend hours watching the carp swimming in the small pond, oblivious to the universe above. Fascinated by their view of the world he would ask himself a question only a child could ask: what would it be like to be a carp?

He considered what a strange world it would be. He imagined that the pond would be an entire universe of its own. Taking a birds-eye view, he considered that the carp would only be able to swim forwards and backwards, and left and right. He imagined that the carp's concept of "up," would be beyond the lily pads and it would be totally alien to them.

He imagined that there would perhaps be carp scientists in the pond who would one day become curious about what lies beyond the lilypads. He imagined what would happen if he reached down from the heavens, beyond the lilypads and grabbed the carp scientist, lifting it up beyond the lilypads into the "hyper-space," before returning it back to the safety of its pond and its old reality. How would the carp scientist explain what he experienced to his carp friends that had never sensed anything beyond their pond?

He imagined that the scientist carp would return back to the pond and ramble on about the phenomenal new laws of physics: beings who could move without fins and breathe without gills. Surely, he would be labeled "a dreamer" or a "pseudoscience theorist" as he tried to communicate the ineffable to others who did not consider life beyond their pond.

The Dalai Lama and Deepak loved listening to his childhood view, and it made sense as to why he became a leading pioneer in his field. He always thought beyond the material, Earthly view.

Michio went on and shared with his friends how one time as a child he was wondering how a carp scientist would know about our human existence beyond the pond. Then it rained. He noticed the raindrops formed gentle ripples on the surface of the pond. It dawned on him. The carp may not be able to see beyond their pond but they could sense it. The ripples would create sensations in the form of vibrations and though they would be invisible (like gravity, ultraviolet light and other universal laws are to us), the vibrations in their pond could be felt.

He imagined the carp may even invent silly concepts to describe this "force." He concluded that in many ways we were like the carp, blissfully unaware of something beyond our little pond. The higher dimensions may not be seen but they can be felt in ripples and waves of gravity and light.

He shared his belief with Deepak and the Dalai Lama saying, "I lean toward the God of Einstein and Spinoza; that is, a God of harmony, simplicity and elegance, rather than a personal God who interferes in human affairs."

They all sat there present, as life's natural, organized and yet seemingly chaotic moments happened around them. Birds flying, bees buzzing, ducks swimming, trees swaying. The natural vibrations and frequencies dancing all around them.

Finally, Michio Kaku, looked to the Dalai Lama and asked what he believed. The Dalai Lama paused and took in a deep breath in as he appeared to empty his mind of any thoughts. He put his hand on his heart and said, "there is no need for temples, or complex philosophy. Our own brain, our heart is our temple: the philosophy is kindness, compassion and empathy."

Silence and awed vibrated around them. And with that they stopped talking and went back to feeding the ducks and watching the bees zoom from flower to flower.

*"The notion that science and spirituality are somehow
mutually exclusive does a disservice to both."*
— **Carl Sagan** —

DEFINE SPIRIT AS MEDICINE

Everything is connected as energy to the "Source." How you connect to this "Source" and what you call it is up to you. Our sense of connection, (spirit) with the energetic "Source" is as important for human well being as our connection to nature.

The "Source" is all around us, but it is felt and acknowledged in many different ways. Some people connect through collective rituals and ceremonies, some by looking at the stars, or planting in the soil, perhaps internal veneration or following virtuous principles for living from influential prophets, gods or deities. No matter how it's done, we all worship this "Source" as our divine benefactor, having supremacy over nature and humans. It provides a sense of peace, comfort, destiny and energy to overcome hardship.

Human beings are wired to seek meaning from life. We have been attempting to define the source of everything for as long as civilisation itself. I don't believe it's possible to capture it in a few words, but a few curious souls come quite close in my opinion. Alfred James in his blog post "Spirituality— What Does it Really Mean?" suggests it is a personal and unique quest.

"Spirituality exists within a personal, unique, unbreakable relationship between the heart (feeling) and the mind (thinking). It is an internal harmony that allows one to endure the most harrowing of circumstances. It gives us hope in a future of unknowns. Even when lacking in material possessions and physical freedoms, this relationship endures and enables its host to continue to offer compassion to others. Spirituality is an internal sanctuary, free of the rules and expectations of the physical world. It is a place where one can submit to one's mortality and rest properly, without worry, anxiety, desire and striving."[1]

This definition allows for those not considering themselves as religious, still consider themselves as spiritual. It even allows us to relabel "God" as a connection with "Mother Nature" or the "Universal Source," or some form of deep knowing. From here our spiritual connection becomes easier to understand and encompasses many different cultures and thoughts processes. However, ultimately, how you define and marinate yourself in Spirit is your business only. As Mother Teresa was attributed as saying, "In the final analysis, it's just between you and God."

Historically, ancient quests for understanding "Spirit" became known as religions, a system to worship and organize our collection of beliefs, cultural nuances and worldviews that relate humanity to an order of existence. There are thousands of religions even to this day. They use narratives, symbols, and sacred histories that are intended to explain the meaning of life and its universal origin. From their beliefs about the cosmos and human nature, people derive morality, ethics, religious laws or a preferred lifestyle from their chosen faith or universal view.

It is contrary to think we are all human with the same physical realities of earth, sun and sky, yet our belief systems about creation, how we should live our lives and what happens after we die, all manifest so differently. These beliefs will continue to adapt and evolve along with humanity as we become ever more conscious and conscientious beings. There are millions of unique beliefs about this subject all operating within the one Earth.

As human beings we will still continue to search for meaning within the three mental constructs that overarch virtually all "religions"—where we came from, why we are here and what happens after we die. This can be expressed in the essence of, "zero–one–infinity."

ZERO
Creation from nothing—How did we end up on this third rock from the sun?

ONE
Connection and meaning—How is everything interconnected as one?

INFINITY
Redistribution to everything—What happens when we die? Elementally, biologically, consciously and soulfully?

For some people, they no longer look to any "source" for guidance or comfort, some don't believe in an omniscient energy at all. I would say to them, if their deep internal compass intuits that there is no source, then who am I to tell them otherwise? Except perhaps I would point them to the benefits of operating in their highest energetic human vibration anyway, good thoughts, good feelings and good relationships are all critical.

If they believe that this is all there is and ever will be, I'm sure they would want to still create the best life possible for themselves! Makes sense, right?

Love, peace and unity are the highest energetic human vibrations. They are the "Source." So whether you call it God, emptiness, nothing, everything or Fred—love, peace and unity are both Divine and human qualities. You can be an atheist and still be an incredible loving and caring person.

Perhaps this is why Lao Tzu's Tao Te Ching is so potent. He begins by reminding us there are no names that can reach "what is."

> *"The Tao that can be told is not the eternal Tao.*
> *The name that can be named is not the eternal name.*
> *The nameless is the beginning of heaven and earth.*
> *The named is the mother of ten thousand things.*
> *Ever desireless, one can see the mystery.*
> *Ever desiring, one can see the manifestations."* [2]
> **— Lao Tzu, Tao Te Ching —**

Life is cyclical and in a constant state of change. We just give it meaning and decide to resist change or find energetic flow in the natural chaos and flux of life. Western cultures have become fixated on celebrating our births (birthdays), but ultimately fearing death as an ultimate end point. What if these mental constructs for life were missing something that would permit a sense of inner peace in all of us? Life is cyclical and infinite.

For me, the Dalai Lama exemplifies the simplicity of this conversation about Spirit as medicine. *"This is my simple religion, there is no need for temples of complex philosophy, our own brain, our own heart is our temple. My philosophy is kindness."*[3]

On creationism:
"However the tea is prepared, the primary ingredient is always water. While we can live with out tea, we can't live with out water. Likewise we are born free of religion, but we are not born free of the need for love and compassion."[4]

On life:
"All religions carry the same basic messages, that is love, forgiveness and compassion. Importantly this should be part of our daily lives."[5]

On death:
"There is no way to escape death, it is just like trying to escape by four great mountains touching sky. There is no escape from these four mountains of birth, old age, sickness and death."[6]

Coming to terms with the fact that one day we will all take our last breath is a powerful insight too. The Dalai Lama shares how to use these insights to live a virtuous life:
"We cannot hope to die peacefully if our lives have been full of violence, or if our minds have mostly been agitated by emotions like anger, attachment, or fear. So if

we wish to die well, we must learn how to live well: Hoping for a peaceful death, we must cultivate peace in our mind, and in our way of life."[7]

LIVE WELL TO DIE WELL

We must learn to live well in order to die well.

What makes you feel "In Spirit?"—"inspired" by life. Is it music or dance that makes you feel most alive inside? Is it serving others and helping out in some special way? Is it through business or mentoring? Do you love meditating or walking in nature?

What is your Soulfood? What makes your soul sing? What inspires you from the inside? What helps you live in a "good spirit"?

List 3 things that makes your spirit sing.

1. ....

2. ....

3. ....

How do you feel connected to "Source" to Universal Intelligence? List three ways that help you feel connected to your source. Is it prayer, mediation, loving your children, sitting in silence, worship, singing, being at the ocean?

List 3 ways you feel connected.

1. ....

2. ....

3. ....

LEGACY

Mahatma Gandhi said, "My life is my message." Is your life your message?

Do you have a legacy that you would like to leave? Make it real and write it down here.

....

....

....

....

....

....

....

....

....

....

ENERGY MEDICINE

"If you want to find the secrets of the universe, think in terms of energy, frequency and vibration."
— **Nikola Tesla** —

ENERGY FLOW

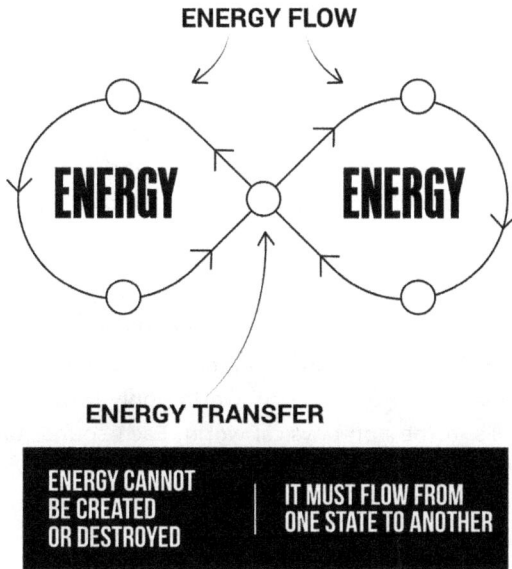

ENERGY TRANSFER

ENERGY CANNOT BE CREATED OR DESTROYED	IT MUST FLOW FROM ONE STATE TO ANOTHER

EVERYTHING IS ENERGY

The whole Universe from the stars in the sky to the atoms that create them, including the world we live on and the bodies we dwell in, is made up of this universal energy at the most fundamental level. Everything is energy originating from "the source," meaning we can tune into the frequency of this energy and channel it into our human vessel to raise our vibration.

We can raise our vibration by tuning into the natural world around us. We can transfer energy from the natural world into our own human vessel through the sun, clean air, clean water and high-density fuel based in plants. We can transfer energy between each other through the environments we create for each other.

It is up to us to sustain and maintain the fine balance so that future generations get the opportunity to experience the gift we are lucky to have. To do this, it's important to familiarize yourself with the 12 Universal Laws of Energy.

12 UNIVERSAL ENERGETIC LAWS

You may have read books about the law of attraction, theories of relativity or cultural concepts like Karma. All of these are constructs, refering to 12 universal laws of energy: the ways in which energy is transferred, shared and circulated from one place to another. Let's explore them together.

1. THE LAW OF ONENESS

Separation is an illusion that we as human beings constructed when we created borders, ethnicity and nations. Oneness helps us to understand that we live in a world where everything is connected to everything else. Everything we do, say, think and believe affects others and the universe around us. Remember that we all come from the same divine source.

2. THE LAW OF VIBRATION

Be the vibe and energy that you wish to see in the world. This Law states that everything in the universe vibrates and moves in circular patterns. The same principles of vibration in the physical world apply to our thoughts, feelings, desires, and wills in the non-physical world. Each sound, thing, and thought has its own vibrational frequency, unique unto itself. Notice how you feel when someone smiles at you, or when you put your favorite song on.

3. THE LAW OF ACTION

Action negates negative emotion. This Law must be applied in order to manifest things and outcomes. Therefore, we must engage in actions that support our thoughts, dreams, emotions and words. Aligned action with consistency is all we need to consciously engineer anything into reality. Believe that anything is possible and find stories that help you believe it to be true.

4. THE LAW OF CORRESPONDENCE

"As above, so below." This Law states that the principles or laws of physics that explain the physical world: energy, light, vibration, and motion, have their corresponding principles in the non-physical realms. Einstein tried to create an equation that explained everything in the universe but the universe cannot be explained with the limited senses and consciousness that we have. Look up at the stars tonight, remembering that every star is a universe just like ours, with planets, and maybe even life.

5. THE LAW OF CAUSE AND EFFECT

Have you ever experienced the unexplainable synchronicities in your life? Opportunities in plain sight, conversations that opened doors you never knew existed? This Law states that nothing happens by chance or outside the Universal Laws. Every action has a reaction or consequence and we essentially "reap what we have sown." If you are attracting a lot of scarcity, pain and low-vibing thoughts. Then go inwards, change your own vibe, heal past traumas, create a new narrative for your life that you believe to be true deep down. Treat people the way you wish to be treated and watch the universe conspire in your favor.

6. THE LAW OF COMPENSATION (ABUNDANCE)

Abundance is so much more than money and success. This is the Law of Cause and Effect applied to blessings and abundance that are provided for us. The visible effects of our deeds are given to us in gifts, money, inheritances, friendships, and unexpected blessings.

7. THE LAW OF ATTRACTION

Ultimately we attract what and who we are. This Law demonstrates how the quality and vibration of our thoughts, feelings, unconscious and conscious energies create the things, events, and people that come into our lives. Like attracts like. Negative energies attract negativity and positive energies attract positivity. Take stock of your energy, thoughts, feelings, health, relationships, bank account, proximity and environment to see what you are currently attracting into your life. At any point in your life, you can choose and act differently.

8. THE LAW OF PERPETUAL TRANSMUTATION OF ENERGY

Remember that energy cannot be created or destroyed, simply transferred from one state to another. We can even transfer/receive energy to other people and nature. Every time we drink water, eat food and breathe, we are tuning into nature's abundance. This Law suggests that all persons have within them the power to change the conditions in their lives. Higher vibrations consume and transform lower ones; thus, each of us can change the energies in our lives by understanding the Universal Laws and applying the principles in a way to effect change. Growth is a natural process in life, welcome it, receive it and share it back with the world.

9. THE LAW OF RELATIVITY

Accepting the full spectrum of the human experience allows us to welcome pain, pleasure and bliss as a natural part of life. Pain can be the greatest motivator when we learn the lesson gain gives us. This Law states that each person will receive a series of challenges or life lessons and we must consider each of these tests as a message to remain connected to our hearts when problems arise. This Law also teaches us to compare our problems to others' problems and put everything into perspective. No matter how bad we perceive our situation to be, there is always someone who is in a worse position. It is all relative. Remember, it only takes 10 seconds of courage to act and rise above and change your internal narrative.

10. THE LAW OF POLARITY

This Law states that everything is on a continuum and has an opposite. We can suppress and transform undesirable thoughts by concentrating on the opposite pole. You may know of people that have experienced the depths of pain, yet still maintain a positive mindset and choose to see the beauty in every moment. It's not that they ignore or suppress their feelings. They feel it all, more than most. Choose to see and think with compassion and empathy.

11. THE LAW OF RHYTHM

Have you ever experienced the flow state? This Law states that everything vibrates and moves to certain rhythms. These rhythms establish seasons, cycles, stages of development, and patterns. Each cycle reflects the regularity of the universe. Masters know how to rise above negative parts of a cycle by never getting too excited or allowing negative things to penetrate their consciousness. You can find your own rhythm by mastering your morning rituals and tuning into the flow of abundance that is present.

12. THE LAW OF GENDER

It is more than male, female or LBGTQI. It is energetic. This final Law states that everything has its masculine (yang) and feminine (yin) principles, and that these are the basis for all creation. Balancing the masculine and feminine energies allows us to be whole and well-balanced. We can each operate from a healthy masculine and feminine energy or an unhealthy one. I'm sure you have met people that have a beautiful sense of compassion, empathy and unconditional love, yet they are bad ass manifestors that can consciously engineer anything into reality. They understand the meaning of WE, not just ME.

You might also notice how these laws of energy combines elements of religion, cultural beliefs, science and even quantum physics and beyond. However, never forget the simplicity. A smile, a hug, a nice gesture or time spent in nature might be all you need to tune into these universal laws.

RECHARGING YOUR ENERGY

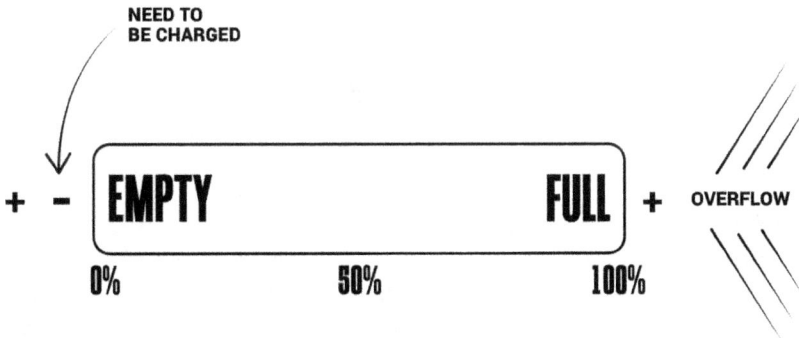

NEED TO BE CHARGED

+ − **EMPTY** **FULL** + OVERFLOW

0%   50%   100%

Have you ever noticed that you might be in an energetic funk? How many times have you wished you could just shake it all off and come back to your highest vibration?

Even if we are living our best life or in our best physical state of being, we can still be mentally or emotionally in an energetic funk. Here are some things we can do to change state. It seems contradictory, but they hold great wisdom.

1. CHANGE YOUR ENVIRONMENT
Environment is stronger than the greatest willpower. Immerse yourself in nourishing environments and transfer the energy from these environments into your own being.

2. SOCIALLY CONNECT
It is probably the last thing you feel like doing in this state. You may even want to isolate yourself from the world. However, connecting with the right people, having fun and keeping it simple can shift your states with ease and simplicity.

3. MOVE YOUR PHYSICAL BODY
Poor physiology reinforces negative feelings. Tony Robbins is well-known for saying, "Motion creates emotion." Change your physiology and your mental state changes automatically. It may sound simple but good physiology

leads to better emotions. This is one easy but effective way to get out of a mental funk. Do something physical like surfing, or an activity you love. Nine times out of ten, you'll feel better.

4. LIVE IN THE PRESENT

One reason we can feel stuck in a rut is because we continually dwell on the past or focus too much on the future. Continual over-thinking about either one isn't productive because when we do this too much, the present moment gets overlooked, and that's the one moment we actually have. The present moment is the only moment we have any control over. Use it well.

HOW TO LIVE IN A HIGH VIBRATION
1. CONNECTION—PEOPLE

Have you ever met someone and straight away you feel better?

Consider what would happen if you spent the majority of your time around people like this. Their thoughts, stories and conversations are more aligned with courageous inspiration, willingness, acceptance, reason, unconditional love, joy, peace, and even enlightenment.

On the flipside, have you ever met someone and you walk away from feeling energetically drained? From how they show up, to what they talk about, or the stories they tell. We need to be mindful of the people we choose to connect with; as Jim Rohn suggests, we are the sum of the five people we spend the most time with.

2. CONNECTION—ENVIRONMENTS

Have you ever been in an environment, either natural, like a waterfall, or a social environment, like a music festival, where the energy felt contagious? One might ground and recharge you, the other might get your feet and every part of your body moving.

On the flipside, have you been in environments where the vibration feels really low, or it just doesn't feel right? Perhaps it's the people, or perhaps it's a work environment in which no one actually wants to be in. Again, this vibration can become contagious.

You have no obligation to be in low vibration environments or continue low vibration connections.

3. CONNECTION—NATURE & FOOD

Consider how you feel energetically after eating and consuming certain foods. Does it make you feel more energized or does it make you feel drained and tired?

Have you ever spent a day or a week consuming low vibration, high-calorie food that may taste really good, but lacks the nutritional energy to give you what you need? Maybe it's fast food or highly processed "food-like" substances. Also consider how you might feel after a day or week of consuming alcohol and other fake sugary drinks. Initially there might be a spark in energy, but notice how you feel later in the day, or the following morning.

Compare this to how you feel when you might take a month or more off of consuming any low vibration foods or drinks and you shift your energy to high vibration plants, water and anything else that energetically feeds your atoms and cellular pathways on every level. Your digestive system is functioning optimally and you're saturating your body with nutrients. Your system feels as though it has flicked a switch; and your whole body lights up. If you have seen the movie *Limitless* it would be akin to showing up, feeling, thinking and operating from this vibration every day.

4. RAISING YOUR VIBRATION: AN INSIDE-OUT APPROACH

Change your energy, vibration and frequency internally, and inquire within, before you start trying to change the external reality. It has been said over and over that our external reality is simply a reflection of our internal world. Energy is transformed from one state to another, so make sure you are finding the high-vibe food sources and getting that into your system daily. Keep your body away from harm, and your digestive and immune systems will keep the body functioning optimally from the inside-out.

It is easier to think more positively if we feel better internally.

This is the reason why committing to your health and wellbeing is the best thing you could ever do. How you wake up tomorrow is a reflection of the choices you made 12 months ago, not last week. The choices you make tomorrow will start a positive shift towards living as your ideal self in 12 months' time. Be the change.

Embody and be it in your daily actions and rituals. Like yoga, you can practice the Asanas on the yoga mat and feel good in that environment, but how do you apply these practices off the mat?

5. RAISING THE COLLECTIVE VIBRATION

How can we raise our collective vibration towards a higher collective frequency of thought; love, peace or unity? In the same way sporting events can mobilize millions of people to support how a piece of leather is kicked or thrown with emotional ferocity, we could mobilize the world towards a higher collective vibration. The world game.

Paraphrasing Martin Luther King Jr.—"Those who love peace, connection and unity must learn to organize as effectively as those who love war, disconnection and isolation."

How do we change the world? By taking a stand for compassion, one person at a time. It only takes one person to inspire others and create widespread change.

In 2015 a Global Meditation event set the Guinness World Record for the largest online meditation gathering in history, where more than 140,000 people from nearly every country in the world came together with Deepak and meditated with one powerful shared intention—to cultivate peace.

The impact was immediate and widespread. Families came together to meditate for the very first time. Neighbors became friends as they gathered in each other's homes. Yoga studios became true community centers, as people all over the world came together and took a stand for peace. SelfCare is a journey of choices. If you can make high-vibrational choices in low-vibrational environments, then making better choices in nourishing environments will be a lot easier. Right now, there is both peace and war existing in the world at the same time. Whilst you experience pleasure someone else is experiencing heart-wrenching pain. Self-care like yoga, becomes a system for reacting and making better choices in the context of any environment or emotional event. Even when certain factors are beyond our control, we still get to choose how we react in any moment.

What takes you into a LOW vibration? Write 5 things that lower your vibration.

1. ....

2. ....

3. ....

4. ....

5. ....

What keeps you in a HIGH vibration? Write 5 things that raise your vibration

1. ....

2. ....

3. ....

4. ....

5. ....

Think about daily practices, maybe it's breath work, yoga, meditation or even a sexual connection with a partner.

SPIRIT IS MEDICINE PRESCRIPTION

» Find time to connect to your Spirit/Soul in whatever way you define it and however feels right for you.

» Make time to experience what makes your soul sing, frequently. And do that more.

» Can you feel or experience "universal ripples" outside of your visual perception? Can you find way to "hear" and be "in tune" with the larger cosmos and beyond?

» Meditate, pray, spend time in nature—whatever feels right for you.

» SHARE one SPIRITUAL practice that connects to the "source" each day

To learn more about this medicine, or to contribute to this medicine, visit **selfcare.global/spirit**. Here you will find blogs, videos and podcasts.

Selfcare.global/spirit

NOTABLE EXPERTS IN THIS CHAPTER:
Michio Kaku, Deepak Chopra, Dalai Lama, Carl Sagan, Mother Teresa, Lao Tzu, Mahatma Gandhi, Nikola Tesla, Tony Robbins, Martin Luther King Jr, Indigenous elders.

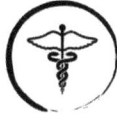

11

MODERN IS MEDICINE

"The person who relies on non-natural medicine
must recover twice; once from the disease and
once from the synthetic medicine."
— William Osler —

THE FISHERMAN AND THE FISHMONGER[1]

Two men make their living from the ocean. The fisherman sails the sea, feeling the currents rolling beneath him, the temperature of the water, and the agitation of the choppy waves. Gradually he learns the behaviors and peculiarities of his catch. Together the fisherman and the fish share a sensory, intrinsic relationship because they experience the same home. So in tune is he to the fishes' vivacity, the fisherman knows whatever disturbs the fishes' plight will ultimately disturb his too.

The fishmonger is the fisherman's closest ally but he lives far removed from the fisherman's boat bobbing amongst the waves. His is a cold, unemotional environment smelling of chemical disinfectant while he wears a thick smock as a shield and welds sharp knives. His forte is the understanding of fish anatomy in order to dismember one efficiently and he excels at this task. The fish he knows are dead or dying and he sees no point in considering the once vibrant elements of their lives.

The original metaphor (from which I have adapted) was written by Dr Emil Kim and reflects his awakening to the intuitive nature of eastern medicine. Where once he was ruled by intellect only, he experienced a shift that impelled him to surrender and simply feel. Finally he sensed the energy waiting within, and his transformation from faceless fishmonger to instinctive fisherman began. He reveals, *"This didn't happen through my academic studies, this occurred for me first on my yoga mat; from this space it spread outward into everything."*[2]

So what is the difference between our fisherman of the East and our fishmonger of the West? Dr Kim says simply that it is the environment in which they work, "one understands it, the other lives it."[3] One treats the disease; the other treats the person and understands their environments. I am compelled to wonder if we cannot do both?!

From its stronghold of the last few centuries, many people are reassessing the dominance of modern western medicine as the world becomes more conscious of ancient wisdom and the interconnectedness of all things, especially with nature.

MODERN MEDICINE HAS ITS PLACE WHEN USED IN THE RIGHT WAY

Modern medicine is ideal in order to support and assist the body's natural healing mechanisms, rather than trying to replace them. With the right approach, modern medicine can intervene to support our natural healing designs. Modern medicine creates sophisticated tools from natural elements to conduct complex surgeries, to test for underlying causes in dis-ease and dys-function.

Ideally modern medicine could be a tool to help us stay healthy and to prevent us from moving down the health spectrum. Also in times of sudden need when accidents and acute trauma occur. Modern medicine can be used to intervene and support the changing conditions of bones, ligaments, tendons and all other biological systems.

Modern medicine should not replace natural healing mechanisms, it should support and enhance. The future of healing is human and nature centric in its approach, integrated and holistic.

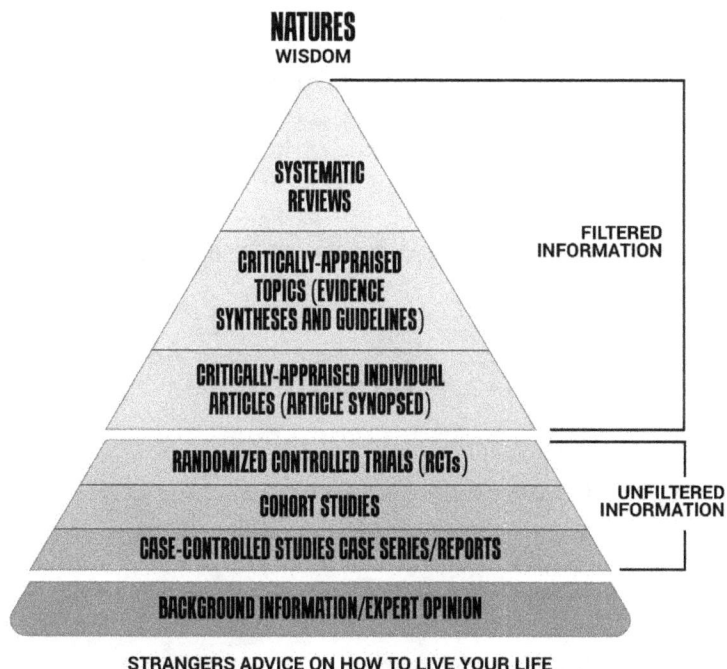

NATURES
WISDOM

SYSTEMATIC
REVIEWS

CRITICALLY-APPRAISED
TOPICS (EVIDENCE
SYNTHESES AND GUIDELINES)

CRITICALLY-APPRAISED INDIVIDUAL
ARTICLES (ARTICLE SYNOPSED)

FILTERED
INFORMATION

RANDOMIZED CONTROLLED TRIALS (RCTs)

COHORT STUDIES

CASE-CONTROLLED STUDIES CASE SERIES/REPORTS

UNFILTERED
INFORMATION

BACKGROUND INFORMATION/EXPERT OPINION

STRANGERS ADVICE ON HOW TO LIVE YOUR LIFE

DEFINE MODERN MEDICINE

Modern medicine is a system in which medical doctors are the "gate-keepers" and other healthcare professionals (such as nurses, pharmacists, and therapists) treat symptoms and diseases using drugs, radiation, surgery or other interventions based on the best available scientific evidence. This approach can also be called allopathic medicine, biomedicine, conventional medicine, mainstream medicine and orthodox medicine.

So is modern medicine making progress in tackling the common health challenges of the 21st century? Well, it depends on what we use as the yardstick.

If we measured:

- The absence of chronic disease—then we find that 1 in 2 people are currently living with a chronic preventable disease and 7 in 10 will have their quality and length of life reduced because of this same burden.
- Longevity and the prevalence of Bluezone communities. Only seven such communities in the world stand out as having truly embodied longevity and quality of living for all in their community, whilst remaining connected to the natural environments they live in.
- Length of life—We would find that globally we have improved our global average to 72 however there are huge locational discrepancies. Some communities' life expectancy is only in the 50's.

- Quality of life—Bhutan may be one of the only countries with the right approach, measuring gross domestic happiness over productivity.
- Life lived free of disability and restriction (DALY'S)—As mentioned previously, our length of life is increasing, it's questionable whether our quality of life is better than our grandparents. What is clear is that 1 in 2 people are living into their old age restricted by one or more chronic and preventable diseases. With an increasing burden. Perhaps the amount of days we live free of disease and restriction over the age of 50 is a better measure for us to consider?

MODERNIZATION OF MEDICINE

Dr Margaret Chan is Director-General of the World Health Organization; in her address at the International Conference on the Modernization of Traditional Chinese Medicine in 2016[4] she explained why we need a modernization of medicine, integrating the best of ancient philosophies such as Chinese medicine with the technological advances of modern science.

I will share some of her insights below.

- **Unsustainable health development**

  When we take a step back and look at our human development as individuals, communities and populations, there is an illusion that we are getting healthier and living longer. Yes, as a whole, our average life expectancy has increased over the centuries. Today the average life expectancy for a human born today is 71.2 years, which gives that child 4,365,984 hours to live, love, laugh, grow and live their own legacy. However, it would be incorrect to say that this is due to modernization of medicine. Hospitals, medication, educated health consultants and specialists have played an amazing role in saving lives. However, the truth is that our health outcomes have improved due to the increased access and distribution of resources globally. This has empowered many children to have access to resources that meet their basic human needs for survival; food, water, safety, security, shelter and connection.

  The challenge today is the polarity and disconnection we face as humanity. Yes, we can send people to outer space, spending trillions of dollars innovating childhood dreams into reality. Yes, I see the benefit for humanity. I too imagine if every child could see the earth from outer space. Even if we just leveraged technology and virtual reality, their young brains would gain the perspective they need. They would see no borders, race, gender or religion; just a beautiful blue planet that is nourishing and sustaining us all. That perspective would expand every young mind to dimensions from which they could never return, reminding them of our oneness and connection with everything.

However, whilst the richest people in the world build spaceships for the few, there are 1 billion people that will go to bed hungry tonight. Hundreds of millions of people were pushed into extreme poverty during the pandemic. The number is set to rise to 750 million by 2021.[5] It is common knowledge that over 170 billion dollars allocated over 20 years towards building nourishing environments, giving access to basic human needs, and creating empowering systems can lift over 15% of the world's population to new heights.[6]

I can't understand how we can spend trillions of dollars on the few, whilst the many go to bed hungry at night. If we have the technology, resources and innovations to reach space, then surely we have the solutions to help create a rising tide that lifts all the boats, not just some. I imagine that there is a young child in a village somewhere in the world that has the drive, passion and ambition that could pivot this world in a new direction. Like the true story of young William Kamkwamba from Malawi, who at age 14, hand-built a windmill out of a bicycle generator and scraps of metal to create a windmill that could generate power and run water pumps and electricity to help his poverty-stricken family. A movie *The Boy Who Harnessed the Wind* was made about his struggles and successes.

The rising cost of passive medication and interventions, aging populations, industrialized toxic environments and lifestyles, chronic stress, and living in scarcity is the real challenge. Self-care, empowering positively geared systems, healthy living environments, and equal access to resources and care is the solution we need to ensure sustainable health and the enduring wellbeing of all people. We need to go first, look after our front doorstep, serve from overflow and build enabling communities and environments that promote longevity.

We already have a working concept available right now in the Blue Zone societies.

- **Integrating ancient practices and medicine with a modern world**
Traditional Chinese Medicine and Indian Ayurvedic medicine as an example, have thousands of years of practice compared to only hundreds of years of modern medicine. These more traditional approaches treat the whole person in the context of their life cycle and environment. They aim to activate the bodies innate wisdom for healing and regeneration, whilst "reminding them" that they have never needed to be fixed. As Hippocrates was attributed as saying—"It is more important to know what sort of person has a disease than to know what sort of disease a person has."

Today we have created a situation where traditional medicine meets a perceived need, yet earns a bad name at the same time. More and more people are losing trust in modern medicine, spending money with complementary, alternative, and traditional medicine approaches. Many are finding the solutions they seek, which is what we should focus on. Solutions, rather than the approach alone.

Modern health care is seen to be passive, over-medicalized and over-specialized, with the patient treated like a collection of specialized body-parts on an assembly line, instead of a whole person. People want more control over what is done to their bodies. They want to regulate their own health with guided support. We need a balance of active empowerment through self-care practices, community, and building healthy environments—integrated with the wonderland and innovations of modern medicine.

In other words, making *self-care* the foundation for modern healthcare, founded in ancient wisdom and integrated with modern science and technology.

- **Science is often mistrusted**
Dr Margaret Chan shares that this can be seen today more than ever: "the movement of vaccine refusal, science is often mistrusted, sometimes even vilified. Rumors spread via social media can carry more weight than hundreds of well-designed, peer-reviewed research studies. People are suspicious that powerful new drugs may have side-effects that have either not yet been detected or were never honestly disclosed."[7]

Why the lack of trust?

Dr Margaret Chan shares: "Some analysts attribute this dissatisfaction and mistrust to the system, the infrastructure, the training, incentives, and the orientation of modern medical care. The public feel like the person has been forgotten and healthcare has become a business."[8]

Imagine a system where those seeking solutions, get access to service providers who only have less than 20 minutes to listen, understand, diagnose and provide a solution for health challenges than someone who may have had for months, years and decades. The challenge with a system like this is that the service provider has a limited ability to "seek to understand." To ensure the patient feels validated, they end up prescribing a band-aid solution, ordering an expensive investigation that may not be necessary, and sending them down a path of confusion as they gather more labels and diagnoses without a solution. This is the modern approach, and is vastly different to the traditional medicine approach that treats the person as whole, within the context of their environment, community and lifestyle. Ordering expensive investigations only if necessary or indicated.

THE RISE IN INTEGRATED PRACTITIONERS
Functional, lifestyle-based, integrated, holistic and medical practitioners are becoming more common. They are training in a specific field of expertise to begin with, and over time are learning to integrate foundational tools into their tool belt, like yoga, nutrition, mind and lifestyle-based therapies, in order to guide people up the health spectrum towards optimal wellbeing, and into lifestyles that help sustain longevity.

These practitioners are also learning to work as collaborative allied teams who eventually become redundant as people within each community become empowered to maintain their own health and wellbeing, supported by the community. We need to take ownership of our own self-care and promote self-governance within our own communities.

EVIDENCE-BASED MEDICINE
Evidence-based medicine (EBM) is, "the conscientious, explicit, judicious and reasonable use of modern, best evidence in making decisions about the care of individual patients."[9]

However it has its limitations. You may recall from an earlier chapter that it was only in 2012 that scientists declared nonhuman animals are conscious![10] This is where science understanding human consciousness is limited. We've all shared a moment of connection with at least one other living animal! Before 2012 when science agreed and told us what we already innately knew and felt to be true! Imagine if we waited on science to rationally confirm what nature has known to be true for millennia? We need to acknowledge that nature is already smarter than us.

There is no such thing as "the science." It is not absolute. Science evolves and adapts as we evolve and adapt to make meaning of the world we live in. Science is about curiosity and exploration with the limited senses and consciousness that we as human beings use to create mental constructs for what has always been. We are meaning-making machines who love to think in terms of linear systems, i.e., "This means that"—whilst remaining willfully ignorant and unconsciously aware of the whole. We are becoming experts at using our pride and ego to argue our differences, polarize conversations, reinforce our beliefs and therefore our own reality, without allowing it to be challenged. Rather than reminding ourselves that we all share the same planet, we all come from the same source and have never been separate from each other, the natural world, and everything else that co-exists here and above.

Science is testing, measuring, proving, disproving. It is *not* finite. It is human curiosity. How can you compare A to B without being mindful of the whole? E.g., Is a biotech man-made (patented—not from nature) vaccine better than natural immunity for long term health and longevity? How can we speak with certainty of the unknown, when the smartest virologists who made it their life's work openly admit that we understand less than 1% of all viral diversity, let alone their implications on human health and wellbeing.

There are 10 million viruses, 1 million bacteria and thousands of protozoans/ algae in just one drop of seawater. According to an outdated germ theory that teaches us to fear the unknown, does that mean we should fear the ocean, when "vitamin sea and sunshine" always makes us feel better, irrespective of the science?

How can we dismiss our bodies' innate wisdom, our thoughts, our emotions and the environments that sustain us? Or the 50-million cells that regenerate you as you read this sentence without conscious attention?

The placebo effect, another "mental construct" created by human beings no smarter than you or I, is scientific proof that we have the ability to heal ourselves. Our thoughts are energy, chemical reactions and intentions for our actions. If we can guide our beliefs, we can change our biology. If we can guide our thoughts, we can change our daily actions, rituals and behaviors. It then holds true that we become what we most think about, we attract what we feel, and we can create and consciously engineer anything we can imagine in our mind. What an amazing thought. It is the reason why leading pain scientists like Dr David Butler have shown that pain is an output of the brain, not an input.[11] Which is the reason why all experience it differently; depending on past experiences, what we think and believe, neural sensitivity and our overall sensitivity.

Look up at the stars tonight and stay curious; those glittering stars are universes just like ours. Stay curious and be open to being evidence-based, but solution-focused. If we focus on the end in mind, we will stop arguing about differences in opinion, science and belief—until someone finds the path of least resistance and a solution for all.

Researchers from the Faculty of Medicine at the University of Sarajevo studied the approaches and challenges and evidence-based medicine, they wrote:

EBM is not a "cookbook" with "how to" recipes, but its application brings cost-effective and better health care. The key difference between evidence-based medicine and traditional medicine is not that EBM considers the evidence while the latter does not. Both take evidence into account; however, EBM demands better evidence than has traditionally been used. One of the greatest achievements of evidence-based medicine has been the development of systematic reviews and meta-analyzes, methods by which researchers identify multiple studies on a topic, separate the best ones and then critically analyze them to come up with a summary of the best available evidence.[12]

The researchers suggest that EBM-orientated clinicians of the future have three specific tasks:

1. To **APPLY** knowledge and use best evidence summaries in clinical practice to help empower, ignite and activate the bodies natural healing mechanisms with their guided support towards harmony.

2. To **HELP** develop and update selected systematic reviews or evidence-based guidelines in their area of expertise; 12 areas of medicine, or specialty. Handing over this wisdom to future generations.
3. To **ENROLL** patients in studies of treatment, diagnosis and prognosis on which medical practice is based.

Perhaps we can integrate the best evidence, taking into account the human within the context of their environment and whilst treating the human as a whole. Treat the person and treat the specific issue.

> *"The cure of many diseases is unknown to physicians...because they are ignorant of the whole. For the part can never be well unless the whole is well."*
> *— Plato —*

A HUMAN AND NATURE CENTRIC APPROACH

Traditional Chinese Medicine (TCM) is rooted in the ancient philosophy of Taoism and dates back more than 2,500 years. Traditional systems of medicine also exist in other East and South Asian countries, including Japan (where the traditional herbal medicine is called Kampo) and Korea.

There are 4 underlying beliefs of TCM.

- **One**—The human body is a miniature version of the larger, surrounding universe.
- **Duality**—Harmony between two opposing yet complementary forces, called yin and yang, supports health, and disease results from an imbalance between these forces. Modern medicine calls this "homeostasis."
- **Cyclical**—Five cyclical elements—fire, earth, wood, metal, and water—symbolically they represent all phenomena, including the stages of human life, and explain the functioning of the body and how it changes over the lifespan and even during disease.
- **Energy**—Qi is a vital energy force that flows through the body and performs multiple functions in maintaining health.

The big question is does TCM work?

For most conditions, there is not enough rigorous scientific evidence to know whether TCM methods work for the conditions for which they are used.[13] How do we measure energy and the interconnectedness of everything as one, within a cyclical existence that is constantly in a state of change?

In spite of the widespread use of TCM in China and its use in the West, rigorous scientific evidence of its effectiveness is limited. TCM can be difficult for researchers to study because it's treatments are often complex and are based on ideas very different from those of modern Western medicine.

Western Doctors like Elizabeth Cohen, Erika Schwartz and Leana Wen have begun to appreciate traditional medicine and how doctors can avoid misdiagnoses, empower their patients and really listen to them Here are some lessons from Eastern practices that are applicable to our Western medical practice:

- Nature is our primary life support system. Traditional Chinese medicine and other philosophies understand that the natural world was here long before humans. Nature and our bodies wisdom is not an alternative, but our primary medicine. The role of health professionals, coaches and healers is to ignite, enable and support these innate mechanisms, not to replace them.

- Listen, really listen to the person. Many traditional Chinese medical professionals will actively listen to the person before measuring vital signs with expensive technological devices. They will become curious and ask about your lifestyle, your relationships, your work, stress, finances and anything that might point towards the origin of the disharmony. Many traditional Chinese medicine practitioners have even been known to diagnose complex conditions just by observing the person as they walk into the room. The color of their eyes, their weight, the black bags under their eyes, their skin and many other signals that can share information and reveal the state of their internal organs symptoms.

- Treat the whole person in the context of their life. Not just the individual parts. A big difference between western and eastern medicine is that western medicine treats people as organs. Eastern medicine treats people as a whole. As mentioned above, traditional medicine practitioners will ask about family, food and life stressors and then treat these underlying causes by offering support and guidance in family planning, food practices, and even managing work, finances and debt. It could even go as far as helping clients choose schools for their child. This is truly "whole person" care! A recent Netflix show *New Amsterdam* shines the light on how we can evolve modern practice; prescribing people nature, connection and even safe home environments, not just medication.

- Health is not just about disease, but also about wellbeing. It is about living in a state of harmony internally in your cells and externally in the environments we choose to live in. There is a term in Chinese that does not have its exact equivalent in English which means "tune-up to remain in balance," it refers to maintaining and promoting wellness. Many choose to see a TCM doctor not because they are ill, but because they want to stay well. Imagine seeing a health professional in order to stay well, rather than waiting until you're in a state of dysfunction, dis-ease and disharmony. We do it with our cars and businesses, so what not with our human bodies and minds?

- Evidence is in the eyes of the beholder. Modern medicine is very new and is largely based on "evidence-based science." However curious souls like Carl Sagan and others that look at the stars realize that "absence of evidence is not evidence of absence." Biocentrism is a limited human construct that thinks we are the center of the universe, rather than a small, yet integral part of the whole. Perhaps this underlying belief drives our desire to fix, rather than to connect, empower and enable healthy people through healthy environments and supportive communities. At university evidence-based medicine was the mantra in my western medical training, so I was highly skeptical of the anecdotes I heard. But then I met so many patients who said that they were able to find a solution from Eastern methodologies where Western allopathic treatments had failed them. Is there a placebo effect? Of course. Is research important? Of course. But research is done on populations, and our treatment should focused on individuals within the context of their lives. However, I have learned that even with the same diagnosis, no two patients are treated in the same way. All in all, there is more evidence for eastern types of medicine. They have four to five thousand years of experience, which must count for something.
- Community, community, community. We were never designed to survive alone. All evidence and wisdom shines light on fact that it takes a community to raise a child, a community to heal the sick and a community to thrive together.

THE FUTURE IS AN INTEGRATED APPROACH

Can we merge ancient wisdom with modern medicine by taking the best of all our approaches, whilst leaving out the ineffective approaches and philosophies?

The World Health Organization looked at this topic at a keynote address at the International Conference on the Modernization of Traditional Chinese Medicine.

Traditional medicine has many critics. Their criticisms must also be addressed if traditional medicine is to perform a legitimate role as an integrated part of a health system. Some critics dismiss the entirety of this ancient art as nothing but pseudoscience, or "snake oil" medicine. They argue that the differences between East and West can never be reconciled.

They point to the difficulty of standardized quality control, especially since the chemical composition of a plant species can vary according to where it was grown and in what type of soil, and when and how it was harvested.[14]

Can we be specific in a non-specific sense?

Any dysfunction or disease has two parts in terms of appearance. Modern medicine is largely aimed to investigate the specificity of the disease or disorder, while traditional medicine mainly explores the disease by looking at the external appearance. One aims to treat the "symptom," the other is more curious about finding a solution to the underlying cause. It is believed that the non-specificity sometimes could influence or change the process of morbidity, and only targeting the specificity is not enough to stop the progress of morbidity.[15]

Treat the person—Non-specific (traditional medicine)—Foundational
Treat the disease—Specific (modern medicine)—Interventional

Could specific treatments be used on a foundation of non-specific or foundational medicine? Or SelfCare?

Many clinical studies have shown the effects of combining modern drugs with herbal medicine (natural food and plants over synthetic derivatives). For example, the effect rate in treating coronary heart disease with modern drugs was 45.5%, while combining with herbal medicine it was up to 87.3%.[16] The key is looking between the gap and exploring how to best combine the two therapies.

The future is to reconcile.

We have 12 integrated systems working together in our bodies, cells are regenerating at a rate of 50 million cells per second, living symbiotically with roughly 370 trillion bacteria both in and on our body. All whilst our mind commands our human body to dance through life in its unpredictable chaos.

Evidence shows that diet, exercise, great environments and a reduction in stress can preventing or delay many diseases and accelerated aging. Ancients have always shown that healthy diets and movement combat ill-health. Yet modern medicine also has its obvious advantages, we can prevent disease and combat a while range of issues with new medicines. Physiotherapy and other modalities.

Returning to some of Dr Margaret Chan conclusion from her speech, *"Countries aiming to integrate the best from traditional and modern medicine would do well to look not only at the many differences between traditional and modern medicine. Instead, they should look at those areas where both converge to help tackle the unique health challenges of the 21st century."* [17]

With an open-mind to both East and West, we can co-create blue zone communities and healthy future generations that thrive together.

THE PIVOT: SYNTHETIC TO NATURAL MEDICINE AS A FOUNDATION FOR HUMAN WELLBEING

To understand how we got to where we are today, we need to look at the way in which modern medicine evolved and how we came to be so reliant on synthetic (not from nature) medicine.

As I write this, and the "pandemic" comes to an end, I can't help but reflect on how we have all been challenged to question the efficacy and trust we have in the modern pharmaceutical industry. Some people willingly took the intervention, some were labeled conspiracy theorists, other anti-vaxxers and prominent people were even censored from sharing their views on social networks that once promoted freedom of speech. I am not going to argue whether the intervention worked or whether viruses exist. Hopefully you can shape your own view from previous sections. However, one thing is clear: the approach to good health and wellbeing was completely contrary to what we shared in this book—isolation, disconnection, financial stress, polarization, fear and some very manipulative marketing tactics. I was also curious to see why more people lived than died in 2020 in places like Australia during this crisis.[18] Usually when something doesn't make sense, doesn't feel right, or for some reason your gut instinct rings alarm bells, then it's important to investigate.

When I was working as a health professional, patients would come to see me with lower back pain. Usually it was an ongoing experience, yet sometimes it was the first time they had felt this type of pain. I noticed how without identifying the cause, the health profession was so willing to provide people with painkillers and anti-inflammatories. For most people, the pain was an inconvenience to their busy lifestyle and rather than listening to the signals from their body and nurturing the body's innate wisdom to restore harmony, they were set on a quick fix.

I'm not sure if you have ever sprained your ankle whilst running or falling down a step? But the pain and swelling that occurs after the event is a normal part of the process. For the most part, if managed well, most of the pain and inflammation will settle within 72 hours. However, if you ignore what your body is trying to tell you and you keep walking, running and weight-bearing on your ankle, then the pain can persist for weeks, months and even years—as you never gave the body a chance to complete its normal healing process.

I am curious why we have learned to ignore the natural signals that we get from our body in favor of interventions that suppress the natural mechanisms and the very processes that actually promote healing.

As an example, we are no longer recommended to give patients anti-inflammatories during the first 72 hours after an injury. Why? Because inflammation is a powerful and necessary process for healing the injured area and suppressing that process is actually detrimental to healing. Which sounds like common sense, right? Yet painkillers, anti-inflammatories and other synthetic medications are available free and willingly from any local pharmacy without the need of a doctor's prescription.

To understand why we moved away from listening to our bodies' innate wisdom and natural healing mechanisms lost in a misinformation minefield of "Red Herrings" (information that distracts us from the actual solution), in favor of silver bullet solutions and quick fixes, it might be worthwhile to understand how the trillion dollar pharmaceutical industry began.

Writer on healthcare and the pharmaceutical industry, Robin Walsh, looked at the origins of our 21st century Biotechnology sector and the history of pharmaceutical interventions.[19] He shows us a general sequence of events and decisions that helped us arrive where we are today.

The pharmaceutical industry can be traced back as far as the middle ages. You may even remember some mid-century marketing material depicting doctors and dentists recommending tobacco and asking people to "smoke a fresh cigarette."[20] The American tobacco industry in the 1920s–1950s, targeted female nurses and healthcare workers to promote the benefits of cigarette smoking as "modern, healthy, fashionable, and safe!"[21] Even cocaine and heroin was once a "health" ingredient in everyday cough syrup, lozenges and toothache mixture.[22]

To understand how we moved away from nature in favor of synthetic alternatives, it is important to recognize that the industry we know today is actually a byproduct of the chemical industry of the late 19th century in the Upper Rhine valley of Switzerland. The place where industry experts noticed that certain chemicals seemed to have antiseptic properties. If you cast your mind back to the section that ran through the 25 elements that a body requires to sustain and maintain itself, and if you reflect on the fact that the majority of the elements available in the world today are mild carcinogens (cause cancer etc.) then you can start to understand why people might be angry if there is mercury in their fish from industrial pollution, and even in modern interventions like vaccines and other over-the-counter "medicines" that contain elements like graphine oxide.

Famous physician William Osler said: "The person who takes medicine must recover twice, once from the disease and once from the medicine." I can't help but wonder what our world could be like if our "medicines" were founded in nature, rather than the laboratory. But as you saw in 2020, if anybody spoke of #naturalimmunity and tried to remind people of their own innate wisdom and nature's free abundance, they were often polarized and gaslighted for being conspiracy theorists.

We must remain curious about things and ask ourselves why? Why are things the way they are?

For example, the founders of Pfizer in the USA were actually two German immigrants, and initially Pfizer was a fine chemicals business. With the onset of the American civil war the "demand for painkillers and antiseptics rocketed."[23]

This led them to evolve their chemical business into a "health" business. Today in 2021 they are the third richest pharmaceutical company in the world.[24] Generating over 3.5 billion in vaccine sales alone in the first 3 months of the 2021 pandemic.

Senator Paul Rand, a medical doctor, was courageous enough to ask whether natural immunity had a place in the pandemic. He shared an Israeli study (among others) where over 2.5 million participants who had already had the virus had natural immunity which was around 7x more effective than the vaccine.[25] [26] Yet, these individuals were still required to have the medical intervention in order to return to work and travel. Even though, throughout history, people who had already had measles were not indicated to have the vaccine as their body already had natural immunity. He too suggested that we can integrate awareness and the efficacy of natural and modern interventions to serve populations.[27]

The conflict is in plain sight, health has become a business and the care for you and your family is measured secondary to the company's bottom line and profit margins. This is all founded on a vision and model that promotes repeat customers and 6-month booster shots.

In the mid 1900s the health industry was booming in the same way the technology sector is now. Innovative companies started to patent their creations. In the same way the coronavirus vaccine was patented years before the virus hit the global stage.[28] How could they have known? What is important to remember is that these companies were founded by chemical industries and patent law classifies physical phenomena as products of nature. Thus, if your invention occurs in nature, it is a physical phenomenon and cannot be patented. Which means that anything patented is not from nature!

Essentially any of these interventions are synthetic chemical derivatives engineered by human beings who openly admit—*the more we come to know, the more we realize we don't know*. The FDA (Food and Drug Administration), World Medical Association and even the World Health Organization (WHO) stepped in to try and create regulations for the research, application, adverse drug reactions and the economic interests of these synthetic chemicals that were about to hit our market with full force, and also with unknown long-term consequences.

A quick internet search will show you that Big Pharma companies, their backers and handful of small people, profiteered trillions of dollars, whilst the rest of the world was in pain.[29] My mom always told me that the same people who sell you the problem, will sell you the solution. If you keep seeking, then you will see that some top companies selling you the 2020 solutions also lost billions of dollars in lawsuits for adverse drug reactions due to opioids and other interventions that they had once reassured the public were safe.[30]

Unfortunately in the "State of Emergency" of 2020, they were able to leverage their power and rush synthetic interventions to the market without any liability or care for the people. Imagine any other company that created a product that resulted in even one death or adverse reaction. Let alone millions. It would be pulled from the shelf and dragged through mainstream media. It would crush a company's reputation. A book called *100,000,000 Guinea Pigs: Dangers in Everyday Foods, Drugs, and Cosmetics* written in 1933 written by Arthur Kallet and F.J. Schlink warned us of the dangers in everyday foods, drugs and cosmetics.[31] However, like most banned books, we suppressed this knowledge as we watched the list of deaths and adverse reactions increase over the decades. Today, we are seeing a shift in the narrative. Initially it was "do the right thing to save other people's lives"...and now the evolving narrative is..."one death is okay, as long as it saves the many." I'm not sure if you have ever been in a traumatic, manipulative or emotionally abusive relationship? But we are all in one now! Leaders are building higher fences rather than longer tables. To see some of the wealthiest people on Earth profited trillions of dollars during the pandemic, whilst the rest of the world struggled to meet their basic needs is a bitter pill to swallow.[32] It is hard to wake up and realize that not everyone has the best interest of you and your family at heart. This is why you need to be empowered to look after yourself, your family, your front door step and be an active supporter of your local community.

In the 2020 vaccine race, tech giants like Bill Gates openly stated in an essay in the *Wall Street Journal* that biotech and vaccines have been "the best investment I have ever made."[33]

Personally, I think if you are generating millions, billions or trillions of dollars in revenue from passive interventions, silver bullets and repeat customers, then it starts to become more clear that it is money, before people. My mom always taught me to trust patterns of behaviors, not the silky words. Even if people are trying to "help" from a good place, a good heart and with good intentions, sometimes it's still harmful. Remember, good intentions are the plastic bags of the future. We need to consider the long-term consequences. Evil can only ever prevail, if good people stand by and watch.

The pharmaceutical industry has boomed during the past two decades with revenues worldwide totaling 1.25 trillion U.S. dollars in 2020.[34] Remembering that with the right allocation of resources it would take less than 200 billion dollars to address the issues affecting the 1 billion human beings that will go to bed hungry tonight.

So why do we not empower ourselves to learn how to care for ourselves and care for others. The simple answer is that there is no profit in what is already abundant and free. And if you want to go a little further, there is a concept called "ideological subversion." It is how prominent leaders with false confidence and values used propaganda and subliminal marketing to control the masses for their own self gain, narcissism and megalomania. In simple terms, you thought you were thinking your own thoughts, but ultimately it had all been planned 20 years before you became aware of it. These are the puppeteers. I'm sure you can reflect back in history on Nazi Germany, communism and the USSR.

The crisis, the chaos, the demoralization, the fear and the control.

I'm sure you can think of some tech giants that became health experts and global saviors in 2020 to understand the point I'm making. High on false confidence, whilst being unconsciously incompetent, willfully ignorant and apathetic to the real needs of the world right now. Isolation, disconnection, financial stress, removing people's purpose, demoralization, fear, polarization (us vs them) and a silver bullet solution being sold by the very people who perpetrated the narrative and the problem, should be enough to start questioning things.

Scientists say that the statistics reveal that "adverse drug reactions (ADR) are far more commonplace than one would think. It is estimated that ADRs represent the fourth leading cause of death in the United States and Canada behind heart disease, cancer, and stroke."[35]

Today these patented chemicals have led to a serious national crisis that affects public health as well as social and economic welfare. There is a growing misuse of and addiction to opioids, including over-the-counter and prescription pain relievers, heroin, and synthetic opioids such as fentanyl.[36] I'm sure there is someone in your proximity that is using these drugs to suppress how they feel, distract their mind, and even avoid the pain of a past trauma and life event.

I also know from my own experience that a quick-fix solution looks appealing when we are in the depths of our pain. We need to remember that the keys have always been in our hands. Pain has also been my biggest teacher in life and it's not always comfortable that's for sure. Perhaps we need to stop suppressing and distracting ourselves from reality. Feel more, suppress less and gain the lessons we need to find harmony once again.

FEEL MORE, SUPPRESS LESS

The Civil War in the USA helped ignite the creation of opioids (painkillers) to help soldiers keep fighting a war that they never started. From this ancestral trauma, conflict and pain, we created a new type of pain to suppress and distract us all from the trauma we were feeling individually and collectively.

The future generations need a new approach. To be encouraged and inspired to feel more, to normalize the aspects of pain, pleasure and every other human emotion, as an essential part of the human experience.

To do this, we must remain curious, seek to understand, not just to be understood. We need to individually and collectively "wake up"—otherwise our subconscious minds will fall victim to clever marketing and propaganda tactics of businesses and people that have trillions of dollars of resources and a new level of power and control that they will not give up easily.

Even as recent as the late 1990s, pharmaceutical companies reassured the medical community that patients would not become addicted to prescription opioid pain relievers, and healthcare providers began to prescribe them at greater rates.[37] Even with good intentions, the end result is that we are left with a widespread diversion and misuse of these medications.

In 2020–21 we have been reassured that Covid-19 vaccines are safe, yet they come with a long list of side-effects and the legal ground for being able to file a law-suit against a company for an adverse reaction gives them basic immunity from liability.[38]

When I am unsure, I listen to my gut and my heart, and rationalize with my mind last. I ask whether I would recommend it to my mother, my family, friends and their children, before considering whether I would do it myself. If it's not a "hell yes," then that's enough for me to stay informed and strong in my own choices. Even in the heat of the polarization and propaganda of unconsciously, incompetent and willfully ignorant leaders with "good intentions."

The future is ours. We need to reconsider what role synthetic "not from nature" medicine plays in the future health and wellbeing of our populations. Perhaps we need more "health companies" founded on nature and community, not just chemical companies that have become part of the problem they are trying to solve. It is clear that many of these synthetic chemicals can disrupt normal cellular function and even lead to adverse reactions and long term health challenges.[39] When we start to consider that 1 in 2 people in 2020 are likely to develop some form of uncontrolled cellular growth or cancer in their lifetime[40] compared to 1 in 10 people in our grandparents era. It is clear to see that the pharmaceutical health boom, industrial revolution, and more recently technological revolution plays a huge role in why we have become so disconnected from ourselves and nature.

I imagine a world where one day we all wake up to see a headline that reminds 422 million people that: **"Type 2 diabetes is reversible for up to 10 years in most people and the solution is plain sight!"** The news article would continue to share that if want to avoid blindness, kidney failure, pancreatic disease and even lower limb amputation, then all you have to do is limit your franken-food and excessive sugar intake, eat real food, eat more plants from natural sources, quit smoking and master the 12 Medicines in your own life.

I imagine a government official supporting this initiative and being quoted to say: *"To ensure that you have a nourishing and supportive environment, a community that cares and leaders who truly stand for you and your family, we are going to disincentivize the problem. Fake food will be taxed, and companies that are part of the problem will be banned from marketing their addictive low-quality food to children. We want to protect the minds and bodies of our children. And... we will also incentivize the solution. Organic produce will have a tax exemption, farmers will have access to everything they need, insulin will be free for those who need it and companies that are doing the right thing to support the health, happiness and connection of our communities will be rewarded for helping us get to the root cause of the problems we are facing today. We understand that addressing the root causes of today's problems will save us time, energy, resources and pain in the long run. Together we are stronger!"*

The article could then add a touch of good science and offer some practical and relevant solutions too.

They would mention that the Counterbalance study published in 2016, demonstrated that Type 2 diabetes remains reversible for up to 10 years in most people.[41] They would shine the light on Professor Roy Taylor from Newcastle University in the UK who has spent almost four decades (his life work!) studying the condition. Here is an overview of his findings at the European Association For The Study Of Diabetes (EASD 2017) in Lisbon.

For the reader, they would share a couple of simple facts and solutions that could save 500 million people and their families from pain.

Avoid excess calories (frankenfood), as they lead to excess fat in the liver. As a result, the liver responds poorly to insulin and produces too much glucose.[42]

Excess fat in the liver is passed on to the pancreas, causing the insulin producing cells to fail. Losing less than 1 gram of fat from the pancreas through diet can restart the normal production of insulin, reversing Type 2 diabetes.[43]

This reversal of diabetes remains possible for at least 10 years after the onset of the condition.[44]

Which means that nearly 500 million people are living with a condition that they could each reverse in 10 years. Imagine how much time, energy and resources it would save. The only issue is that the profit margins on insulin would disappear. Do you see the point and what we are fighting?

The number of people with diabetes rose from 108 million in 1980 to 422 million in 2014[45] and the cost of the four most popular types of insulin has tripled over the past decade[46], and the out-of-pocket prescription costs patients now face have doubled.[47] By 2016, the average price per month rose to $450[48]—and costs continue to rise, so much so that as many as one in four people with diabetes are now skimping on or skipping lifesaving doses. If vaccines can be free, then perhaps insulin can be too?

We need more people like Frederick Banting who discovered insulin in 1923 to stand up and be counted! He refused to put his name on the patent. He felt it was unethical for a doctor to profit from a discovery that would save lives. For every one "idealistic," heart-centered leader like this, there are a handful of people who think otherwise.

*"A single bee is often ignored. But when millions
come together, even the bravest run in fear."*
— Unknown —

I look forward to the day we all stand together and be the change we wish to see in the world. It is clear that something needs to change. True health interventions should not have collateral damage, they should not be expensive and limited, they should be empowering, not passive.

It is also clear that modern medicine is necessary too. If you find yourself in a traumatic accident, then modern medicine is amazing. The best herbs and natural remedies may not save you there!

The simplicity of the 80–95% is in 12 Medicines of SelfCare; many which are free and readily available to you right now. Where modern medicine and biotechnology are secondary. They are here to support, but never to replace your body's innate wisdom. Nature, community, and daily lifestyle choices, truly are the foundation for good health and wellbeing.

Perhaps we need to start listening and taking advice from global longevity hotspots living in the Blue Zones and less advice from global chemical and bio-technology companies that are more interested in profit margins than global health and longevity.

Whatever you believe to be true. It is clear that if our current approach was working, then the statistics in this book would not be a reality. But they are. Let's pivot together and change the way we do things. Let's focus on moving as many people as possible out of the red zone and orange zone and into the green and blue zone. By doing so, we can free up 47-trillion dollars in resources to help address larger issues for humanity. Imagine what we could co- create together for future generations!

⚕ MODERN IS MEDICINE PRESCRIPTION

» Nature and natural remedies are the foundation for good health and wellbeing, not alternative or secondary. AGREE / DISAGREE?

» Community and connection is the elixir to longevity. Name one community that empowers and enables your health and wellbeing.

» Modern medicine is here to support and intervene when we find ourselves in desperate need. It is a secondary intervention that needs to be utilized to support our bodies innate wisdom. But never to replace.

» How has modern medicine/interventions helped you restore harmony, health and homeostasis in your body in the past? Eg. After an accident or an acute injury?

....

....

....

....

....

....

....

» HOW many prescription drugs are you currently taking?

» HOW many prescriptions drugs were you taking 10 years ago?

» HOW would it feel to no longer need synthetic medication to feel better? Or to manage whatever symptoms, dysfunctions, pains or diseases you currently have?

To learn more about this medicine, or to contribute to this medicine, visit **selfcare.global/modern**. Here you will find blogs, videos and podcasts.

Selfcare.global/modern

NOTABLE EXPERTS IN THIS CHAPTER:
Dr. Emill Kim, Dr Margaret Chan, World Health Organization, Hippocrates, Elizabeth Cohen, Erika Schwartz, Leana Wen M.D.

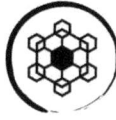

12

TECHNOLOGY IS MEDICINE

"Make Healthcare delightful, personalised,
and ultimately preventive."
— Koan Kan, Healthcare futurist —

ALL TECHNOLOGY IS A PRODUCT OF THE NATURAL WORLD

Technology can support our health, wellbeing, happiness and sense of connection.

The long-running TV show Star Trek has a knack for predicting the future of technology. Just some of the program's pioneering inventions include tablet computers, the communicator (enter the mobile phone), voice interface computers (hello Siri!) as well as cloaking devices. Of all the space-age gadgets used in the plot, there is one that, if replicated in reality, would far surpass any medical tool we have imagined so far. These galactic doctors used the Tricorder; a handheld device they simply pointed at the patient, human or otherwise, to instantly diagnose any galactic disorder or dysfunction!

Technology has been trying to catch up to the imaginings of Star Trek for decades but it's only in recent times that the dream of such a device has seemed possible. Its creation could help address numerous medical challenges faced today by millions; wait times, doctor expenses, uncertainty and even remote locations. Running between 2011 and 2017, the chipmaker Qualcomm sponsored the Tricorder X Prize, generating global interest and competition in developing groundbreaking medical hardware around the Tricorder concept. The call was to invent a machine that could diagnose a set list of 13 medical conditions as well as monitor five vital signs.

The strongest performing device in the competition, designed by Basil Leaf Technologies was called Dxter™, a small yet sophisticated diagnostic engine for conditions such as; diabetes, atrial fibrillation, chronic obstructive pulmonary disease, urinary tract infection, sleep apnea, leukocytosis, pertussis, stroke, tuberculosis, and pneumonia.[1] The competition was trailblazing and Dxter™ was just the beginning as advancements and testing continues for all companies now pioneering the forefront of this incredible medical technology that one day will hit the market and change the lives of millions.

Technology is the application of knowledge to serve a practical purpose.

The human factor in helping to heal will never be replaced, nor should be, however if we consider the above definition, technology has the potential to enable and enhance human health and connection on a global scale. Imagine the influence digital technology could have on underdeveloped regions where medical practitioners are often scarce. It should not substitute for medical supervision, but when there is none, mobile devices designed to measure a person's vital signs could prove life-saving. Technology could also manifest the full potential of the digital health age: allowing the patient's home environment, wherever it may be, to be the point-of-care. Thus combining the benefits of human and nature centric technology.

The 12 Medicines began with Nature as Medicine and it is fitting that we finish with Technology as Medicine, because as the opening sentence suggests, **Technology *is* Nature, there is no separation.** This is no doubt surprising to many who might consider technology as a heartless army of sterile robots however technology is not the bad guy, far from it, it is inherently part of human nature.

We are an organic species that has learnt to manipulate inorganic elements into tools and technology, which has enabled and empowered our long-term survival and success; technology has been our evolutionary friend in fact. For thousands of years, medicines and treatment principles have depended on the technology at hand; such as scalpels, probes and materia medica. Today, this has evolved into hospitals that rely on complex, computerized machines to either analyze the body or support its function.

In this chapter, we explore the upside and dark side of Technology as Medicine. I will share how it can be effectively utilized towards longevity and more abundance of health, energy, time and even resources. We just need to understand how best to apply our knowledge. The challenge is that technology, like many mind altering substances such as alcohol or synthetic drugs, is often used to numb our mind and escape our reality.

The 12 Medicines aim to recreate a natural reality that you love and never want to escape from. Modern technology allows you to do this more than ever, supporting your natural mechanisms towards self-care and freeing your time and location to do what you love, to live your purpose and ideal lifestyle at the same time.

DEFINE TECHNOLOGY AS MEDICINE

Technology, like our human vessel, finds its origin in nature. Philosopher and poet, Blaire Ostler contends that technology is an essential and natural part of human evolution.[2] It can be seen all around us being applied in nature. "The use of technology is a pattern well established in the natural world," Ostler explains, "for example, when a spider spins a web she is using the natural elements of her environment and body to produce a piece of technology to serve the practical purpose of catching her food. The web functions as a net, a common technology also used by humans to capture food."[3]

Imagine back when Early Man first used sticks and primitive stone implements to hunt and build basic dwellings, he was the earliest "technologist" using nature and his increasing cognition to gain his desires.[4] This adaption of the natural elements around us has expanded into the rapid-fire developments we see in modern times, however the cause of our adaptations hasn't changed! Our desires and aims motivate our actions each day, just as we invent increasingly sophisticated levels of "natural" technology to fulfill them.

Therefore there is no need to look for a moral distinction between what is technology and what is nature, because just as Ostler asserts, technology *is* nature.[5] Even when we are surpassing the boundaries of our known limits, we are effectively doing what comes naturally!

The same natural elements used to make your human vessel and the ones that keep nourishing it over your lifespan, are the same base elements used to create the book or device that you are reading, the smartphone in your pocket, the Wi-Fi and internet that enables you to connect with social media platforms and the technology that operates your businesses.

Technology has enabled these practical purposes for us, empowering us in this reality. Technology is not meant to take us away from reality or to replace nature or human connection. It shouldn't be designed that way. As discussed previously, our environments, our cultures and the communities that support us govern the reality we create in our mind. Together these factors guide our willpower, our thoughts and importantly our actions.

The danger emerges when the principles that drive our environments, cultures and communities move our actions away from nature and collectively become stronger than our convictions, subverting our realities into false digital lives. **Technology can empower the human experience but should never replace it.** We wield its control; it should not control us.

You could say nature and technology are the same medicine, just in a different configuration. The distinction to be aware of is that technology is a natural extension of nature, due to human manipulation of those basic tools we used as cave dwellers right through to spaceships and beyond in the modern era.

The dual nature of technology challenges us to create technology from nature, whilst remaining connected to it. Technology's use must promote harmony and interconnectedness of all the systems; healthy circular economies and the human and earth biomes inclusively. In the same way that astronaut Piers Sellers on his deathbed, utilized technology to create a system to monitor climate change. A living legacy that will help future generations inform their decisions on this beautiful planet.

4 WAYS THAT HUMANS, NATURE AND TECHNOLOGY ARE INTEGRATED

The lines separating humans, nature and technology are blurred to say the least. History shows advances and retreats on each side just like the ebb and flow of the tide or an age-old battle between superpowers. Technology certainly seems to have supremacy as we've hit the 21st century. As the developments keep coming thick and fast, the values and desires of human nature are often difficult to reconcile in the modern world.

On the one hand we attempt to protect remote and exotic places from the spread of wifi, yet we contend that Internet access should be a human right all over the world. We lament the continuing decline of rare wildlife even as we unwittingly support the industries that have a hand in their decline. Most disingenuous of all are the modern expectations to be able to fly to any destination on Earth, while shopping around for unsustainably cheap flights to get us there.[6]

A similar challenge is the perpetual, ever onward and upward nature that propels technology into new realms. So many interrelated systems around the world have created a reliance on each other and an energy that impels them to constantly increase and expand into new territory, just like nature and human evolution. The technologist Kevin Kelly even declares that technology is in fact, "A force of nature! That it is an extension and an acceleration of natural evolution." The two fields become more interconnected with every new approach; let's look at them in action.

#1: TECHNOLOGY MIMICS NATURE

The field of biomimetics is where elements and processes in nature are used as a model for new technological developments. The structure of a spider's web was the inspiration behind a new neonatal surgical tape design that is more suited to peeling off the fragile skin of premature babies.[7] An imitation virus was created to mimic self-assembling nanoparticles, an effective way of sending medication straight into cancer cells.[8] While a full-color, reflective, e-reader screen was created using the principles of a butterfly's iridescent wings that shimmer in the sunlight.[9] Enhancing our limited human senses to see the unseen.

#2: TECHNOLOGY CONNECTS HUMANS

Technology can be used for incredible good as seen when Google created a Person Finder to reunite relatives after natural disasters such as during 2011's Japanese tsunami.[10] There are also government apps that allow citizens to photograph and upload disaster scenes and their GPS location can then be plotted in order to help with recovery and relief operations.[11]

#3: TECHNOLOGY AND NATURE COMBINE TO CO-CREATE "GREEN CITIES"

Technology can even offer great respite from our concrete jungles with innovative ways to incorporate green plantings and vegetation into urban settings. Rooftop crops and gardens, vertical farms, cultivating algae-based biofuels and trees as street lamps using bioluminescence are some of the revolutions we can look forward to. Even London's Garden Bridge project, despite being fraught with bureaucracies that ultimately led to its undoing, was a dynamic vision towards this fusion of urban-rural landscape.

#4: THE DOWNFALL

We are becoming increasing aware that technology has the potential to disconnect us from each other and the natural world. Research continues into the addictive nature of digital platforms[12] and the related, dysfunctional pattern of a life indoors. Even when we do try and immerse ourselves in nature, we still "wear" technology that keeps us more attached to our virtual status than to reality.

The interconnection of nature and humans will be enabled and empowered through the right technology used the right way. We can wield the technology sword for a positive future vision that is connected and more sustainable, or for a world that is more disconnected, isolated and detrimental to the natural world that ultimately sustains all life. We need to find the intricate balance and harmony of all the elements.

ARE GOOD INTENTIONS ENOUGH?

I was once asked whether a good intention behind an action is enough. Let's consider the development of a tool designed by Sten Gustaf Thulin in the 1960s that fulfilled a need he saw around him; a tool to help people carry food and other needs back to their house. That sounds like a positive, helpful application of his knowledge. He even thought he was alleviating a problem he saw from the current method he wanted to replace.

Thulin designed the plastic bag to save the planet from the tree-destroying paper bags he saw multiplying around the world. So he had a good intention when creating the plastic bag however 60 years later it has become our biggest problem. Thulin would be astonished if he knew that today plastic bags were used and simply thrown away into the environment, to the extent that we are heading towards the day when plastic bags will outweigh fish in the sea!

I believe it is not just the intention and creation that matters. It is important to cast a vision of integrity that accounts for the future repercussions for that creation and holds to the values that underpin its conception. When we create a solution to a problem of the day, we need to ask ourselves whether it is the root cause of the problem or just another band-aid solution.

Anyone at any time can use technology as a tool for good, promoting connection and harmony internally and externally. Or it can be wielded to disconnect us and promote disharmony. Imperative is the character of the person that wields the sword of technology and how they ultimately choose to use it. Perhaps only time will tell if we can self-govern holistically for all, or if our lower egos will prevail.

> Good intentions, with the wrong underlying values, and
> creations built on unconscious unawareness or
> incompetence are the plastic bags of the future.

There is a fine line between using technology to fulfill a perceived need such as providing supportive healthcare, and the disservice of undermining the key message that 80–95% of who we are is within our control, especially for those living in environments with opportunity and education. This is the objective of the message, to reconnect with the fundamentals of self-care first, and then use technology to continue to promote these values.

The task for our modern, enlightened human species is to maintain the balance of our evolutionary legacy whilst promoting harmony with the natural world. Hopefully we never need to inhabit the desert planet of Mars because we forgot to nourish this beautiful blue planet we call home. In the same way, I hope that we never need transplants for our human body or even our very consciousness, because we forgot to look after this amazing human vessel that is home to us each day.

HUMAN 3.0 MEETS MACHINE

According to one man, linking technology and the human brain is a real and positive possibility for the future and is on the mind of Elon Musk, the South African born, American entrepreneur and CEO of Tesla, a world leader in creating sustainable energy solutions.

Tesla's ultimate purpose is to help the world transition away from its reliance on fossil fuels and toward the embrace of sustainable energy sources.[13] Musk believes that technology can help us take a large step towards co-creating healthier environments for all humans to live in.

From sustainable energy, Musk has expanded his quest for development and in the essence of ironman, he now believes in linking human brains with computers! He founded Neuralink Corporation in 2016 and is developing "neural lace" technology that would allow people to connect directly with machines without the need for a physical interface.[14]

Imagine—if you can—electrodes planted in the brain that can upload or download your thoughts! Musk envisions humans achieving new levels of perception through this synergy with machines. The biological human could integrate and become a biological machine without the mind becoming ruled by artificial intelligence.

The potential of Musk's vision is really exciting because we're not talking about the lure and addiction of virtual reality games, rather some of the aims up for discussion include using the technology for internally treating disorders such as epilepsy or major depression. There is even research in the US into brain computer interface technology that could one day allow people with paraplegia to walk again![15] So there is a highly admirable incentive for **humans, technology and nature all working together as one.**

Virtual reality is also a burgeoning field that could be used to treat neurological conditions and assist with intense rehabilitation for those that need it. Day to day activities such as making a cup of tea can be lived first through virtual reality as a way to remember, retrain and prepare our body, our balance and attention for daily tasks again. VR can also be used to address people's fear of heights; the possibilities are exponential![16]

PRACTICAL WAYS TECHNOLOGY CAN SUPPORT HEALTH AND WELLBEING

Technology as medicine already supports our natural healing mechanisms when we think of acute surgery needed to treat victims of serious trauma, or investigative scans (like the Tricorder in star trek) that are used to enable evidence-based practice for healing in the context of a person's life.

The time is approaching when wearable technology and smart data can monitor our internal harmony (heart rate, breathe rate, blood pressure etc.) and let us know when things are in balance and when they are not.

Such live data could then guide us towards immediate strategies to reduce the stress we are experiencing and empower us to make better informed choices minute-by-minute in the context of our daily lives. The Apple watch is pioneering internal health connectivity through the blood flow detected in the wrist it's worn on. Wearing such a device also seems likely to make you want to keep better track of your health as well!

Just like the digital assistants we're becoming used to in Alexa and Siri, these applications could evolve one day to tell us when we are dehydrated or deficient in some element. Then how quick could our response be to refuel our body in a way that supports our normal function!

Perhaps they could tell us our physical body or cardiovascular system is deconditioning due to our sedentary lifestyle, and we can again be empowered to embrace strategies that pivot our health and wellbeing back in the right direction, in the context of our environments.

If we choose, digital assistants could become full-time healthcare companions; patient conditions, results, medications and past history can be tracked, virtual or real appointments can be made. Doctor alerts and advice can be provided in real time and this connection could even help reduce the feelings of loneliness for isolated or older people.

Technology could also help us to monitor our personal ecological footprint each day and ensure we are consuming and operating at less than 1.0 Earths. This enables the evolution of our individual and collective behaviors as we go, promoting harmony between nature, technology and a healthy populace that continues to swell!

HOW ARTIFICIAL INTELLIGENCE WILL IMPROVE HEALTHCARE

AI is generally defined as the capacity for a computer or machine to exhibit or simulate intelligent behavior. Examples such as Tesla's self-driving car and our much-loved digital assistants illustrate this fast-advancing field that is attracting much dedicated research and investment. How could AI actually improve healthcare in the future?

One surprising example of the benefit of AI systems and models for predictive medicine is the removal of current systemic healthcare inequalities that are linked with social inequalities. In other words, AI takes away human bias when using algorithms to analyze data. Fair and just application could be a life or death matter.

Further imagine the vast amounts of human information that AI can store, analyze and correlate with existing research and procedures. Allowing for the ethical and legal issues that will need to be resolved, AI could one day generate individually customized advice and treatments for anyone anywhere! Utilizing mobile solutions could help reach people in remote areas considering the increasing uptake of mobile phones in developing nations.

AI has even traversed into robot doctors. Yes, there is an AI robot in China that downloaded information from countless medical textbooks, millions of medical records and hundreds of thousands of articles in order to "sit" the medical exam; its results were faster and more precise than real students. The robot even achieved a much higher mark than the required 360 to pass, 456 out of a possible 600. Don't worry though this AI doctor won't be treating you or anyone you know any time soon, rather it's designed to assist doctors by retrieving information as they attend to patients.[17]

In a positive step forward, AI is also contributing to reducing deaths due to medical errors. It is heartbreaking to know that thousands of people die each year from the incorrect administration of treatment drugs.[18] AI is being aimed at monitoring the entire process, from prescription to correct dosage for the patient, minimizing the chance of human error.

Artificial intelligence also gives doctors a run for their money when diagnosing skin cancers. Even "out-detecting" real doctors in one study where the human specialists detected 87% correctly while the AI achieved 95% detection success.[19] The help of these modern examinations could eventually reduce the number of false positives, meaning less stress, less unnecessary treatment and shorter wait times for those needing surgery.

DECENTRALIZATION BENEFITS ALL

Decentralized Autonomous Organizations (DAOs) are a new concept in governance but are already creating a ripple of change. They are both at the forefront of global technology in that they are governed by computer codes and programs, and yet they operate on the simple premise of no central authority or bureaucratic hierarchies. They function autonomously by executing commands based on the protocols and rules of its founding and the external data that the stakeholders input.

Most effective of all, is that the rules and transaction records are stored transparently on the "blockchain" (a unique type of database where it's virtually impossible to alter records). DAOs are revolutionary in being a system for open, transparent collaboration and privacy!

These DAOs can be applied to the health and wellness systems globally. *Medicalchain* and *Healthchain* are examples of this. Imagine health and wellness systems that are truly human centric, decentralized, transparent and work with a common vision to keep all of us in a state of good health and wellbeing, whilst reducing costs and collateral damage to the world around us, and each other. This becomes even more powerful when it is solution focused and collaborative, without competition.

Medicalchain (medicalchain.com)—decentralized healthcare. Imagine all of your health records in one place over your lifespan, integrated and secure. *Medicalchain* uses blockchain technology to securely store health records and maintain a single version of the truth. The different organizations such as doctors, hospitals, laboratories, pharmacists and health insurers can request permission to access a patient's record to serve their purpose and record transactions on the distributed ledger.

Healthchain (healthchain.io)—efficient systems that reduce wastage. Patient centric healthcare: imagine saving your precious time by seeing the right people at the right time. *Healthchain* aims to improve healthcare by providing software solutions that integrate with existing healthcare management systems to make outdated technologies and paper-based processes more efficient. Their mission is to make medication management more accurate and patient-focused by using innovative technologies and building strategic partnerships.

Integration of all this information will allow you to move freely with your collected, up-to-the-minute information adjusting to your location. For example, your mobile phone or wearable device might alert you and your doctor when it detects a serious change in your internal harmony. The doctor (located anywhere) can contact you to discuss remedial treatment or prescriptions. This system can incorporate local allied health professionals and virtual assistants in achieving this flow of information and prompt response no matter where you are in the world. Technology supporting our self-care in action!

WHERE TO FROM HERE?

When thinking about the future of healthcare, the potential is immense. With the right intention, we can leverage technology to enable and empower human beings, however there are a few values we need to embody with this advanced level of connection and data flow. From an organizational standpoint we should be:

- Developing rules of integrity and security in the collection and storage of data
- Preserving strong ethical foundations for the intended purpose of any medical technology, particularly so the message is clear for the patient to understand when decisions are based on algorithms or internal processes as with AI.
- Casting big visions to eradicate many of the world's diseases, just as we did with polio and smallpox in many parts of the world. A world without sickle cell anemia, without cancer is possible!

With the responsible use of all this integrated information, an efficient, sustainable health and wellbeing system for all, not just the lucky few, *is* possible; a human and nature centric system where self-care is the foundation. As the ground workers, the new generation of allied health professionals are collaborative, not competitive. Their role is to support your body's natural mechanisms and guide you back on the right track using this evolving technology whenever necessary.

Collectively we need to be headed toward:

- Understanding technology and how it can be used to co-create healthy environments to support healthy humans
- Promoting good health and wellbeing as a human right for all
- Practices that support global community "bluezones" becoming the new normal
- Encouraging the synergy of human, nature and technology working as one
- Each wellness pathway being personalized to our uniqueness
- **Professional approaches that are integrated, holistic solutions, embodying the best of ancient wisdom and modern science.**

We know that technology has the potential to lead us down a virtual path of "unreality." If we keep in tune with our internal harmony there are simple practical examples of getting the balance right.

In a pertinent tale about the hazards of virtual reality, the savior at the end of the movie *Ready Player One* turns the "system" off every Tuesday (natural connection Tuesday) and Sunday (SelfCare Sunday). He knew that promoting more human connection and connection to nature in the real world, would ultimately promote the health, wellbeing and happiness of everyone who had suffered under the virtual regime for so long.

Imagine if the Internet or social media platforms turned off for one or two days a week. Reminding people that reality is the only place that you can get a good meal, share an intimate moment with a partner or watch the sunset with a group of friends. Creating those experiences that are felt, not just consciously created. *Feeling* is an underestimated ingredient of maintaining our health.

The Balinese culture already has a day like this. They call it "Nyepi Day." It is a day of silence around March 25th every year. Mobile data is turned to 3G, Wi-Fi is off, airports are shut and the local Banjar (community police) ensure that everyone stays at home. For many people it is the first time they switch off from work, share a meal with friends, or perhaps even look up at the stars again after too long.

Modern culture needs a weekly day of silence, a weekly "Nyepi Day" in the essence of SelfCare Sunday; a day to connect inwards with ourselves and outwardly with each other and the natural world. Filling our cup with all the abundant natural medicine we need to serve from overflow in the coming week.

The time is now to modernize and integrate our approaches towards good health and wellbeing. We live at the cross roads of an age of information and a millennium of ancient wisdom. We can utilize the best of each approach by focussing on the collective solution and a common vision to reduce the burden of chronic preventable disease in this generation for future generations. Ultimately good health and wellbeing is a universal human right that people in both developing and developed parts of the globe do not have access to or are simply not choosing.

TECHNOLOGY IS MEDICINE PRESCRIPTION

Consider how you can leverage modern medicine to support (not replace) the body's natural healing and regenerative mechanisms, intervening only as necessary. Remember prevention is the best cure, we know now that technology can support our self-care practices and therefore we are fully in control as the driver, not the passenger of our health journey.

Consider how you can integrate technology into your modern lifestyle and own self-care in principle or practice. Here are some final questions to guide you.

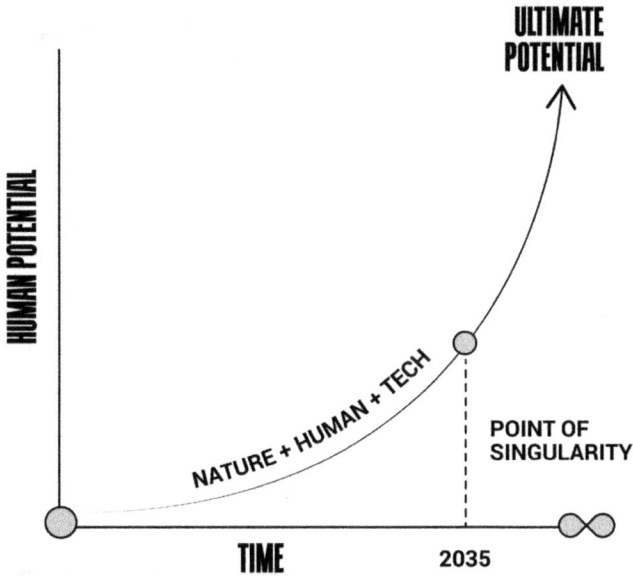

- Can you use technology as a tool to free your time or location? Public transport? Zoom software for remote meetings? Mobile education?
- Can you work remotely from a nice outside area or get technology to do some work for you?
- Do you have a holistic allied health professional to help you on your health journey? Do they draw from both modern and ancient practices?
- Can technology help you access the world's wisdom to inspire you to surmount those health dysfunctions you are experiencing? Is it movement or diet related that you can research and learn more about? Knowledge is power.
- Are you supporting the right value structure that endorses real and healthy solutions? Unlike the unintentional creation of the plastic bag?
- Are you using technology to ultimately tune into a lifestyle that nourishes your soul?

You have the information; now it is time to use it.

⚙ TECHNOLOGY AS MEDICINE PRESCRIPTION

» Limit social media use to 30 minutes a day.

» Have a digital detox weekend every couple of months.

» The recommended amount of screen time depends on a child's age. Children under 2 years should not have any screen time and those under 5 years should have less than two hours a day.

» Use technology to enhance your wellbeing—connect to some health apps and listen to podcasts and audiobooks about good health and longevity.

To learn more about this medicine, or to contribute to this medicine, visit **selfcare.global/tech**. Here you will find blogs, videos and podcasts.

Selfcare.global/tech

NOTABLE EXPERTS IN THIS CHAPTER:
Elon Musk, Kevin Kelly, Koan Kan, Blaire Ostler.

THE 12 MEDICINES AND BEYOND

The whole intention of this book is to ignite a global self-care revolution, founded on ancient wisdom, longevity hotspots, centenarian lifestyles and global blue zone communities, in the hope that we can all thrive together as one amazing human race on this fragile blue planet.

Now, that you have finished the 12 Medicines, I am sure you can ascertain how you too can fill your own cup with good health and wellbeing each day, so that you can serve from overflow in every aspect of your life.

Now, I must confess, this manuscript was originally double in size and some valuable content was edited out in order to fit it into a printable book. However, the **selfcare.global** ecosystem online is an extension of this conversation. So have fun tuning into the podcasts, blogs and social content.

What you do with the information, tools and resources is totally up to you. Take what you need and embody it into your own beliefs, thoughts and actions. Give yourself permission to put your own oxygen mask on before trying to save the world. If you are lucky enough to live a life where you have more than you need then hopefully this book can inspire you to build longer tables, rather than higher fences. Remembering that anyone who has access to read this book is already part of the top 20% of people who have been born into environments and communities where opportunities are plenty.

In this book, I have been inspired by 1000s of the world's leading experts and have leveraged 100,000 + years of wisdom in ancient texts. I have researched some of the best modern evidence-based medicine and science. Hopefully I have succeeded in simplifying much of the complexity so you can easily make small changes along the way.

Give yourself a break too. You don't need to arrive at your end vision tomorrow. By just growing one percent each day from the person you were yesterday compounds your health, wellbeing and lifestyle exponentially.

I haven't told you to trust me, but I want you to trust this—commit to growing just 1% each day. One change in thought, one change in action, and one change in connection is all we need to change the direction of your life and the world.

Everyone has the ability to be healthy, happy and connected in a unified and sustainable existence. If we treat this as a WE game, not just a ME game then life becomes about all of us, not just some of us.

IF IT'S OKAY, I WILL LEAVE YOU WITH A CALL TO COURAGE...

If the systems we have co-created to live in no longer serve us or future generations; then let's innovate new ones that make the old obsolete. If you find yourself being a victim of circumstance. Go inwards and take back the keys, stop being and be the driver.

If a challenge keeps repeating itself, then seek guidance, mentorship and support to move outside your comfort zone and into the unknown.

If you find that you are your own worst enemy. Then find compassion and empathy for yourself, then give that to the world around you.

If you find a solution in the context of your own life, then share it. You never know who is watching and seeking an answer to the very problem you just solved.

If you find yourself like I was unhealthy, unhappy and disconnected. Then tune into the 12 Medicines and change just one thing, anything.

Naturally, if you implement these changes, you really become your own SelfCare Doctor. Not in a medical way that endorses you self-diagnosing ailments or anything radical like that. But in a way that you can stay healthy and happy for many long and wonderful years.

One day when I was surfing, it occurred to me that I really needed a take-home summary of the 12 Medicines.

A way to embody the SelfCare revolution and create a positive disruption in the world of passive "sickcare" largely driven by business motifs more than human ones. So I decided to summarize this book into 9 simple steps that you can use immediately to ignite your own SelfCare revolution.

AS WE DO, LET'S KEEP THE END IN MIND

Our 100-year vision Is to simply remind people that they have never needed to be fixed, simply nourished; to co-create environments and empowering systems that enable the health and wellbeing of all people, irrespective of geographical, cultural and social context.

We stand against the "normal" where 19 in 20 of the people do not live free of disease or dysfunction. We stand to be part of the solution, by empowering the rising billions to move up the health and wellbeing spectrum. Even If I do not see this come to fruition in my lifetime, I am happy to plant trees that I never sit under, in the hope that future generations will bring this vision to life. The vision is simple. I want us all to win. To chase a feeling. Something that can be felt in any moment. It's not about money, success and status. It's about living a life that ignites your human potential and enables you to live your ultimate human experience. Just make sure you do it in a way that lives by the golden rule: treat others along the way, as you would like to be treated. This includes animals and the natural world. If we all adhered to this one belief alone, it would change our entire biology individually and collectively.

LET'S HAVE FUN AND GAMIFY HEALTH AND WELLNESS

We have created a SelfCare ecosystem that goes beyond this book: We wanted to make sure that anytime YOU DO SOMETHING GOOD FOR YOURSELF: SOMETHING GOOD HAPPENS IN THE WORLD.

To make this measurable we have aligned with the 2030 UN Sustainable Development Goals: So...help us reach 1 billion + impacts before **selfcare.global/ why-we-exist**

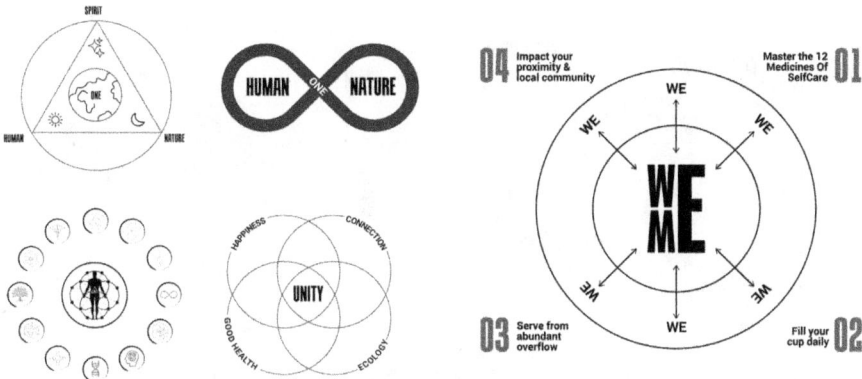

There are 3 crucial steps to creating a positive change in our own lives.

1. **Self-awareness**—This is the thinking , learning, assessing and self-realizing dynamic
2. **Self-mastery**—This is the action dynamic, doing, growing by 1% per day and discipline
3. **Self-expression**—This is the embodiment dynamic, where we become what we repeatedly think and do.

If you would like a structured workbook and course to take action on everything that you have learned in 8 simple steps, click the EMPOWER link in the previous section. If you would like to do-it-yourself with community support, then use the workbook tools and assessments below.

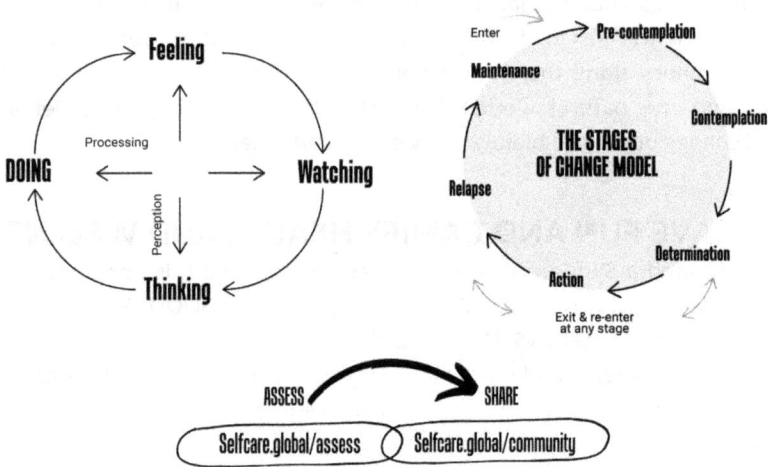

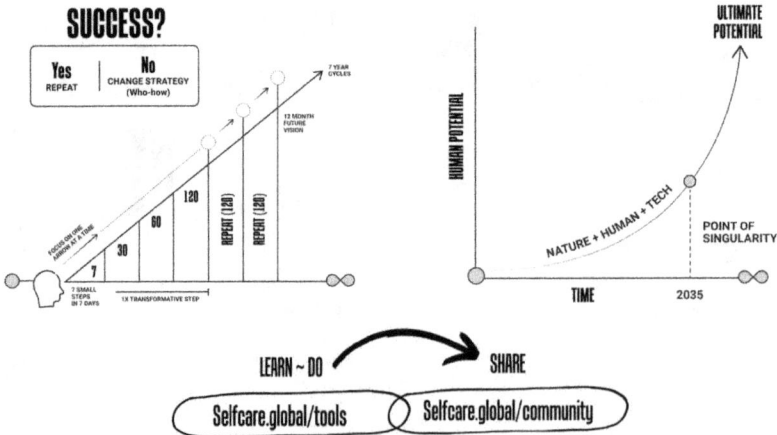

BE EMPOWERED: 8 STEPS TO EMPOWER YOUR SELFCARE REVOLUTION

1. Be evidence-based, solutions-focused: Blue Zones
2. Start with your why, an inspiring future vision: your True North
3. Create a personal and meaningful goal: What by When
4. Align your internal compass with your True North
5. Choose your normal; minimize self-harm and find a balance of healthy moderation
6. Master SelfCare and the 12 Medicines
7. Fill your cup each day and serve from overflow
8. Self-mastery, power of small and 1% growth per day.

BONUS STEP: THANKYOU, IMPACT AND RIPPLE EFFECT

Selfcare.global/courses Selfcare.global/empower

1

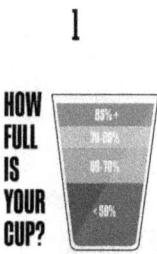

4 Zones

2

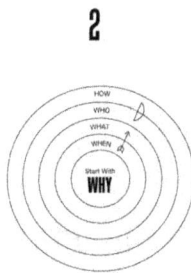

Start with Why

3

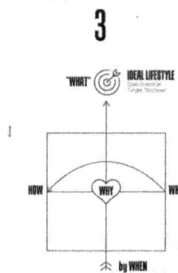

What by When?

4

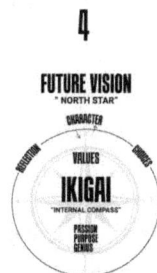

True North

5

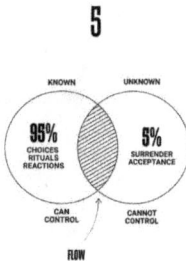

Self Harm

6

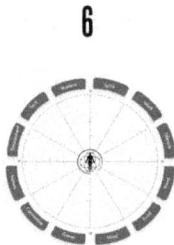

SelfCare

7

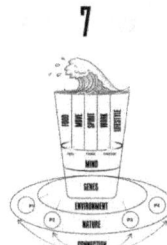

Fill Your Cup

8

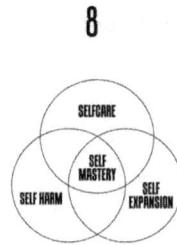

Self Mastery

STEP 1: BLUE ZONES: EVIDENCE BASED, SOLUTIONS FOCUSED

4 ZONES	100 PEOPLE
BLUE ZONE	1
GREEN ZONE	4
ORANGE ZONE	45
RED ZONE	50

IDENTIFY

1. Which of the 4 zones you are starting in? (radical responsibility)

....

....

....

....

....

2. Which zone you are moving to next?

....

....

STEP 2: START WITH WHY; AN INSPIRING FUTURE VISION: "TRUE NORTH"

Remember, you are the author of your own biological story! Choose your true north and find your own unique north star! It's something that you will be able to see and feel, even in the stormiest days.

WHAT does your ideal lifestyle look like? Why is this meaningful to you?

....

....

....

....

....

PAST EVENTS

NOW

FUTURE VISION

12 MONTHS   7 YEAR

HOW
WHO
WHAT
WHEN

Start With
WHY

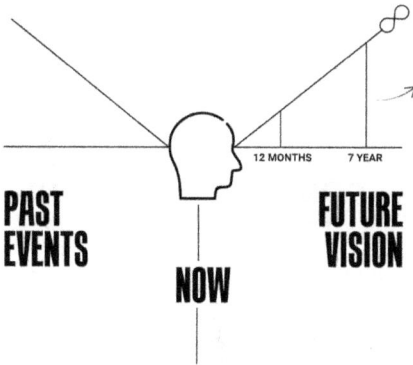

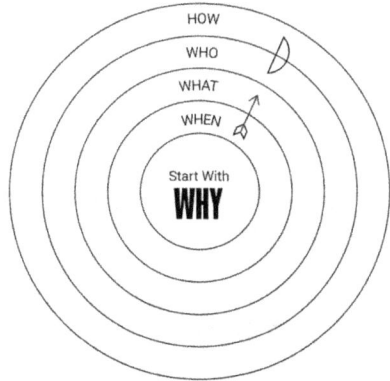

STEP 3: CREATE A MEANINGFUL GOAL "WHAT BY WHEN"

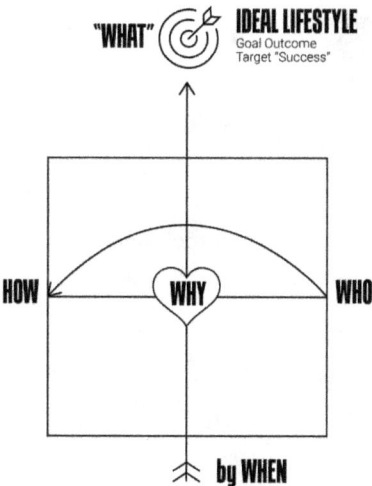

"WHAT"

IDEAL LIFESTYLE
Goal Outcome
Target "Success"

HOW   WHY   WHO

by WHEN

Remember an action without vision and clarity will leave you running in circles. So, let's get intentional. Create a goal that is meaningful to you in the context of your life right now. No comparison or self-judgment needed. This is just for you.

WHAT?

WHEN?

....

....

Link to your WHY? E.g., Run 1km–10km (what) by 25th July (when) for cancer research (why) fun run with 2 friends (who).

....

....

STEP 4: ALIGN YOUR INTERNAL COMPASS WITH YOUR TRUE NORTH

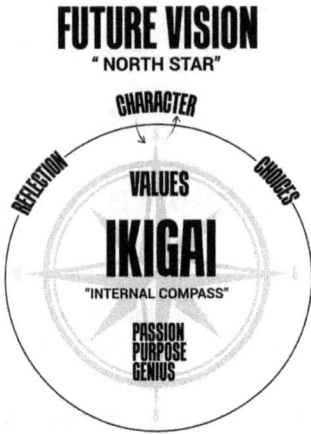

FUTURE VISION
" NORTH STAR"

CHARACTER

REFLECTION VALUES CHOICES

IKIGAI
"INTERNAL COMPASS"

PASSION
PURPOSE
GENIUS

Alignment is queen, it's the nurturing energy to the lower ego's desires. If Mother Earth has its own way of aligning itself to find balance and homeostasis, then so do you.

Compass = Values + Passion + Purpose + Unique Genius + Skills

1. What do you love to do? (Passion: when does time stand still?)

....

....

2. GENIUS: What are you naturally good at? Take the genius test tools and share you results below.

....

....

3. PURPOSE: What does the world need right now? (timing) Take the purpose test and share which of the sustainable development goals you align with most.

....

....

4. SKILLS: What is the world willing to pay you for solving? What skills do you have to do that?

....

....

5. VALUES: What do you value? Take the values test and share your top 5 values below.

....

....

....

....

....

STEP 5: SELF HARM AND HEALTHY MODERATION

HEALTHY MODERATION

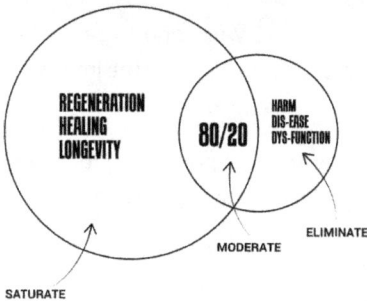

REGENERATION
HEALING
LONGEVITY

80/20

HARM
DIS-EASE
DYS-FUNCTION

ELIMINATE

MODERATE

SATURATE

Add 14 years to your life and reduce the risk of chronic preventable disease by over 80%! How? By stopping or swapping or moderating these 4 behaviors:

1. Not smoking, or at least quitting
2. Not being obese or living in a body that you feel comfortable with.
3. Move for at least half-hour a day in a way that is meaningful to you.
4. Eat more plants: fruits, vegetables, whole grains, less meat. Avoid sugar and processed "franken-foods."

What are 3 habits that you are willing to START, STOP or SWAP?

....

....

....

STEP 6: MASTER THE 12 MEDICINES OF SELFCARE

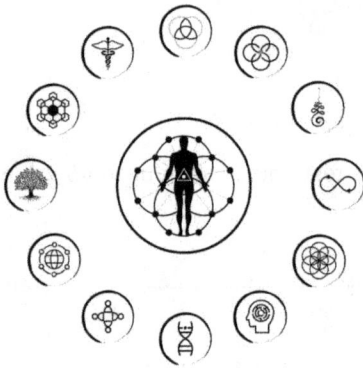

NATURE: Spend 30 minutes in nature per day. (90 min is preferable). Connect to nature's life support system every day in every way. Look after and support your front doorstep.

CONNECTION: Keep frequent connection with two people you can confide in and 5 high-vibing, like-minded people that you can grow with. Set boundaries for energy vampires. Find a mentor that shows you where to look without telling you what to see!

GENES: Find new ways to empower yourself as a "driver" not as a passenger in your life. Ignite your human potential each day with your beliefs, thoughts and daily actions. Believe that anything is possible and find stories of people that reinforce this belief.

ENVIRONMENT: Keep a record of the hours you spend in nourishing environments geographically, socially, culturally and in your home and workplace. Remember that the environment you spend the most time in is often stronger than your willpower. Limit places that you feel are toxic or negative to you.

MIND: Learn how your subconscious and conscious mind work and begin to use their power in your life. Develop a positive mental attitude and silence the imposter.

FOOD: Eat more plants! Be a compassionate omnivore and remember that every time you breathe air, drink water or eat food, you are either promoting longevity or disease and dysfunction. Choose no-compromise sources and buy from regenerative farmers.

MOVEMENT: Move that beautiful body of yours for a minimum 30 minutes per day. Motion is lotion and the healing stimulus for all your organs. Make movement meaningful and a lifestyle, rather than a chore.

WORK: Do what you love each day and you will never work a day in your life. Seek your ikigai and plan de veda and live your legacy from a passionate heart.

LIFESTYLE: Cast a positive future vision to live your ideal lifestyle and be courageous enough to live this dream in reality. Live a life worth living. Live a story worth sharing.

SPIRIT: Make time to connect with your own soul and sense of spirit each day. Live by the golden rule and dissolve any construct that creates separation. Everything is interconnected as one. If you get time to stargaze, then do so and remain curious.

MODERN: Find natural ways to support and optimize your human vessel, boost your immunity and intervene only when necessary. Use modern medicine as a tool for prevention and as a way to stay healthy and happy. Use it as a tool to support the body's natural healing mechanisms, never to replace it.

TECHNOLOGY: Use technology to free your time, monitor your health and free your location to help optimize your human experience. Limit your time on devices to less than two hours per day.

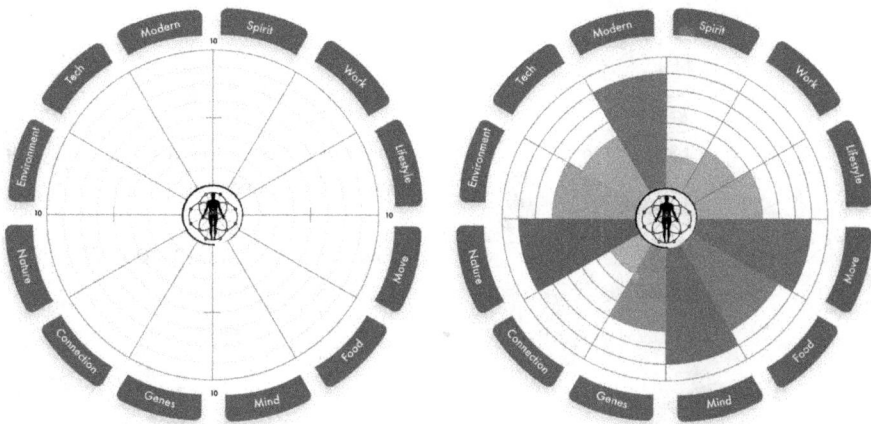

Give yourself a score from 0–100 (add them up) ....

What are your top 3 Medicines (the areas you are nourishing already)?

....

....

....

What are your bottom 3 Medicines (the areas you are currently neglecting)?

....

....

....

STEP 7: THE FILLYOURCUP METHOD

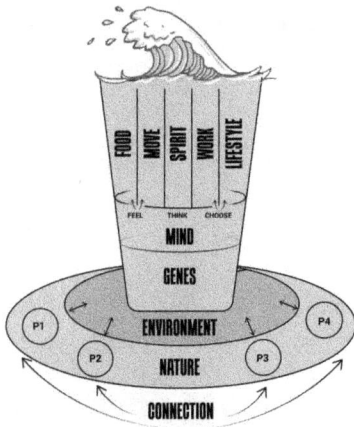

Add up your scores from the previous section "SelfCare & the 12 Medicines" quiz.
0–100 for each of 12 Medicines

....

Use these scores to DRAW and fill your own cup (get creative!)

How full is your cup (0–100%)?

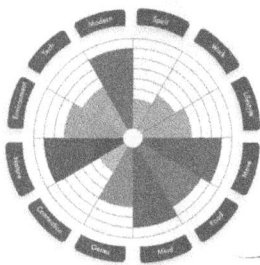

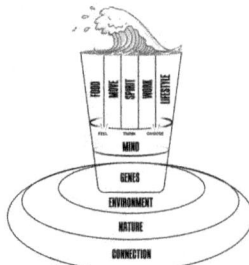

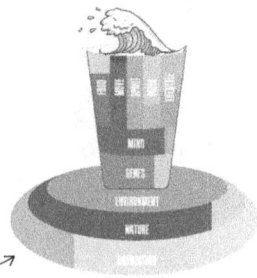

STEP 8: SELF MASTERY & MORNING RITUALS

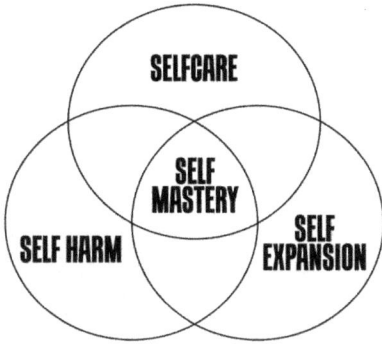

SELFCARE

SELF MASTERY

SELF HARM

SELF EXPANSION

1 HOUR MORNING MASTERY

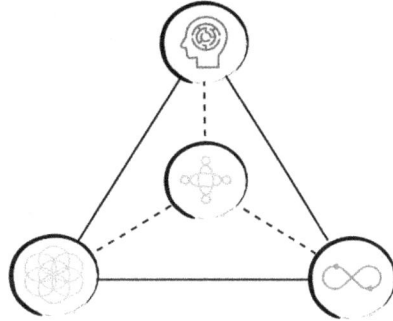

What are 3 morning rituals you would like to commit to?

1. Positive MIND (e.g., podcast, scripting, gratitude list)

2. MOVE in a meaningful way (walk, surf, run, gym, yoga)

3. FOOD (hydrate, nourish with a smoothy bowl, breathing exercises)

HOW TO MASTER YOUR MORNING IN 1 HOUR

MIND 20" Mindfullness Practice

FOOD Hydrate, Breathe, Saturate

MOVE 30" Motion is Lotion

CONNECTION
Together is better, find your tribe

THE POWER OF SMALL HABITS COMPOUNDED DAILY: 1% RULE

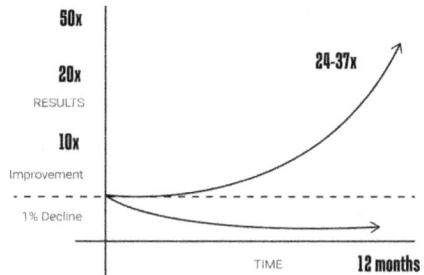

50x

24-37x

20x
RESULTS

10x
Improvement

1% Decline

TIME 12 months

THANKYOU STEP: GIVE FORWARD AND CREATE YOUR OWN RIPPLE EFFECT

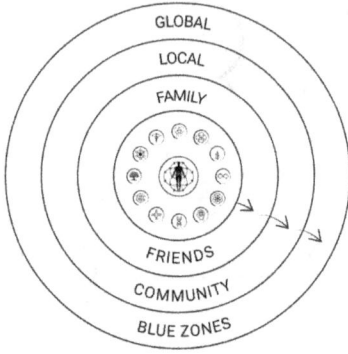

"THE RIPPLE EFFECT"

IMPACT SCALE

10,000+	GLOBAL COMMUNITY
1000	NATIONAL COMMUNITY
100	LOCAL COMMUNITY
10	FAMILY COMMUNITY
1	YOU, GO FIRST

ONE TO MANY

IF WE ALL DID JUST THIS! TOGETHER WE COULD MAKE THE WORLD WORK FOR ALL OF US!

1. Go first—Be courageous
2. Master the 12 Medicines
3. Fill your own cup every day
4. Serve from overflow
5. Create a ripple effect of positive change that starts by Impacting your own front doorstep
6. Do something good in your local community aligned with your purpose or the Sustainable Development Goals.

And here is the framework of what these 12 Medicines look like in your everyday life:

Focus on the 95% within your control.

	Out of your control (5–20%)	In your control (80–95%)
Hours in the day	x	
How you spend them		x
Your genes	x	
How your beliefs, thoughts and daily choices express them		x
Where you were born and opportunities available	x	
How you choose to lean into the opportunities available		x
The family, culture and society you were born into	x	
The 5 people you spend most of your time with		x
Your human potential	x	
What you do with it over your lifespan		x
Life's natural chaos and change	x	
Your human experience and how you act and react in any moment		x
Your age	x	
Your choices, behaviors, habits and biological age		x
Passive healthcare and "sickcare" systems	x	
Active and empowered self-care and daily lifestyle choices		x

PLAN YOUR OWN SELFCARE REVOLUTION TODAY

Nothing changes until you decide to do something different. I don't want this book to be put back on the shelf until you make a plan that is going to benefit you. Write down your PLAN for living true to you. How will you keep these natural, free and life-affirming medicines alive and growing in your life?

What Will You Decide? What Type of "Old Person" Do You Want to Be?

YOUR NAME ....

I would love to live until .... (Write the age you would like to live until).

My ideal day would be

....

....

....

....

....

....

....

To do that I will need to have a happy, healthy and connected human vessel. I will do this by making an agreement with myself to grow just 1% per day, focusing on being better than who I was yesterday.

HEALING WITH THE 12 MEDICINES

Your body has innate wisdom for healing, regeneration and even your human potential. Think of this...the moment your body gets cut or hurt; the body goes into instant self-repair mode. It has a huge capacity to regenerate; it is designed to fight and repair disease and illness. Naturally, we don't always "win" the fight against some diseases or illnesses, but I believe if we can enhance our natural immunity, our overall wellness, adapt to be more resilient—then we can increase our capacity to heal and rejuvenate.

By using the 12 Medicines (alongside whatever else you need to do medically) you can put the body in a receptive state for repair and one day, an inner sense of harmony; mentally, physically, biologically and even emotionally.

Now, don't get me wrong, I'm not offering quackery or new-age methods that have no science backing. I am talking about the natural innate building blocks your body already has. It's surprising that many people don't even know how amazing their bodies are. That's all this book is. A reminder to trust yourself. Trust your bodies innate wisdom and do everything you can to support it, so that it continues to do its job with ease and flow.

I'd like to offer you a ***FREE chapter on Healing With the 12 Medicines.***

You can begin your own healing revolution too. I'm so blessed to be surrounded by some incredible people who are experts in this subject, and I also get the chance to interview many leading changemakers about our ability to lead happy, healthy lives free from the pitfalls of modern-day ailments. Throughout my years of working as an allied healthcare practitioner, I have seen so many perplexing and often paradoxical situations. The monk I mentioned at the beginning of this book dying from a cowardly unprovoked punch to the head; countless young people with everything to live for suffering from depression and anxiety; people who were "supposed" to die miraculously recovering from late-stage cancer.

Healing and rejuvenation are complex and multi-faceted topics filled with many breakthroughs and many opportunities for further breakthroughs. Let's be honest, most of us now know someone who has died from cancer, heart disease or lives with chronic physical or mental health conditions. I know many. And it's because of this that I am burning with a passion to find new ways, to help adjust our collective focus to empower our wellness and wellbeing and collapse old paradigms that perhaps don't serve us anymore.

I believe we are creating a new paradigm of healthcare, with SelfCare as a foundation. Sure, we don't have all the answers yet, but one thing is for certain, we mustn't sit idle and believe our health will be handed to us on a silver platter or in a magic longevity pill.

Some people's healing stories already break the old paradigm. Harvard-trained and published neuroanatomist, Dr Jill Bolte Taylor is one such paradigm-shifter. Her revealing and fascinating story about how she suffered from a severe stroke and took eight years to rebuild her brain, often in the most surprising ways, highlights the opportunities still available to us when we combine science, healing, nature's life support system, community support and nourishing environments.

The opportunities for us to live longer, healthier, happier lives is abundant, and I believe we are part of the leading-edge pioneering movement to BE THE CHANGE we want to see in this generation, for future generations.

SO, WHAT DO YOU WANT TO SEE FOR THE FUTURE GENERATIONS?

I believe in a world where people live without the burden of chronic pain, suffering and disease. I want to run and play with my future kids and grandkids and hear their laughs and watch their somersaults and cartwheels.

Max Planck said, "A new scientific truth does not triumph by convincing its opponents and making them see the light, but rather because its opponents eventually die, and a new generation grows up that is familiar with it."[1] Wouldn't it be even better if we didn't have to wait for the next generation to do it for us. What if we didn't have to die off and wait for new paradigms to be lived out in our wake. Let's trailblaze a world where health isn't complex and full of prescriptions but full of natural wellbeing and joy.

LET'S 10X OUR IMPACT!

Before I say *thank you* for taking the time to read this book, I would like to ask you a favor. Would you like to help us 10x our collective impact? Here are some ideas below (but don't let this dampen your innate and unique creativity).

IMPACT SCALE

10,000 +	GLOBAL COMMUNITY
1000	NATIONAL COMMUNITY
100	LOCAL COMMUNITY
10	FAMILY COMMUNITY
1	YOU, GO FIRST

ONE TO MANY

IF WE ALL DID JUST THIS! TOGETHER WE COULD MAKE THE WORLD WORK FOR ALL OF US!

SOCIETY

5.0	AGE OF ... ?
4.0	INFORMATION AGE
3.0	INDUSTRIAL AGE
2.0	AGRARIAN
1.0	HUNTER/GATHERER

What type of legacy do we want to live? What type of world do we want to hand to future generations? This is our final exam as Buckminster Fuller described it; "Humanity is taking its final examination. We have come to an extraordinary moment when it doesn't have to be you or me. There is enough for all. We need not operate competitively any longer. If we succeed, it will be because of youth, truth and love."

What will you decide? Would you like to be the change that we all hope and wish for, or do we continue to run off the edge of the cliff together towards the 6th mass extinction and lifestyles that would require four earths to sustain us? I will go first, with you.

1. Take a photo with *SelfCare* in the favorite place that you read it. Tag us and share it on your favorite social media channel. We would love to see where this consciousness reaches!
2. Invite 10 people that you care about into the SelfCare online communities with permission.

3. Once you finish reading the book, pay it forward to someone else. If you want to gift it to them and keep your copy, then feel free to do so too.
4. If you have any other ideas, we are open to them...reach out.

For anyone that helps us get this message out there, we will continue to create a giving impact on your behalf. I am also inspired to give gifts and opportunities to join our courses and retreats to anyone that wishes to help us 10x our collective impact. I would rather give that value to you than social media marketing algorithms. I hope to show the power of value, solutions and human beings helping each other. I am open to receive any support that is out there. This book is not about me, it's about you and the people you care about. Let's thrive together!

TO CONNECT WITH RORY GO TO: **selfcare.global**

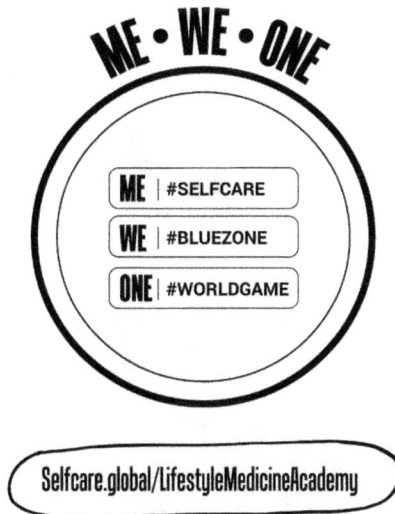

ME • WE • ONE

ME | #SELFCARE
WE | #BLUEZONE
ONE | #WORLDGAME

Selfcare.global/LifestyleMedicineAcademy

WOULD YOU LIKE TO JOIN OUR LIFESTYLE MEDICINE COACHING ACADEMY?

Are you a......

- Health, well-being or lifestyle medicine professional who would love to apply these SelfCare frameworks into your patient care?
- Health and wellness coach, ambassador or influencer that would like to magnify these frameworks and add value to your networks and customers?
- Health, wellbeing and.or lifestyle-based business owner who would like to integrate these frameworks into your workplace or your business models, workshops and retreats? Knowing that healthy and happier staff are more productive.

- Health and wellbeing enthusiast or simply a curious soul that would love to learn how to use the SelfCare frameworks in your family or community?
- APPLY to be an accredited Lifestyle Medicine Practitioner orSelfCare coach in the link on the previous page.
- The numbers are limited, but we have unique "smart contracts" that enable you to share and circulate your spot once you have learned, embodied and become empowered to utilize and integrate all of the frameworks shared. We understand that this has always been a WE game, not just a me game. Help us have a bigger impact!

ABOUT THE AUTHOR

FACILITATOR | ALLIED INTEGRATED HEALTH CONSULTANT | SOCIAL ENTREPRENEUR

Rory is an author, speaker, health futurist, digital nomad, and Allied Health professional based in Bali "the island of the gods." He takes a "big picture" approach to good health and wellbeing and has a passion for helping people ignite their human potential and optimize their human experience.

He decided to create **selfcare.global** as a platform to help people help themselves: reminding everyone that our human vessels have the amazing innate wisdom to thrive, not just survive. He believes that we don't need to be fixed by gurus or expensive coaches/consultations; we simply need to be nourished by healthy environments and connected as communities (Blue Zones). In the same way, it takes a village to raise a child, it takes a community to heal the sick and thrive together.

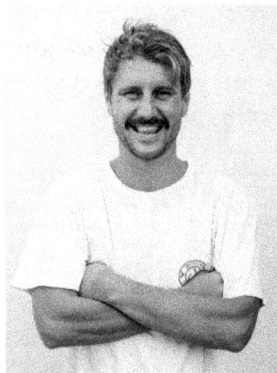

Click on the link below to subscribe and receive Rory's weekly lifestyle medicine tools, tips, stories and frameworks.

rorycallaghan.com

He uses the #fillyourcup method as a way to help people fill their own cup with daily self-care rituals that empower each individual to learn, do and embody so they too can serve from abundant

357

overflow. He advocates for empowering others to create a ripple effect of positive social impact starting at their front door.

By empowering people to go first, he hopes to inspire them to influence their proximity to family and friends. Rory believes that if we each had the courage to go first and impact our local community, together, we could create a ripple effect that changes the world.

Rory hopes to help people raise their individual and collective consciousness so that we can co-create a world that is healthy, happy and connected. He imagines a world where good health and wellbeing is a human right for all people, not just some. Where we all live as global #bluezone communities connected as one. #wemeone

This is more than just a book! selfcare.global

Rory has created an online SelfCare ecosystem and community that you can engage and interact with as you read this book.

He envisioned everyone, anywhere with Wi-Fi, having access to empowering SelfCare education, tools, resources, mentors and a real community with real people on a similar journey together.

Behind the scenes: **deanpublishing.com/selfcare**

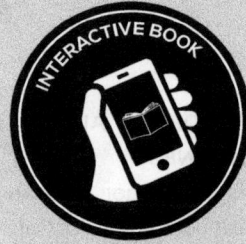

CAN I ASK A FAVOR?

If anything in this book or platform has helped you on your personal journey, would it be okay if you take two minutes and write a review? We value honesty, trust and transparency. Plus, we would genuinely love to hear your feedback and whether this has had an impact in your life. Click on the REVIEW tab and by doing so, you will help us impact more people. Lastly, if you love the vision and values of this movement and are called to reach out to us, there is an opportunity to grow with us and even work with us. We are open to all good people, ideas and ways that we can help more people. Click on the GROW tab if you feel called.

Selfcare.global/review   Selfcare.global/grow

ACKNOWLEGMENTS

Throughout history it has become a collective realization that none of us got to where we are right now, alone. It took a community (a village) to raise us as a child. I am grateful for every single person in my life that has nourished, supported, challenged and inspired me to give this gift to the world. Let's do this together! We were never meant to go this path alone.

I would love to acknowledge my family (Mum, Dad, my brother, aunties, uncles, nieces and nephews). You have been "my why," this whole time. When I wanted to give up on the project and throw in the towel, I thought of all of you.

To my friends and the local community in Fremantle "Freo" and the south west of Australia; thank you for everything. Truly. Home is where my young mind and heart was nourished and supported. You gave me the opportunity to do this, and in many ways I felt that it was my duty to ensure that I finished it.

To my global family and friends in Bali and beyond. Thank you for guiding me through the depths and successes as I sought out the mentors and the consciousness that was needed to curate this book. SelfCare is a lesson that I too needed to first learn (and am still learning!) so that I could share this with you.

To all the people that I have crossed paths with, whether it was for a simple reason, a season, or a lifetime: thank you for the lessons and shared experiences.

You made me realize what life is truly about. As Professor R.C. Henry, from Johns Hopkins University said, "A fundamental conclusion of the new physics also acknowledges that the observer creates the reality. As observers, we are personally involved with the creation of our own reality. Physicists are being forced to admit that the universe is a 'mental' construction." I honour this realization.

To everyone that helped me bring this book to life: Natalie, Susan and Jazmine (Dean Publishing) , Paul Dunn (mentor), Jampal and Mic (@saltywings), Lo who became a senior editor and anyone that joined or supported this journey along the way. Those small messages along the way, meant the world to me and kept me going. I can't express in words how grateful I am.

In 1159, John Salisbury wrote *Metalogicon* and shared that, "We are like dwarfs sitting on the shoulders of giants. We see more, and things that are more distant than they did, not because our sight is superior or because we are taller than they, but because they raise us up, and by their great stature add to ours."

To everyone that has shared their wisdom over the centuries. Thank you for helping shape the human consciousness and collective mind-stream of energy. These thoughts are not simply my own, they are ours.

Johann Wolfgang von Goethe reminded me that "All truly wise thoughts have been thought already thousands of times; but to make them truly ours, we must think them over again honestly, until they take root in our personal experience."

To the scientists and evidence-based health professionals quoted in this book and to those working behind the scenes to do their best to support our community health and wellbeing: I thank you. This is for us and the people we are driven to help and serve. Let's seek solutions and explore the unknown together, as Donald Rumsfeld shared, "The absence of evidence is not evidence of absence, or vice versa." We have a world of unknowns to explore together.

To all the individuals working tirelessly behind the scenes. To the light workers illuminating the darkness; I see you and thank you. Let's keep going. We are just getting started. The world needs you more now than ever. As Helen Keller reminded us —"We live by each other and for each other. Alone we can do so little. Together we can do so much."

To the future leaders, innovators and change-makers. Use this to inspire and ignite your journey and bring your unique insights and passions into the world.

This for you and the people you care about. Free medicine for the people!

Selfcare.global/Impact

We have created an IMPACT on your behalf, simply by being here! That's our way of saying thank you. If you would like to do something nice for someone else, the book link is below too. Feel free to give this book to someone else, or use that link to send a copy to someone who may need this message right now.

Selfcare.global/book

REFERENCES

THE MEANING AND THE MISSION

1   True Health Initiative, accessed online 29 November 2021, https://www.truehealthinitiative.org

2   Katz, D. L., Frates, E. P., Bonnet, J. P., Gupta, S. K., Vartiainen, E., & Carmona, R. H. (2018). "Lifestyle as Medicine: The Case for a True Health Initiative." *American journal of health promotion : AJHP, 32*(6), 1452–1458. https://doi.org/10.1177/0890117117705949

INTRODUCTION

1   Adapted from The State of the Village Report, original version by Donella H. Meadows. https://thevillage.org

2   Clinton Global Initiative, "Empowering Girls & Women." Accessed online December 3 2020. https://www.un.org/en/ecosoc/phlntrpy/notes/clinton.pdf

CHAPTER 1

1   Campbell, Joseph, 1904–1987, Phil. Cousineau and Stuart L. Brown. 1990. *The Hero's Journey: The World of Joseph Campbell : Joseph Campbell On His Life and Work.* San Francisco: Harper & Row.

CHAPTER 2

1   https://mokokoma.com

2   Alexander, Bruce K. Professor Emeritus, Simon Fraser University (2010) "Addiction:

The View from Rat Park," available from https://www.brucekalexander.com/%20 articlesspeeches/rat-park/148-addiction-the-view-from-rat-park

Alexander, Bruce K. "Towards Controlling the Drugs and Alcohol Problem in Scotland: Going Up the Down Staircase. " Available from http://www.brucekalexander.com/ articles-speeches/treatmentarecovery/216-scotland-aberdour-1

Alexander, B.K. *The Globalization of Addiction: A study in poverty of the spirit*, Oxford Univ. Press, 2010.

3   Hyman, Mark Dr. The Doctor's Farmacy with Mark Hyman, M.D. [podcast] "The Most Important Medicine for your Health and Longevity with Radha Agrawal." https:// podcasts.apple.com/us/podcast/most-important-medicine-for-your-health-longevity-radha/id1382804627?i=1000423382942

4   Hari, Johann. Ted Global London. TED.com. "Everything you think you know about addiction wrong." Accessed June 2nd 2021.
https://www.ted.com/talks/johann_hari_everything_you_think_you_know_about_addiction_is_wrong/transcript?language=en

5   Cohen, Peter (1990), Table of contents. In: Peter Cohen (1990), *Drugs as a social construct*. Dissertation. Amsterdam, Universiteit van Amsterdam. pp. I–IV. Accessed http://www.cedro-uva.org/lib/cohen.drugs.toc.html

CHAPTER 3

1   Silicon Valley Historical Association, "Steve Jobs Secrets of Life," Oct 6, 2011, YouTube. https://www.youtube.com/watch?v=kYfNvmF0Bqw

2   What Is Epigenetics. Website accessed 3rd December 2020. https://www. whatisepigenetics.com

3   Palagini, L., Biber, K., & Riemann, D. (2014). "The genetics of insomnia--evidence for epigenetic mechanisms?" *Sleep medicine reviews*, 18(3), 225–235. https://doi. org/10.1016/j.smrv.2013.05.002

4   Sleiman, S. F., Henry, J., Al-Haddad, R., El Hayek, L., Abou Haidar, E., Stringer, T., Ulja, D., Karuppagounder, S. S., Holson, E. B., Ratan, R. R., Ninan, I., & Chao, M. V. (2016). "Exercise promotes the expression of brain derived neurotrophic factor (BDNF) through the action of the ketone body ß-hydroxybutyrate." *eLife*, 5, e15092. https:// doi.org/10.7554/eLife.15092

5   Iradj Sobhani, Emma Bergsten, Séverine Couffin, Aurélien Amiot, Biba Nebbad, Caroline Barau, Nicola de'Angelis, Sylvie Rabot, Florence Canoui-Poitrine, Denis Mestivier, Thierry Pédron, Khashayarsha Khazaie, Philippe J. Sansonetti. "Colorectal cancer-associated microbiota contributes to oncogenic epigenetic signatures." *Proceedings of the National Academy of Sciences*, 2019; 201912129 DOI: 10.1073/ pnas.1912129116

6   Global Burden of Disease Study 2013 Collaborators (2015). "Global, regional, and national incidence, prevalence, and years lived with disability for 301 acute and chronic diseases and injuries in 188 countries, 1990–2013: a systematic analysis

for the Global Burden of Disease Study 2013." *Lancet (London, England)*, 386(9995), 743–800. https://doi.org/10.1016/S0140-6736(15)60692-4

CHAPTER 4

1   Armenta, Christina N., Megan M. Fritz, and Sonja Lyubomirsky. "Functions of Positive Emotions: Gratitude as a Motivator of Self-Improvement and Positive Change." *Emotion Review 9*, no. 3 (July 2017): 183–90. https://doi.org/10.1177/1754073916669596

2   Csikszentmihalyi, Mihaly (1990). "Flow: The Psychology of Optimal Experience." New York: Harper and Row. p.4. https://www.researchgate.net/publication/224927532_Flow_The_Psychology_of_Optimal_Experience

3   SAVE — Suicide Awareness Voices of Education, "Suicide Facts," https://save.org/about-suicide/suicide-facts

4   Maslow, A.H. (1943). "A theory of human motivation." *Psychological Review.* 50 (4): 370–6. CiteSeerX 10.1.1.334.7586. doi:10.1037/h0054346 – via psychclassics.yorku.ca.

5   Frankl, Victor (1992). *Man's Search for Meaning.* (4th ed.). Boston, MA: Beacon Press.

6   Frankl 1992, p. 143.

7   Baumeister, Roy & Vohs, Kathleen & Garbinsky, Emily. (2012). "Some Key Differences between a Happy Life and a Meaningful Life." *The Journal of Positive Psychology.* 8. 10.2139/ssrn.2168436.

8   Ibid.

9   Ibid.

CHAPTER 5

1   WHO (1946) Preamble to the Constitution of the World Health Organization. WHO, New York, USA

2   World Health Organization, The Ottawa Charter for Health Promotion. First International Conference on Health Promotion, Ottawa, 21 November 1986. https://www.who.int/healthpromotion/conferences/previous/ottawa/en

3   McKinley Health Center—Illinois. Online post: "Understanding Wellness." Accessed December 2020. https://www.mckinley.illinois.edu/health-education/wellness

4   Pozhitkov, A. E., Neme, R., Domazet-Lošo, T., Leroux, B. G., Soni, S., Tautz, D., & Noble, P. A. (2017). "Tracing the dynamics of gene transcripts after organismal death." *Open biology*, 7(1), 160267. https://doi.org/10.1098/rsob.160267

5   Australian Institute of Health and Welfare 2016. *Australia's health 2016.* Australia's health series no. 15. Cat. no. AUS 199. Canberra: AIHW.

6   The Lancet, Global Burden of Disease (GBD) Resource Centre, https://www.thelancet.com/gbd

7   Karma-gliṅ-pa, Padma Sambhava, Gyurme Dorje, Graham Coleman, and Thupten

Jinpa. 2005. *The Tibetan book of the dead (English title): the great liberation by hearing in the intermediate states (Tibetan title)*. London: Penguin, pp.

8 Coleman, Graham. *The Tibetan Book of the Dead: First Complete Translation (Penguin Classics) Kindle Edition*, 6 November 2008, Penguin

9 The World Bank, Data: "Mortality rate, under-5 (per 1,000 live births)" [online], https://data.worldbank.org/indicator/SH.DYN.MORT
Estimates developed by the UN Inter-agency Group for Child Mortality Estimation (UNICEF, WHO, World Bank, UN DESA Population Division) at childmortality.org

10 World Health Organization (WHO), 9 December 2020, "The top ten causes of death." https://www.who.int/news-room/fact-sheets/detail/the-top-10-causes-of-death

11 Ibid.

12 Scully J. L. (2004) "What is a disease?" *EMBO reports*, 5(7), 650–653. https://doi.org/10.1038/sj.embor.7400195

13 Max Roser and Hannah Ritchie (2016 "Burden of Disease." Published online at OurWorldInData.org. Retrieved from: 'https://ourworldindata.org/burden-of-disease' [Online Resource]

14 Ibid.

15 World Health Organization (WHO), "Noncommunicable diseases," 13 April 2021, accessed June 3, 2021, https://www.who.int/news-room/fact-sheets/detail/noncommunicable-diseases

16 Max Roser and Hannah Ritchie (2016 "Burden of Disease." Published online at OurWorldInData.org. Retrieved from: 'https://ourworldindata.org/burden-of-disease' [Online Resource]

17 Ford, E. S., Bergmann, M. M., Kröger, J., Schienkiewitz, A., Weikert, C., & Boeing, H. (2009) "Healthy living is the best revenge: findings from the European Prospective Investigation Into Cancer and Nutrition-Potsdam study." *Archives of internal medicine*, 169(15), 1355–1362.

18 Liu L, Johnson HL, Cousens S, Perin J, Scott S, Lawn JE, Rudan I, Campbell H, Cibulskis R, Li M, Mathers C, Black RE; Child Health Epidemiology Reference Group of WHO and UNICEF. "Global, regional, and national causes of child mortality: an updated systematic analysis for 2010 with time trends since 2000." *External Lancet.* 2012;379(9832):2151-61.

19 Centers for Disease Control and Prevention, "Global Diarrhea Burden: Diarrhea: Common Illness, Global Killer." https://www.cdc.gov/healthywater/global/diarrhea-burden.html#one

20 https://drhyman.com

21 Scully J. L. (2004) "What is a disease?" *EMBO reports*, 5(7), 650–653. https://doi.org/10.1038/sj.embor.7400195

22 World Health Organization (WHO), "Mental health" https://www.who.int/mental_health/management/depression/daly/en

23 GBD 2016 Disease and Injury Incidence and Prevalence Collaborators (2017). "Global,

regional, and national incidence, prevalence, and years lived with disability for 328 diseases and injuries for 195 countries, 1990–2016: a systematic analysis for the Global Burden of Disease Study 2016." *Lancet* (London, England), 390(10100), 1211–1259. https://doi.org/10.1016/S0140-6736(17)32154-2

24 GBD 2016 Disease and Injury Incidence and Prevalence Collaborators (2017). "Global, regional, and national incidence, prevalence, and years lived with disability for 328 diseases and injuries for 195 countries, 1990–2016: a systematic analysis for the Global Burden of Disease Study 2016." *Lancet* (London, England), 390(10100), 1211–1259. https://doi.org/10.1016/S0140-6736(17)32154-2

25 Ibid.

26 Scafoglieri, Aldo, and Jan Pieter Clarys. "Dual energy X-ray absorptiometry: gold standard for muscle mass?." *Journal of cachexia, sarcopenia and muscle* vol. 9,4 (2018): 786–787.

27 Mayo Clinic. "Hyperglycemia in diabetes", [online], accessed June 3 2021. https://www.mayoclinic.org/diseases-conditions/hyperglycemia/symptoms-causes/syc-20373631

28 Davis, Kathleen. Medical News Today, Medically reviewed by Dr. Payal Kohli, M.D., FACC — (July 15, 2019) "What to know about hyperlipidemia." Accessed June 2 2021, https://www.medicalnewstoday.com/articles/295385

29 World Health Organization, 13 April 2021, "Noncommunicable diseases." https://www.who.int/news-room/fact-sheets/detail/noncommunicable-diseases

30 OECD Better Life Index, "Health" accessed online June 3, 2021. http://www.oecdbetterlifeindex.org/topics/health

31 Ibid.

32 GBD 2016 Disease and Injury Incidence and Prevalence Collaborators (2017). "Global, regional, and national incidence, prevalence, and years lived with disability for 328 diseases and injuries for 195 countries, 1990–2016: a systematic analysis for the Global Burden of Disease Study 2016." *Lancet (London, England)*, 390(10100), 1211–1259. https://doi.org/10.1016/S0140-6736(17)32154-2

33 Ibid.

34 Statista "Global health – Statistics & Facts" (November 12 2020), accessed Jun 3 2021. https://www.statista.com/topics/4274/global-health

35 The World Bank, Data, "Population ages 80 and above." https://data.worldbank.org/indicator/SP.POP.80UP.MA.5Y

36 WorldAtlas, "Countries with the most centurians." https://www.worldatlas.com/articles/countries-with-the-most-centenarians.html

37 Ibid.

38 Guinness World Records. "Guinness World Records News." Published online 27 February 2013. Accessed February 2020. https://www.guinnessworldrecords.com/news/2013/2/japans-misao-okawa-confirmed-as-oldest-living-woman-aged-114-years-359-days-47249

39 Guinness World Records. "Guinness World Records News." Published online 31 March 2020. https://www.guinnessworldrecords.com/news/2020/3/englishman-bob-weighton-confirmed-as-the-worlds-oldest-man-living-at-112-years-o-613615

CHAPTER 6

1 The Sloan Digital Sky Survey, SDSS, "The Elements of Life Mapped Across the Milky Way by SDSS/APOGEE." Published online January 5 2017. Accessed February 2020. https://www.sdss.org/press-releases/the-elements-of-life-mapped-across-the-milky-way-by-sdssapogee

2 David, Bohm. *Wholeness and the Implicate Order* (Routledge & Kegan Paul, London, 1980; Ark, London, 1983). It reproduces Bohm's articles in *Found. Phys.* 1, 111 (1971) and *Found. Phys.* 3, 139 (1973). See in this context also D. Bohm, "Quantum theory as an indication of a new order in physics," in: *Rendiconti della Scuola Internazionale di Fisica "Enrico Fermi," Course 49, Foundations of Quantum Mechanics*, B. D'Espagnat, ed. (Academic Press, New York, 1971).

3 Lovelock, J. E. (1989), "Geophysiology, the science of Gaia." *Rev. Geophys.*, 27(2), 215–222, doi:10.1029/RG027i002p00215.

CHAPTER 7

1 Johnson, Ian. *The Independent.* "What is the human body made of?" Published online Friday 05 August 2016, retrieved December 2020. https://www.independent.co.uk/news/science/what-human-body-made-a7173301.html

2 Ibid.

3 Liana Fasching, Yeongjun Jang, Simone Tomasi, Jeremy Schreiner, Livia Tomasini, Melanie V. Brady, Taejeong Bae, Vivekananda Sarangi, Nikolaos Vasmatzis, Yifan Wang, Anna Szekely, Thomas V. Fernandez, James F. Leckman, Alexej Abyzov, Flora M. Vaccarino. "Early developmental asymmetries in cell lineage trees in living individuals." *Science,* 2021 DOI: 10.1126/science.abe0981

4 Mokili, John L et al. "Metagenomics and future perspectives in virus discovery." *Current opinion in virology* vol. 2,1 (2012): 63–77. doi:10.1016/j.coviro.2011.12.004

5 Cobian Guemes, A. "EXPLORING THE GLOBAL VIROME AND DECIPHERING THE ROLE OF PHAGES IN CYSTIC FIBROSIS." *UC San Diego.* (2019). ProQuest ID: CobianGuemes_ucsd_0033D_18986. Merritt ID: ark:/13030/m5wh7x7k. Retrieved from https://escholarship.org/uc/item/1103w639

6 Nature [article], 08 MAY 2019, "These 19 viruses live in human lungs and mouths." https://www.nature.com/articles/d41586-019-01470-6

7 Ed Yong, https://edyong.me/i-contain-multitudes

8 Chopra, Deepak. Tanzi, Rudolph. *Super Genes: Unlock the Astonishing Power of Your DNA for Optimum Health and Well-Being.* (10 November 2015) Harmony; 1st edition.

9   Segerstrom, Suzanne C, and Gregory E Miller. "Psychological stress and the human immune system: a meta-analytic study of 30 years of inquiry." *Psychological bulletin* vol. 130,4 (2004): 601-30. doi:10.1037/0033-2909.130.4.601

10 CK12.org, "The Smarter Way to Learn", [online] https://www.ck12.org/book/ck-12-biology-advanced-concepts/section/17.3

CHAPTER 8

1   Stony Brook University. "New research of oldest light confirms age of the universe." ScienceDaily. www.sciencedaily.com/releases/2020/07/200715170541.htm (accessed December 2, 2021).

2   National Geographic Research Library Collection, "The Age of the Earth" [online] National Geographic. https://www.nationalgeographic.org/topics/resource-library-age-earth/?q=&page=1&per_page=25

3   Ibid.

4   California Academy of Sciences. "Landmark study on the evolution of insects." ScienceDaily. www.sciencedaily.com/releases/2014/11/141106143709.htm (accessed December 2, 2021).

5   Malaspinas, AS., Westaway, M., Muller, C. et al. "A genomic history of Aboriginal Australia." *Nature* 538, 207–214 (2016). https://doi.org/10.1038/nature18299

6   Max Roser, Esteban Ortiz-Ospina and Hannah Ritchie (2013) - "Life Expectancy." Published online at OurWorldInData.org. Retrieved from: https://ourworldindata.org/life-expectancy

7   Parry, Wyne, September 19, 2013, "How Much Longer Can Earth Support Life?" Live Science @ Livescience.com, https://www.livescience.com/39775-how-long-can-earth-support-life.html

8   Strawson, Galen. *The Guardian*. "Sapiens: A Brief History of Humankind by Yuval Noah Harari – review." Published online Thursday 11 September 2014. Retrieved December 2020. https://www.theguardian.com/books/2014/sep/11/sapiens-brief-history-humankind-yuval-noah-harari-review

9   Malaspinas, A. S., Westaway, M. C., Muller, C., Sousa, V. C., Lao, O., Alves, I., Bergström, A., Athanasiadis, G., Cheng, J. Y., Crawford, J. E., Heupink, T. H., Macholdt, E., Peischl, S., Rasmussen, S., Schiffels, S., Subramanian, S., Wright, J. L., Albrechtsen, A., Barbieri, C., Dupanloup, I., ... Willerslev, E. (2016). "A genomic history of Aboriginal Australia." *Nature*, 538(7624), 207–214. https://doi.org/10.1038/nature18299

10 Joy of Museums Virtual Tour, Australian Aboriginal Sayings, retrieved online Dec 2020. https://joyofmuseums.com/museums/australasia-museums/australian-museums/australian-aboriginal-sayings-quotes

11 Ibid.

12 Djiniyini, Terry. "The Land Is My Mother." *Aboriginal and Islander Health Worker Journal9*, no. 2 (July 1985): 6–7. https://search.informit.org/doi/10.3316/

ielapa.096141427116198.

13 Dispenza, Joe. 2015. *You are the placebo: making your mind matter*, Carlsbad, California : Hay House.

14 Hirshkowitz, M., Whiton, K., Albert, S. M., Alessi, C., Bruni, O., DonCarlos, L., Hazen, N., Herman, J., Katz, E. S., Kheirandish-Gozal, L., Neubauer, D. N., O'Donnell, A. E., Ohayon, M., Peever, J., Rawding, R., Sachdeva, R. C., Setters, B., Vitiello, M. V., Ware, J. C., & Adams Hillard, P. J. (2015). National Sleep Foundation's sleep time duration recommendations: methodology and results summary. *Sleep health*, 1(1), 40–43. https://doi.org/10.1016/j.sleh.2014.12.010

CHAPTER 9

1 Poulain M, Pes GM, Grasland C, et al. "Identification of a geographic area characterized by extreme longevity in the Sardinia island: the AKEA study." *Experimental Gerontology*. 2004;39(9):1423–1429.

2 "Longevity, The Secrets of Long Life." *National Geographic Magazine*. November 2005.

3 Buettner, Dan (21 April 2009) [2008]. "Contents". *The Blue Zones: Lessons for Living Longer From the People Who've Lived the Longest* (First Paperback ed.). Washington, D.C.: National Geographic. p. vii. ISBN 978-1-4262- 0400-5. OCLC 246886564. Retrieved 15 September 2009.

CHAPTER 10

1 Blue Zones®Bluezones.com "Blue Zones Project Results." Published online, retrieved Dec 2020. https://www.bluezones.com/blue-zones-project-results/#beach-cities-ca

2 Ibid.

3 Senthilingam, M. (2018, March) CNN News. https://www.cnn.com/2018/03/02/health/hong-kong-world-longest-life-expectancy-longevity-intl/index.html

4 Ibid.

5 HKJC Centre for Suicide Research and Prevention, HKU *Provisional figures for 2018 (registration death date up to 31 Jul 2019) https://csrp.hku.hk/statistics

6 Ibid.

7 Catsnake (catsnake.com) "Secrets of Food Marketing." https://catsnake.com/our-videos/compassion-in-world-farming

CHAPTER 11

1 *Time Magazine*. "This Baby Could Live to 142 Years Old." February 12, 2015. https://time.com/3706775/in-the-latest-issue-23

2   World Health Organization. The Global Health Observatory. "Global Health Estimates: Life expectancy and leading causes of death and disability." Published online. https://www.who.int/data/gho/data/themes/mortality-and-global-health-estimates

3   Clark, William. *A Means to an End: The Biological Basis of Aging and Death.* New York: Oxford University Press, 1999. Pp. 234. Material sourced @ Martin, George M.. "A Means to an End: The Biological Basis of Aging and Death." *American Journal of Human Genetics* vol. 65,5 (1999): 1477–1478.

4   Jerry W. Shay, Woodring E. Wright. "Senescence and immortalization: role of telomeres and telomerase." *Carcinogenesis*, Volume 26, Issue 5, May 2005, Pages 867–874, https://doi.org/10.1093/carcin/bgh296

5   Hekimi Lab — http://hekimilab.mcgill.ca

6   Montgomery, Mark. Radio Canada International. "How long is the potential life expectancy of humans?" July 4, 2017. https://www.rcinet.ca/en/2017/07/04/how-long-is-the-potential-life-expectancy-of-humans

7   Gregor, Michael. "How to Protect Our Telomeres with Diet." April 26th, 2016. https://nutritionfacts.org/2016/04/26/how-to-protect-our-telomeres-with-diet

8   Glassman, Alanna. *Chatelaine.* "How to live to 100 years old as shared by a centenarian." Published online September 11, 2014. https://www.chatelaine.com/health/how-to-live-to-100-years-old-as-shared-by-a-centenarian

9   Kahan, Scott. Blog post — "Genes load the gun, environment pulls the trigger." Published online October 18 2010. http://scottkahan.com/genes-load-the-gun-environment-pulls-the-trigger

10 Campisi J. (1997). "The biology of replicative senescence." *European journal of cancer* (Oxford, England : 1990), 33(5), 703–709. https://doi.org/10.1016/S0959-8049(96)00058-5

11 Ibid.

12 Clear, James. 2018. *Atomic Habits: Tiny Changes, Remarkable Results : An Easy & Proven Way to Build Good Habits & Break Bad Ones.* New York: Avery, an imprint of Penguin Random House.

12 MEDICINES
1 CONNECTION

1   *Foresting Life.* 2013 Documentary. Humanity Watchdog. Directed By: Aarti Shrivastava. https://web.archive.org/web/20140509044350/http://www.humanitywatchdog.org/films/foresting-life-2013

2   Global Footprint Network — https://www.footprintnetwork.org

3   Ibid.

4   B1G1.com

5   Global Footprint Network — https://www.footprintnetwork.org

6   Ibid.

7   His Holiness the 14th Dalai Lama of Tibet. Official website www.dalailama.com. Published online "Universal Responsibility and the Environment." Source indicated from website: *Excerpt from My Tibet by H.H. the Fourteenth Dalai Lama*: Thames and Hudson Ltd., London, 1990 (p 79–80). https://www.dalailama.com/messages/environment/universal-responsibility

8   Isack, H. A., & Reyer, H. U. (1989). "Honeyguides and honey gatherers: interspecific communication in a symbiotic relationship." *Science* (New York, N.Y.), 243(4896), 1343–1346. https://doi.org/10.1126/science.243.4896.1343

9   Peglar, Tom. Yellowstone Park. "1995 Reintroduction of Wolves in Yellowstone." Published online June 30, 2020. https://www.yellowstonepark.com/park/yellowstone-wolves-reintroduction

10 Ibid.

11 Ripple, W.J.; Beschta, R.L. 2012. "Trophic cascades in Yellowstone: The first 15 years after wolf reintroduction." Biol. Cons. 145: 205–213.

12 https://rebellion.global

13 Bar-On, Yinon M. and Phillips, Rob and Milo, Ron (2018) "The biomass distribution on Earth." *Proceedings of the National Academy of Sciences of the United States of America*, 115 (25). pp. 6506–6511. ISSN 0027-8424. PMCID PMC6016768. https://resolver.caltech.edu/CaltechAUTHORS:20180521-155526693

14 Ibid.

15 *Living Planet Report 2018*. World Wide Fund for Nature. https://livingplanet.panda.org

16 Carrington, Damian - Environmental editor. "Humanity has wiped out 60% of animal populations since 1970, report finds." *The Guardian*. Published online October 30, 2018. https://www.theguardian.com/environment/2018/oct/30/humanity-wiped-out-animals-since-1970-major-report-finds

17 Ibid.

18 Tipper R., Forestry and the Clean Development Mechanism, *Edinburgh Centre for Carbon Management*, 12th May 2000. Pederson T. 2000. Climate Change Fore and Aft: Where on Earth are We Going. IGBP Newsletter 44.

19 Nepstad, D., McGrath, D., Stickler, C., Alencar, A., Azevedo, A., & Swette, B. et al. (2014). "Slowing Amazon deforestation through public policy and interventions in beef and soy supply chains." *Science,* 344(6188), 1118–1123. doi:10.1126/science.1248525
    Fearnside, P. M. (2005). Deforestation in Brazilian Amazonia: history, rates, and consequences. *Conservation biology*, 19(3), 680–688.
    Boucher, D., Elias, P., Lininger, K., May-Tobin, C., Roquemore, S., & Saxon, E. (June 2011). The Union of Concerned Scientists (UCS), "The root of the problem: what's driving tropical deforestation today?" Cambridge, MA. https://www.ice.ucdavis.edu//files/ice/UCS_RootoftheProblem_DriversofDeforestation_FullReport.pdf [This report is available online (in PDF format) at www.ucsusa.org/whatsdrivingdeforestation]

20 Handcrafted Films, *The Reunion*. https://vimeo.com/112387515

21 United Nations Development Programme. UNDP. "The Answer Is in Nature."
    Published online https://www.undp.org/content/undp/en/home/stories/the-answer-
    is-in-nature.html.

22 Maeterlinck, Maurice. *The Life of the Bee.* Translated by Alfred Sutro. New York. May
    1901.

23 Twenge, Jean M, and W Keith Campbell. "Associations between screen time and
    lower psychological well-being among children and adolescents: Evidence from a
    population-based study." *Preventive medicine reports* vol. 12 271–283. 18 Oct. 2018,
    doi:10.1016/j.pmedr.2018.10.003

24 Lile, Christopher, May 18 2018. Jane Goodall Organisation. "Good news for all: The
    Greatest Danger to Our Future is Apathy for Endangered Species." https://news.
    janegoodall.org/2018/05/18/greatest-danger-future-apathy-endangered-species

25 Morrow, Julian. ABC Australia, Sunday Extra, "Doctors in Scotland are prescribing
    nature as a treatment." Broadcast Sun 22 Nov 2020. https://www.abc.net.au/
    radionational/programs/sundayextra/doctors-in-scotland-are-prescribing-nature-as-
    a-treatment/12897268

26 Fleischer, Evan. World Economic Forum. "Doctors in Scotland can now prescribe
    nature." October 15, 2018. https://www.weforum.org/agenda/2018/10/doctors-in-
    scotland-can-now-prescribe-nature?fbclid=IwAR2h17w

27 Bond, Michael. BBC article "How extreme isolation warps the mind." Published online
    May 14, 2014. https://www.bbc.com/future/article/20140514-how-extreme-isolation-
    warps-minds

28 *Before The Flood.* Documentary film directed by Fisher Stevens. Produced by Fisher
    Stevens, Leonardo DiCaprio, Jennifer Davisson, James Packer, Brett Ratner and Trevor
    Davidoski. October 21, 2016. Distributed by National Geographic Documentary Films.

29 Herrero, Mario & Havlík, Petr & Valin, Hugo & Notenbaert, An & Rufino, Mariana &
    Thornton, Philip & Blümmel, Michael & Weiss, Franz & Grace, Delia & Obersteiner,
    Michael. (2013). "Biomass use, production, feed efficiencies, and greenhouse gas
    emissions from global livestock systems." *Proceedings of the National Academy of
    Sciences of the United States of America.* 110. 10.1073/pnas.1308149110.

30 Goodall, Jane. Blog article "Dr Jane Goodall's Message For Peace." Published online
    September 20, 2017. https://news.janegoodall.org/2017/09/20/dr-jane-goodalls-
    message-for-peace

32 footprintcalculator.org

33 Silverstone, Michael. *Blinded by Science.* Lloyds World Publishing 2011. United
    Kingdom.

2 ENVIRONMENT

1   Baggini, Julian. *Freedom Regained: The Possibility of Free Will.* University of Chicago
    Press, London, 2015.

2   Ibid.

3   Ibid.

4   Ibid.

5   Benjamin, Emelia J et al. "Heart Disease and Stroke Statistics-2019 Update: A Report From the American Heart Association." *Circulation* vol. 139,10 (2019): e56–e528. doi:10.1161/CIR.0000000000000659

6   UNICEF. "World Water Day: Nearly 750 million people still without adequate drinking water – UNICEF." NEW YORK, 20 March 2015. https://www.unicef.org/media/media_81329.html

7   Food and Agriculture Organization of the United Nations. "World hunger falls, but 805 million still chronically undernourished." 16 September 2014, Rome. http://www.fao.org/news/story/en/item/243839/icode

8   Pantsios, Anastasia. EcoWatch. "Solar Light Solution for 1.6 Billion People Living Without Electricity." Jan. 09, 2015. https://www.ecowatch.com/solar-light-solution-for-1-6-billion-people-living-without-electricity-1881999519.html

9   Do Something.Org. "11 Facts about global poverty. 10% of the world's population lives on less than $1.90 a day." https://www.dosomething.org/us/facts/11-facts-about-global-poverty

10 FAO, IFAD and WFP. "The State of Food Insecurity in the World 2014. Strengthening the enabling environment for food security and nutrition." Food and Agriculture Organization of the UN, 2014. Web Accessed February 25, 2015.

11 Do Something.Org. "11 Facts about global poverty — 10% of the world's population lives on less than $1.90 a day." https://www.dosomething.org/us/facts/11-facts-about-global-poverty

12 *South China Morning Post.* "Joko Widodo completes rise from slum to Indonesia's presidential palace." 21 Oct, 2014. https://www.scmp.com/news/asia/article/1620817/joko-widodo-completes-rise-slum-indonesias-presidential-palace

13 Dummer, Trevor J B. "Health geography: supporting public health policy and planning." *CMAJ : Canadian Medical Association journal = journal de l'Association medicale canadienne* vol. 178,9 (2008): 1177–80. doi:10.1503/cmaj.071783

14 United Nations Development Programme. Human Development Index (HDI) http://hdr.undp.org/en/content/human-development-index-hdi

15 Swing, William Lacy — Director-General, International Organization for Migration (IOM). World Economic Forum. "How migrants who send money home have become a global economic force." Published 14 Jun 2018. https://www.weforum.org/agenda/2018/06/migrants-remittance-global-economic-force

16 United Nations Development Programme. *Human Development Report 2016: Human Development for Everyone.* New York 2016. http://hdr.undp.org/sites/default/files/2016_human_development_report.pdf

17 Durrani, Hammad. "Healthcare and healthcare systems: inspiring progress and future prospects." *mHealth* vol. 2 3. 2 Feb. 2016, doi:10.3978/j.issn.2306-9740.2016.01.03

18 Ibid.

19 Ibid.

20 Malala Yousafzai, https://malala.org/malalas-story

21 Bado, Aristide Romaric, and A Sathiya Susuman. "Women's Education and Health Inequalities in Under-Five Mortality in Selected Sub-Saharan African Countries, 1990–2015." *PloS one* vol. 11,7 e0159186. 21 Jul. 2016, doi:10.1371/journal.pone.0159186

22 Ibid.

23 Clinton Global Initiative, "Empowering Girls & Women." Accessed online December 3 2020. https://www.un.org/en/ecosoc/phlntrpy/notes/clinton.pdf

24 Rine, Christine M. "Social Determinants of Health: Grand Challenges in Social Work's Future." *Health & social work* vol. 41,3 (2016): 143–145. doi:10.1093/hsw/hlw028

25 Cockerham, William C et al. "The Social Determinants of Chronic Disease." *American journal of preventive medicine* vol. 52,1S1 (2017): S5–S12. doi:10.1016/j.amepre.2016.09.010

26 Australian Institute of Health and Welfare. "Deaths in Australia." Last update August 7, 2020. https://www.aihw.gov.au/reports/life-expectancy-death/deaths/contents/life-expectancy

27 Robert Wood Johnson Foundation, "Life Expectancy: Could where you live influence how long you live?" January 2020. https://www.rwjf.org/en/library/interactives/whereyouliveaffectshowlongyoulive.html

28 Bahreynian, Maryam et al. "Association between Obesity and Parental Weight Status in Children and Adolescents." *Journal of clinical research in pediatric endocrinology* vol. 9,2 (2017): 111–117. doi:10.4274/jcrpe.3790

29 Weissman, Myrna & Wickramaratne, Priya & Nomura, Yoko & Warner, Virginia & Pilowsky, Daniel & Verdeli, Helen. (2006). "Offspring of Depressed Parents: 20 Years Later." *The American journal of psychiatry*. 163. 1001–8. 10.1176/appi.ajp.163.6.1001.

30 Weissman, M., P. Wickramaratne, M. Gameroff, V. Warner, D. Pilowsky, Rajni Gathibandhe Kohad, H. Verdeli, Jamie Skipper and A. Talati. "Offspring of Depressed Parents: 30 Years Later." *The American journal of psychiatry* 173 10 (2016): 1024–1032.

31 Peele, Stanton. "My Genes Made Me Do It: Misunderstanding the role of genes fosters myths about mental illness." Psychology Today. June 9, 2016. https://www.psychologytoday.com/us/articles/199507/my-genes-made-me-do-it

32 Ibid.

33 New England Complex Systems Institute. "RE-THINKING PSYCHOLOGY RESEARCH WITH JEROME KAGAN: A Complex Systems Problem?". https://necsi.edu/rethinking-psychology-research-with-jerome-kagan

34 Connor, Steve. "Do Your Genes Make You A Criminal?" The Independent. Sunday 12 February 1995. https://www.independent.co.uk/news/uk/do-your-genes-make-you-criminal-1572714.html

35 Baginni, Julian. "Do your genes determine your entire life?" The Guardian. 19th March, 2015. https://www.theguardian.com/science/2015/mar/19/do-your-genes-

determine-your-entire-life

36   Ibid.

37   The Economic and Social Commission for Asia and the Pacific (ESCAP) – Chapter 9
     [online] – accessed September 2021https://www.unescap.org/sites/default/files/
     CH09.PDF

3 CONNECTION

1   Neil de Grasse Tyson, https://www.haydenplanetarium.org/tyson

2   Cacioppo, J. T., Berntson, G. G., & Decety, J. (2010). "SOCIAL NEUROSCIENCE AND ITS
     RELATIONSHIP TO SOCIAL PSYCHOLOGY." *Social cognition*, 28(6), 675–685. https://
     doi.org/10.1521/soco.2010.28.6.675

3   Ceballos, Gerardo & Ehrlich, Paul & Dirzo, Rodolfo. (2017). "Biological annihilation
     via the ongoing sixth mass extinction signaled by vertebrate population losses and
     declines." *Proceedings of the National Academy of Sciences*. 114. 201704949. 10

4   Lieberman, M.D., *Why Our Brains Are Wired to Connect*. OUP Oxford, 10 October
     2013.

5   Lieberman, M. D. (2007). Social cognitive neuroscience: A review of core processes.
     Annual Review of Psychology.

6   Lieberman, M. D., Berkman, E. T., & Wager, T. D. (2009). "Correlations in social
     neuroscience aren't voodoo: A reply to Vul et al." *Perspectives on Psychological
     Science*.
     Lieberman, M. D., Chang, G. Y., Chiao, J., Bookheimer, S. Y., & Knowlton, B. J. (2004).
     "An event-related fMRI study of artificial gram- mar learning in a balanced chunk
     strength design." *Journal of Cognitive Neuroscience*, 16, 427–438.
     Lieberman, M. D., & Eisenberger, N. I. (2009). "Pains and pleasures of social life."
     Science, 323, 890–891.

7   Holt-Lunstad, Julianne, Timothy B. Smith, Mark Baker, Tyler Harris, and David
     Stephenson. "Loneliness and Social Isolation as Risk Factors for Mortality: A Meta-
     Analytic Review." *Perspectives on Psychological Science* 10, no. 2 (March 2015):
     227–37. https://doi.org/10.1177/1745691614568352.

8   Bond, Michael. BBC. "How Extreme Isolation Warps Minds." Published online 14th
     May 2014. https://www.bbc.com/future/article/20140514-how-extreme-isolation-
     warps-minds

9   Lile, Christopher, May 18 2018. Jane Goodall Organisation. "Good news for all: The
     Greatest Danger to Our Future is Apathy for Endangered Species." https://news.
     janegoodall.org/2018/05/18/greatest-danger-future-apathy-endangered-species

10   Gilbert. P. (2015). "The evolution and social dynamics of compassion." *Journal of
     Social & Personality Psychology Compass*, 9, 239–254. DOI: 10.1111/spc3.12176

11   De Waal, Frans. Greater Good Science Center. *Greater Good Magazine*. "The Evolution
     of Empathy." Published online Sept 1, 2005. https://greatergood.berkeley.edu/article/

item/the_evolution_of_empathy

12 Ibid.

13 Lynch, Patrick. NASA. Dec 25, 2016. Nasa People. "Piers Sellers: A Legacy of Science." Nasa.org. https://www.nasa.gov/feature/goddard/2016/piers-sellers-a-legacy-of-science

14 The Charles Chaplin Film Corporation. *The Great Dictator*. [New York, N.Y.] : Jewish Media Fund, 1997.

4 GENES

1   Chopra, Deepak. Tanzi, Rudolph. *Super Genes: Unlock the Astonishing Power of Your DNA for Optimum Health and Well-Being*, Harmony; 1st edition, 10 November 2015

2   https://nickvujicic.com

3   Zelia Gregoriou & Marianna Papastephanou (2013) "The utopianism of John Locke's natural learning." *Ethics and Education*, 8:1, 18–30, DOI: 10.1080/17449642.2013.793959

4   National Human Genome Research Institute, "The Human Genome Project," https://www.genome.gov/human-genome-project

5   Collins, Dr. Francis S. Director, National Human Genome Research Institute. "Remarks at the Press Conference Announcing Sequencing and Analysis of the Human Genome." February 12, 2001. https://www.genome.gov/10001379/february-2001-working-draft-of-human-genome-director-collins

6   The Chimpanzee Sequencing and Analysis Consortium., Waterson, R., Lander, E. et al. "Initial sequence of the chimpanzee genome and comparison with the human genome." *Nature* 437, 69–87 (2005). https://doi.org/10.1038/nature04072

7   23&Me Blog post, "Genetic Similarities of Mice and Men." April 20, 2012. https://blog.23andme.com/23andme-and-you/genetics-101/genetic-similarities-of-mice-and-men

8   National Human Genome Research Institute. "Genetics Versus Genomes Fact Sheet." https://www.genome.gov/about-genomics/fact-sheets/Genetics-vs-Genomics

9   MacArthur, D. "Superheroes of disease resistance." *Nat Biotechnol* 34, 512–513 (2016). https://doi.org/10.1038/nbt.3555

10 Ibid.

11 Chen, R., Shi, L., Hakenberg, J. et al. "Analysis of 589,306 genomes identifies individuals resilient to severe Mendelian childhood diseases." *Nat Biotechnol* 34, 531–538 (2016). https://doi.org/10.1038/nbt.3514

12 Deloukas, P., Schuler, G. D., Gyapay, G., Beasley, E. M., Soderlund, C., Rodriguez-Tomé, P., Hui, L., Matise, T. C., McKusick, K. B., Beckmann, J. S., Bentolila, S., Bihoreau, M., Birren, B. B., Browne, J., Butler, A., Castle, A. B., Chiannilkulchai, N., Clee, C., Day, P. J., Dehejia, A., ... Bentley, D. R. (1998). "A physical map of 30,000 human genes." *Science* (New York, N.Y.), 282(5389), 744–746. https://doi.org/10.1126/

science.282.5389.744

13   Marc A. Shampo, Robert A. Kyle, J. Craig Venter—The Human Genome Project, Mayo Clinic Proceedings, Volume 86, Issue 4, 2011,Pages e26–e27,ISSN 0025-6196, https://doi.org/10.4065/mcp.2011.0160. http://www.sciencedirect.com/science/article/pii/S0025619611600232.

14   Silverman, Paul H. "Rethinking genetic determinism: with only 30,000 genes, what is it that makes humans human?" *The Scientist*, vol. 18, no. 10, 24 May 2004, p. 32+. *Gale Academic OneFile*, https://link.gale.com/apps/doc/A117605464/AONE?u=googleschol ar&sid=AONE&xid=4fb01c6c. Accessed 14 Dec. 2020.

15   Kahan, Scott. Blog post —"Genes load the gun, environment pulls the trigger." Published online October 18 2010. http://scottkahan.com/genes-load-the-gun-environment-pulls-the-trigger

16   Williamson, R., Anderson, W., Duckett, SJ., Frazer, IH., Hillyard, C., Kowal, E., Mattick, JS., McLean CA., North, KN., Turner, A., Addison, C., (2018). *The Future of Precision Medicine in Australia. Report for the Australian Council of Learned Academies*, www.acola.org.au

17   Lipton, Bruce. Blog article "How Our Thoughts Control Our DNA." Published online June 10, 2014. https://www.brucelipton.com/blog/how-our-thoughts-control-our-dna

18   ETH Zurich. "Controlling genes with your thoughts." ScienceDaily. www.sciencedaily.com/releases/2014/11/141111111317.htm (accessed December 14, 2020).

19   Robson, David. "The secrets of living to 200 years old." BBC, Published online 17th September 2015. https://www.bbc.com/future/article/20150915-the-secrets-of-living-to-200-years-old

20   Caulin, Aleah F, and Carlo C Maley. "Peto's Paradox: evolution's prescription for cancer prevention." *Trends in ecology & evolution* vol. 26,4 (2011): 175–82. doi:10.1016/j.tree.2011.01.002

21   Robson, David. "The secrets of living to 200 years old." BBC, Published online 17th September 2015. https://www.bbc.com/future/article/20150915-the-secrets-of-living-to-200-years-old

22   Hatfield, Dolph L. "Redox Pioneer: Professor Vadim N. Gladyshev." *Antioxidants & redox signaling* vol. 25,1 (2016): 1–9. doi:10.1089/ars.2015.6625

23   Lipton, Bruce. Blog article "How Our Thoughts Control Our DNA." Published online June 10, 2014. https://www.brucelipton.com/blog/how-our-thoughts-control-our-dna

5 MIND

1   Brand, Russell. Russell Brand YouTube video, "The 12 Steps According To Russell Brand." February 7, 2018. https://www.youtube.com/watch?v=lK083EvyiMl

2   Brand, Russell. *Recovery: Freedom from Our Addictions*, Pan Macmillan, 26th September 2017.

3   Bértholo, Joanna. *Shadow Working in Project Management:* Understanding and

Addressing the Irrational and Unconscious in Groups, Routledge, July 20, 2017.

4   Justin, James. *Mindset: How To Transform Your Life From Ordinary To Extraordinary.* Orlando, 2016.

5   Bértholo, Joanna. *Shadow Working in Project Management:* Understanding and Addressing the Irrational and Unconscious in Groups, Routledge, July 20, 2017.

6   Durkheim, Emile. *The Division of Labor in Society.* Translated by W.D. Halls. New York: The Free Press, 1984.

7   Jung, Carl. *Collected Works of C.G. Jung, Volume 8: Structure and Dynamics of the Psyche:* 008 Hardcover – Princeton University Press; 1 edition, 15 January 1970.

8   E. Stanley Jones. *The Christ of the Indian Road (1925).* New York, Abingdon Press, p193–194, 195–196.

9   Smetham, G. P, *Journal of Consciousness Exploration & Research,* November 2010 | Vol. 1 | Issue 8 | pp. 1048–1069 1056. Quantum Mind: Matrix of the Universe

10 Laura Lee Colgin, Tobias Denninger, Marianne Fyhn, Torkel Hafting, Tora Bonnevie, Ole Jensen, May-Britt Moser & Edvard I. Moser. "Frequency of gamma oscillations routes flow of information in the hippocampus." *Nature*, 2009; 462 (7271): 353 DOI: 10.1038/nature08573

11 Ibid.

12 Hawkins, David. *Power vs. Force: The Hidden Determinants of Human Behavior.* Veritas Publishing; 1st edition, May 15, 2012.

13 Smithsonian National Museum of Natural History. "What does it mean to be human?" January 16, 2019. https://humanorigins.si.edu/human-characteristics/brains

14 Ananthaswamy, Anil. "What separates us from other animals?" *New Scientist.* 22 January 2014. https://www.newscientist.com/article/mg22129531-100-what-separates-us-from-other-animals
    Suddendorf, Thomas. (2013). *THE GAP — The Science of What Separates Us From Other Animals.* http://thegap.psy.uq.edu.au

15 Hofman, Michel A. "Evolution of the human brain: when bigger is better." *Frontiers in neuroanatomy* vol. 8 15. 27 Mar. 2014, doi:10.3389/fnana.2014.00015

16 Hofman M. A. (2014). "Evolution of the human brain and intelligence: from matter to mind." *Handbook of Intelligence: Evolutionary Theory, Historical Perspective and Current Concepts*, eds Goldstein S., Naglieri J. A., Princiotta D. (Berlin, Springer Verlag:).

17 Buzsáki G, Logothetis N, Singer W. "Scaling brain size, keeping timing: evolutionary preservation of brain rhythms." *Neuron.* 2013;80(3):751-764. doi:10.1016/j.neuron.2013.10.002

18 Damasio, Antonio. *Descartes' Error: Emotion, Reason, and the Human Brain.* Putnam Publishing, 1994, hardcover.

19 Damasio, Antonio. *Descartes' Error: Emotion, Reason, and the Human Brain.* Putnam Publishing, 1994, hardcover.

20 Graves, Christopher. Institute for Public Relations, Part One: "We Are Not Thinking

Machines. We Are Feeling Machines That Think." March 17, 2015. https://instituteforpr.org/part-one-not-thinking-machines-feeling-machines-think

21 Virginie Sterpenich, Arnaud D'Argembeau, Martin Desseilles, Evelyne Balteau, Geneviève Albouy, Gilles Vandewalle, Christian Degueldre, André Luxen, Fabienne Collette and Pierre Maquet, "The Locus Ceruleus Is Involved in the Successful Retrieval of Emotional Memories in Humans." *Journal of Neuroscience* 12 July 2006, 26 (28) 7416–7423; DOI: https://doi.org/10.1523/JNEUROSCI.1001-06.2006. https://www.jneurosci.org/content/26/28/7416

22 Nielson, K. A., Yee, D., & Erickson, K. I. (2005). "Memory enhancement by a semantically unrelated emotional arousal source induced after learning." *Neurobiology of learning and memory*, 84(1), 49–56. https://doi. org/10.1016/j.nlm.2005.04.001

23 Ibid.

24 Gardner, Howard. *Frames of Mind: The Theory of Multiple Intelligences.* Basic Books; 3 edition, March 29, 2011.

25 Robinson, Ken. "Do schools kill creativity?" TED2006. https://www.ted.com/speakers/sir_ken_robinson

26 Bhajan. Yogi. PhD. *The Mind: Its Projections and Multiple Facets.* Kundalini Research Institute; 1st edition June 15, 1998.

27 Ibid.

28 Rankin. Lissa. M.D. *Mind Over Medicine: Scientific Proof That You Can Heal Yourself,* Hay House Inc.; Reprint edition December 1, 2014.

29 Butler, David. G, Moseley Lorimer. *Explain Pain,* NOI Group; 2nd edition September 25, 2013.

30 Ibid.

31 Doidge, Norman, M.D. *The Brain's Way of Healing,* Bolinda Publishing, Tullamarine, Australia. 01 Apr 2015

32 Ibid.

6 FOOD

1 Gunders, Dana. "Wasted: How America is Losing Up to 40 Percent of Its Food from Farm to Fork to Landfill." *Natural Resources Defense Council,* 2017. Retrieved June 2021. from https://www.nrdc.org/sites/default/files/wasted-2017-report.pdf

2 markbittman.com

3 Dr Igor Tabrizian, *Visual Textbook of Nutritional Medicine.* NRS Publications, January 1, 2007.

4 "Overfed but Undernourished," by H. Curtis Wood, Jr. (Exposition Press. Inc., New York. 1959. Pp. 95. *Health Education Journal* 17, no. 2 (May 1959): 152–152. https://doi.org/10.1177/001789695901700218.

5 Morgan, Heather. Blog Talk Radio with Heather Morgan. https://podcast.

bodytalkradio.com/tag/heather-morgan

6   The Nutrition Society, "Nutrigenomics. The basics." https://www.nutritionsociety.org/blog/nutrigenomics-basics

7   Pollan, Michael. "How to Eat - Diet secrets from Michael Pollan (and your great-grandma)" January 23, 2010 https://michaelpollan.com/reviews/how-to-eat

8   Statistics Canada. List of other Canadian Health Measures Survey (CHMS) documents available external icon. Carroll MD, Navaneelan T, Bryan S, Ogden CL. "Prevalence of obesity among children and adolescents in Canada and the United States." NCHS data brief, no 211. Hyattsville, MD: National Center for Health Statistics. 2015.

9   Ibid.

10   Bancej, C., Jayabalasingham, B., Wall, R. W., Rao, D. P., Do, M. T., de Groh, M., & Jayaraman, G. C. (2015). "Evidence Brief--Trends and projections of obesity among Canadians." *Health promotion and chronic disease prevention in Canada : research, policy and practice*, 35(7), 109–112. https://doi.org/10.24095/hpcdp.35.7.02 Public Health Agency of Canada and Canadian Institute for Health Information . Obesity in Canada: a joint report from the Public Health Agency of Canada and the Canadian Institute for Health Information [Internet] Ottawa (ON): Public Health Agency of Canada; 2011 [cited 2014 Feb 25]. pp 29–30. Joint publication of Canadian Institute for Health Information. Available from: http://www.phac-aspc.gc.ca/hp-ps/hl-mvs/oic-oac/assets/pdf/oic-oac-eng.pdf.

11   William Prout M.D. F.R.S. (1828) IX. "On the ultimate composition of simple alimentary substances; with some preliminary remarks on the analysis of organized bodies in general." *The Philosophical Magazine*, 3:13, 31–40, DOI: 10.1080/14786442808674540

12   Arnold, David. "British India and the "beriberi problem", 1798–1942." *Medical history* vol. 54,3 (2010): 295–314. doi:10.1017/s0025727300004622

13   Shyamala Iyer. "Atoms & Life". ASU – Ask A Biologist. 27 Sep 2009. ASU – Ask A Biologist, Web. 15 Dec 2020. https://askabiologist.asu.edu

14   Thone, Frank. (1936). "Nature Ramblings: 'Chnops,' Plus", *Science News Letters* (CHNOPS, pg. 110; protoplasm, pg. 110), 30(801), Aug 15.

15   Helmenstine, Anne Marie. "What are the Elements In the Human Body?" Feb 24, 2020. https://www.thoughtco.com/elements-in-the-human-body-p2-602188

16   Rahim Biad, Abder. *Restoring the Bioelectrical Machine*, Lulu Publishing. 12 November 2019.

17   Helmenstine, Anne Marie. "Elements in the Human Body and What They Do." *Science Notes*. Feb 7, 2019. https://sciencenotes.org/elements-in-the-human-body-and-what-they-do

18   Vannucci, Letizia & Fossi, Caterina & Quattrini, Sara & Guasti, Leonardo & Pampaloni, Barbara & Gronchi, Giorgio & Giusti, Francesca & Romagnoli, Cecilia & Cianferotti, Luisella & Marcucci, Gemma & Brandi, Maria. (2018). "Calcium Intake in Bone Health: A Focus on Calcium-Rich Mineral Waters." *Nutrients*. 10. 1930. 10.3390/nu10121930.

19   Jaishankar, M., Tseten, T., Anbalagan, N., Mathew, B. B., & Beeregowda, K. N. (2014).

"Toxicity, mechanism and health effects of some heavy metals." *Interdisciplinary toxicology*, 7(2), 60–72. https://doi.org/10.2478/intox-2014-0009

20 Wolfe, David. *Longevity Now: A Comprehensive Approach to Healthy Hormones, Detoxification, Super Immunity, Reversing Calcification, and Total Rejuvenation*, North Atlantic Books; 1st edition, 12 November 2013.

21 The Department for Environment, Food & Rural Affairs, United Kingdom.

22 Project Organic. "Organic – What does it actually mean?" Published online. https://projectorganic.com.au/what-to-expect. Sourced from The Department for Agriculture and Rural Affairs, United Kingdom.

23 White, D. L., Savas, L. S., Daci, K., Elserag, R., Graham, D. P., Fitzgerald, S. J., Smith, S. L., Tan, G., & El-Serag, H. B. (2010)." Trauma history and risk of the irritable bowel syndrome in women veterans." *Alimentary pharmacology & therapeutics*, 32(4), 551–561. https://doi.org/10.1111/j.1365-2036.2010.04387.x

24 Whitehead WE, Palsson O, Jones KR. "Systematic review of the comorbidity of irritable bowel syndrome with other disorders: what are the causes and implications?" *Gastroenterology*. 2002;122:1140–1156.

25 Harvard Health Publishing. "Stress and the sensitive gut. Psychotherapy may help ease persistent gastrointestinal distress." *The Harvard mental health letter* vol. 27,2 (2010): 6.

26 Clapp M, Aurora N, Herrera L, Bhatia M, Wilen E, Wakefield S. "Gut microbiota's effect on mental health: The gut-brain axis." *Clin Pract*. 2017;7(4):987. Published 2017 Sep 15. doi:10.4081/cp.2017.987 https://www.ncbi.nlm.nih.gov/pmc/articles/PMC5641835

27 Carabotti M, Scirocco A, Maselli MA, Carola S. "The gut-brain axis: interactions between enteric microbiota, central and enteric nervous systems." *Ann Gastroent* 2015;28:203-9.

28 Monash University. "FODMAPS and Irritable Bowel Syndrome." Retrieved Dec 2020. https://www.monashfodmap.com/about-fodmap-and-ibs

29 Lee, H., Kim, S., & Kim, D. (2014). "Effects of exercise with or without light exposure on sleep quality and hormone reponses." *Journal of exercise nutrition & biochemistry*, 18(3), 293–299. https://doi.org/10.5717/jenb.2014.18.3.293

30 Zhang, Jim & Wei, Yongjie & Fang, Zhangfu. (2019). "Ozone Pollution: A Major Health Hazard Worldwide." *Frontiers in Immunology*. 10. 2518. 10.3389/fimmu.2019.02518.

31 Ramasamy, Kannamani & S., Jayakumar & M., Somasundaram. (2020). "Enchanted Improvements in Air Quality across India – A Study from COVID-19 Lockdown Perspective." *SSRN Electronic Journal*. 10.2139/ssrn.3596001.

32 EPA. Overview of the Clean Air Act and Air Pollution. https://www.epa.gov/clean-air-act-overview

33 Bada, Ferdinand. "Which Cities Have the Cleanest Air?" WorldAtlas. Published online May 9 2018. https://www.worldatlas.com/articles/the-cleanest-major-cities-in-the-

world.html

34 Barrington, Mitch. "The Cleanest Water On Earth? Hint: It's Not Rainwater!" Food Matters. Published online October 12, 2018. https://www.foodmatters.com/article/cleanest-water-on-earth

35 Novak, Sara. "What's the best type of water to drink?" Organic Authority. April 11, 2019. https://www.organicauthority.com/energetic-health/whats-the-best-type-of-water-to-drink

36 Weidman, Joseph et al. "Effect of electrolyzed high-pH alkaline water on blood viscosity in healthy adults." *Journal of the International Society of Sports Nutrition* vol. 13 45. 28 Nov. 2016, doi:10.1186/s12970-016-0153-8

37 Novak, Sara. "What's the best type of water to drink?" Organic Authority. April 11, 2019. https://www.organicauthority.com/energetic-health/whats-the-best-type-of-water-to-drink

38 Katz, David. "The Case for Eating 'Mostly Plants,' in 260 Words." Huffington Post article. Published online 04/09/2012. Updated June 9, 2012. https://www.huffpost.com/entry/healthy-diet_b_1410803

39 Pollan, Michael. "How to Eat - Diet secrets from Michael Pollan (and your great-grandma)" January 23, 2010 https://michaelpollan.com/reviews/how-to-eat

40 Friend, Catherine. *The Compassionate Carnivore: Or, How to Keep Animals Happy, Save Old MacDonald's Farm, Reduce Your Hoofprint, and Still Eat Meat.* Capo Lifelong Books; 1 edition, 28 April 2009.

7 MOVEMENT

1 https://bethanyhamilton.com

2 https://nickvujicic.com

3 Edwards, S. (2002) *Neurological Physiotherapy: A Problem Solving Approach.* Second Edition. Churchill Livingstone, London.

4 Anne Shumway-Cook Marjorie Hines Woollacott. *Motor Control: Translating Research into Clinical Practice* – Lippincott Williams and Wilkins; 4th revised North American ed edition (1 February 2011)

5 Kathleen Haywood, Nancy Getchell. *Life Span Motor Development With Web Study Guide* 6ed Hardcover, Human Kinetics, Inc.; 6 edition (15 July 2014)
Raine, Sue. Meadows, Linzi. Lynch-Ellerington, Mary. *Bobath Concept Theory and Clinical Practice in Neurological Rehabilitation*, Wiley-Blackwell, July, 2009.

6 Nieman, David. *The Exercise-Health Connection: How to Reduce Your Risk of Disease and Other Illnesses by Making Exercise Your Medicine*, Human Kinetics, 1998.

7 Constance G. Bacon, Murray A. Mittleman, Ichiro Kawachi, et al. "Sexual Function in Men Older Than 50 Years of Age: Results from the Health Professionals Follow-up Study." *Ann Intern Med.*2003;139:161–168. [Epub ahead of print 5 August 2003]. doi:10.7326/0003-4819-139-3-200308050-00005

8   Nieman, David & Wentz, Laurel. (2018). "The compelling link between physical activity and the body's defense system." *Journal of Sport and Health Science*. 8. 10.1016/j.jshs.2018.09.009.

9   Akil, Luma, and H Anwar Ahmad. "Relationships between obesity and cardiovascular diseases in four southern states and Colorado." *Journal of health care for the poor and underserved* vol. 22,4 Suppl (2011): 61–72. doi:10.1353/hpu.2011.0166
    Hill, James. Wyatt, Holly R. "Role of physical activity in preventing and treating obesity." *Journal of Applied Physiology* 2005 99:2, 765–770

10 Pilates, Joseph H., and William John Miller. 1960. *Return to life through contrology.*

11 Ibid.

12 TheBox, "Origins of CrossFit." Published online October 9, 2012. https://www.theboxmag.com/training/origins-of-crossfit-9629

13 SCHMIDT, R. A., &WRISBERG, C. A. *Motor learning and performance: A problem-based learning approach.* 2000 (2nd ed.). Champaign, IL: Human Kinetics.

14 Martin, Suzanne. Kessler, Mayr. *Neurologic Interventions for Physical Therapy* 3rd Edition, Saunders; 3 edition July 8, 2015.

15 Ibid.

16 Ibid.

17 Seidler RD, Bo J, Anguera JA. "Neurocognitive contributions to motor skill learning: the role of working memory." *J Mot Behav.* 2012;44(6):445–453. doi:10.1080/00222895.2012.672348

18 Gladwell, Malcolm. *Outliers: The Story of Success.* New York :Little, Brown and Company, 2008.

19 Fitts, Paul Morris, and Michael I. Posner. 1967. *Human performance.* Belmont, Calif: Brooks/Cole Pub. Co.

20 Ibid.

21 Weaver, Janelle. "Motor Learning Unfolds over Different Timescales in Distinct Neural Systems." *PLoS biology* vol. 13,12 e1002313. 8 Dec. 2015, doi:10.1371/journal.pbio.1002313

22 Vansant, A. F. (1995). "Development of posture." In. D. Cech & S. T. Martin (Eds.), *Functional movement development across the life span* (pp.276–291).

23 Cech, Donna & Martin, S.T.. (2012). *Functional Movement Development Across the Life Span.* 10.1016/C2009-0-60730-3.

24 http://www.idoportal.com

25 http://www.idoportal.com/blog

26 National Research Council (US) and Institute of Medicine (US) Panel on Musculoskeletal Disorders and the Workplace. *Musculoskeletal Disorders and the Workplace: Low Back and Upper Extremities.* Washington (DC): *National Academies Press* (US); 2001. Available from: https://www.ncbi.nlm.nih.gov/books/NBK222440

27 American Psychological Association. "How stress affects your health." 2013, January 1. https://www.apa.org/topics/stress-health

28 Janig, W. (2003). The autonomic nervous system and its coordination by the brain. In Davidson, R. J., Scherer, K. R., & Goldsmith, H. H. (Eds.), *Handbook of affective sciences* (pp. 135–187).3 Oxford: Oxford University Press.

8 WORK

1   Hanalei Swan. https://hanaleiswan.com

2   McCormack, Mark. (1984) *What They Don't Teach You at Harvard Business School.* Section 3: Running a Business, Chapter 11: Building a Business, Section: Charge for Your Expertise, pp 169, Bantam Books, New York.

3   *World Cash Report 2018.* Jesus Rosano Divisional CEO, G4S Global Cash Solutions. https://cashessentials.org/app/uploads/2018/07/2018-world-cash-report.pdf

4   The Survey of Consumer Finances (CSF). Federal Reserve. https://www.federalreserve.gov/econres/scf-previous-surveys.htm

5   The Global Economy. "Percent people with credit cards – Country rankings." https://www.theglobaleconomy.com/rankings/people_with_credit_cards

6   Frank, Robert. "The Perfect Salary for Happiness: $75,000." *The Wall St Journal.* Sept. 7, 2010. https://www.wsj.com/articles/BL-WHB-3576

7   Bennett, Roy. *The Light in the Heart: Inspirational Thoughts for Living Your Best Life.* Roy Bennett, 25 February 2016.

8   Rohn, Jim. "Rohn: 6 Essential Traits of Good Character." *Success,* October 9, 2016 https://www.success.com/rohn-6-essential-traits-of-good-character

9   Eisenstein, Charles. "The Ascent of Humanity." Published online February 2007. https://charleseisenstein.org/essays/the-ascent-of-humanity

10 Demartini, John. The Demartini Value Determination Process. https://drdemartini.com/values

11 Covey, Stephen R. *The Seven Habits of Highly Effective People: Restoring the Character Ethic.* New York: Simon and Schuster, 1989.

12 Ibid.

13 Ferriss, Timothy., Ray Porter, and OverDrive Inc. *The 4-hour Workweek: Escape 9–5, Live Anywhere, and Join the New Rich.* Expanded & updated ; unabridged. Ashland, Or.: Blackstone Audio, 2009.

14 World Wildlife Fund. https://wwf.panda.org/discover/our_focus/forests_practice/deforestation_fronts2/deforestation_in_the_amazon/?

15 Brady, Jeff. NPR, "Teen Climate Activist Greta Thunberg Arrives In New York After Sailing The Atlantic." Published online August 28, 2019. https://www.npr.org/2019/08/28/754818342/teen-climate-activist-greta-thunberg-arrives-in-new-york-after-sailing-the-atlan

9 LIFESTYLE

1   High On Life. https://www.youtube.com/user/sundayfundayz/about

2   Grace Hopper Fullstack Academy. "Grace Hopper: 8 Interesting Facts About the Computer Science Pioneer." https://www.gracehopper.com/8-facts-about-grace-hopper

3   Hunter S. Thompson, *The Proud Highway: Saga of a Desperate Southern Gentleman, 1955–1967, (Gonzo Letters Book 1)*. Ballantine Books (1 August 2012)

4 Steiner, R. (1919/1996). The foundations of human experience (R. F. Lathe, Trans.). Great Barrington, MA: Anthroposophic Press. Based on Steiner Lectures (1919).

5   Kraut, Richard, "Aristotle's Ethics." *The Stanford Encyclopedia of Philosophy* (Summer 2018 Edition), Edward N. Zalta (ed.). https://plato.stanford.edu/archives/sum2018/entries/aristotle-ethics

6   Ibid.

7   Ibid.

8   Ibid.

9   Dooley, Mike. *Notes From The Universe*. Atria Books/Beyond Words; 1 edition. 18 September 2007.

10 Mihaly Csikszentmihályi. *Flow: The Psychology of Optimal Experience*. 1990. Harper & Row.

11 Frankl, Viktor E. (Viktor Emil), 1905–1997. *Man's Search for Meaning; an Introduction to Logotherapy*. Boston :Beacon Press, 1962.

12 Mihaly Csikszentmihályi. *Flow: The Psychology of Optimal Experience*. 1990. Harper & Row, Page 271.

13 Mihaly Csikszentmihályi. *Flow: The Psychology of Optimal Experience*. 1990. Harper & Row, Page 68.

14 Greger, Michael Dr. https://nutritionfacts.org. https://drgreger.org/products/how-not-to-die

15 Greger, Michael Dr. Nutrition Facts. "Eliminate Most of Your Chronic Disease Risk in Four Steps." September 22nd, 2015. https://nutritionfacts.org/2015/09/22/eliminate-most-of-your-chronic-disease-risk-in-four-easy-steps

16 Wahls, Terry L. "The seventy percent solution." *Journal of general internal medicinevol.* 26,10 (2011): 1215-6. doi:10.1007/s11606-010-1631-3

17 Willett, Walter C. "Balancing life-style and genomics research for disease prevention." Science (New York, N.Y.) vol. 296,5568 (2002): 695-8. doi:10.1126/science.1071055

18 Greger, Michael Dr. Nutrition Facts. "Eliminate Most of Your Chronic Disease Risk in Four Steps." September 22nd, 2015. https://nutritionfacts.org/2015/09/22/eliminate-most-of-your-chronic-disease-risk-in-four-easy-steps

19 Ford, Earl S et al. "Healthy lifestyle behaviors and all-cause mortality among adults in the United States." *Preventive medicine* vol. 55,1 (2012): 23-7. doi:10.1016/j.ypmed.2012.04.016

20 Greger, Michael Dr. Nutrition Facts. "Turning the Clock Back 14 Years." Video, June 2nd, 2014 Volume 19 https://nutritionfacts.org/video/turning-the-clock-back-14-years

21 Greger, Michael Dr. Nutrition Facts. "Eliminate Most of Your Chronic Disease Risk in Four Steps." September 22nd, 2015. https://nutritionfacts.org/2015/09/22/eliminate-most-of-your-chronic-disease-risk-in-four-easy-steps

22 Ibid.

23 Dr David Katz. https://www.truehealthinitiative.org

24 Katz, David & Williams, Anna-Leila & Girard, Christine & Goodman, Jonathan & Comerford, Beth & Behrman, Alyse & Bracken, Michael. (2003). "The evidence base for complementary and alternative medicine: methods of Evidence Mapping with application to CAM. Alternative therapies in health and medicine." 9. 22–30.

25 Egger, Garry & Binns, Andrew & Rossner, Stephan. (2009). "The emergence of "lifestyle medicine" As a structured approach for management of chronic disease." *The Medical journal of Australia*. 190. 143-5. 10.5694/j.1326-5377.2009.tb02317.x.

26 The IQVIA Institute for Human Data Science. https://www.iqvia.com/insights/the-iqvia-institute

27 Ibid.

28 Egger, Garry & Binns, Andrew & Rossner, Stephan. (2009). "The emergence of "lifestyle medicine" As a structured approach for management of chronic disease." *The Medical journal of Australia*. 190. 143-5. 10.5694/j.1326-5377.2009.tb02317.x.

29 Barbour KA, Edenfield TM, Blumenthal JA. "Exercise as a treatment for depression and other psychiatric disorders: a review." *J Cardiopulm Rehabil Prev* 2007; 27: 359-367.

10 SPIRIT

1 James, Alfred. Blog article, "Spirituality – What Does it Really Mean?" Pocket Mindfulness. https://www.pocketmindfulness.com/definition-of-spirituality

2 Tzu, Lao. *The Tao Te Ching*. Legge translation of the Tao Teh King at Project Gutenberg. https://www.gutenberg.org/ebooks/216

3 Dalai Lama XIV. *Policy of Kindness: An Anthology of Writings by and about the Dalai Lama*. Snow Lion; 2nd edition (12 August 2012).

4 Ibid.

5 Ibid.

6 Ibid.

7 Ibid.

11 MODERN

1 Original story by Dr. Emill Kim. Mind Body Green. "What's the Difference Between Eastern & Western Medicine?" https://www.mindbodygreen.com/0-5860/Whats-the-Difference-Between-Eastern-Western-Medicine.html

2   Ibid.

3   Ibid.

4   *Zhongguo Zhong xi yi jie he za zhi Zhongguo Zhongxiyi jiehe zazhi = Chinese journal of integrated traditional and Western medicine* vol. 33,9 (2013): 1157.
     World Health Organization. Address at the International Conference on the Modernization of Traditional Chinese Medicine in 2016.

5   Lakner, Christoph, Daniel Gerszon Mahler, Mario Negre, and Espen Beer Prydz. 2020. "How Much Does Reducing Inequality Matter for Global Poverty?" Global Poverty Monitoring Technical Note 13 (June), World Bank, Washington, DC

6   Sachs, Jeffrey. *The End of Poverty: Economic Possibilities for Our Time*. 2006. New York: Penguin Books

7   *Zhongguo Zhong xi yi jie he za zhi Zhongguo Zhongxiyi jiehe zazhi = Chinese journal of integrated traditional and Western medicine* vol. 33,9 (2013): 1157.
     World Health Organization. Address at the International Conference on the Modernization of Traditional Chinese Medicine in 2016.

8   Ibid.

9   Masic, I., Miokovic, M., & Muhamedagic, B. (2008). "Evidence based medicine – new approaches and challenges." Acta informatica medica : AIM : *journal of the Society for Medical Informatics of Bosnia & Herzegovina* : casopis Drustva za medicinsku informatiku BiH, 16(4), 219–225. https://doi.org/10.5455/aim.2008.16.219-225. https://www.ncbi.nlm.nih.gov/pmc/articles/PMC3789163

10   Mountain, Michael. "Scientists Declare: Non-Human Animals Are Conscious." Earth In Transition. July 30, 2012. http://www.earthintransition.org/2012/07/scientists-declare-nonhuman-animals-are-conscious

11   Butler DS, Moseley GL 2003 *Explain Pain Second edition* (2013) Noigroup Publications, Adelaide.

12   Masic, I., Miokovic, M., & Muhamedagic, B. (2008). "Evidence based medicine – new approaches and challenges." Acta informatica medica : AIM : *journal of the Society for Medical Informatics of Bosnia & Herzegovina* : casopis Drustva za medicinsku informatiku BiH, 16(4), 219–225. https://doi.org/10.5455/aim.2008.16.219-225

13   Manheimer E, Wieland S, Kimbrough E, Cheng K, Berman BM. "Evidence from the Cochrane Collaboration for Traditional Chinese Medicine therapies." *J Altern Complement Med.* 2009;15(9):1001-1014. doi:10.1089/ acm.2008.0414

14   *Zhongguo Zhong xi yi jie he za zhi Zhongguo Zhongxiyi jiehe zazhi = Chinese journal of integrated traditional and Western medicine* vol. 33,9 (2013): 1157.
     World Health Organization. Address at the International Conference on the Modernization of Traditional Chinese Medicine in 2016.

15   Lu AP, Jia HW, Xiao C, Lu QP. "Theory of traditional Chinese medicine and therapeutic method of diseases." *World J Gastroenterol.* 2004;10(13):1854-1856. doi:10.3748/wjg. v10.i13.1854, https://www.ncbi.nlm.nih.gov/pmc/articles/PMC4572216

Tsokos GC, Nepom GT. "Gene therapy in the treatment of autoimmune diseases." *J Clin Invest.* 2000;106:181–183.

16 Wang, X., Chen, K., & Wang, W. (1998). Zhongguo Zhong xi yi jie he za zhi Zhongguo Zhongxiyi jiehe zazhi = *Chinese journal of integrated traditional and Western medicine*, 18(7), 399–401.

17 Ibid.
World Health Organization. Address at the International Conference on the Modernization of Traditional Chinese Medicine in 2016.

18 Australian Bureau of Statistics, October 23 2020. "Causes of Death, Australia." https://www.abs.gov.au/statistics/health/causes-death/causes-death-australia/latest-release

19 Walsh, Robin. October 1, 2010. "A History of The Pharmaceutical Industry." SCRIBD, accessed online June 17, 2021. https://www.scribd.com/document/378721439/A-History-of-the-Pharmaceutical-Industry

20 Soine, Aeleah, and Sioban Nelson. "Selling the (Anti-) Smoking Nurse: Tobacco Advertising and Commercialism in the American Journal of Nursing." *Journal of Women's History* 30, no. 3 (2018): 82–106. doi:10.1353/jowh.2018.0031.

21 Ibid.

22 Holland, Brynn, History. April 1 2019. "7 of the Most Outrageous Medical Treatments in History: Why were parents giving their children heroin in the 1880s?" https://www.history.com/news/7-of-the-most-outrageous-medical-treatments-in-history

23 Walsh, Robin. October 1, 2010. "A History of The Pharmaceutical Industry." SCRIBD, accessed online June 17, 2021. https://www.scribd.com/document/378721439/A-History-of-the-Pharmaceutical-Industry

24 Ipharmacenter. Updated May 5 2021. "Top pharmaceutical companies by revenues in 2021." https://www.ipharmacenter.com/post/top-pharmaceutical-companies-by-revenues-in-2021

25 Sivan Gazit, Roei Shlezinger, Galit Perez et al. "Comparing SARS-CoV-2 natural immunity to vaccine-induced immunity: reinfections versus breakthrough infections." *medRxiv* 2021.08.24.21262415; doi: https://doi.org/10.1101/2021.08.24.21262415

26 Hall, V. J., Foulkes, S., Charlett, A., Atti, A., Monk, E., Simmons, R., Wellington, E., Cole, M. J., Saei, A., Oguti, B., Munro, K., Wallace, S., Kirwan, P. D., Shrotri, M., Vusirikala, A., Rokadiya, S., Kall, M., Zambon, M., Ramsay, M., Brooks, T., ... SIREN Study Group (2021). "SARS-CoV-2 infection rates of antibody-positive compared with antibody-negative health-care workers in England: a large, multicentre, prospective cohort study (SIREN)" *Lancet* (London, England), 397(10283), 1459–1469. https://doi.org/10.1016/S0140-6736(21)00675-9

27 Wolff, Mark. Oct 1, 2021, "Powerful Natural Immunity Debate in the Senate this is Power," - Senator Rand Paul debates natural immunity with Xavier Becerra United States Secretary of Health & Human Services, YouTube. https://www.youtube.com/watch?v=vPsjH-FJFww

28   United States Patent
     https://patentimages.storage.googleapis.com/a8/c0/6a/0584dd67435ef2/US7279327.
     pdf
     https://patentimages.storage.googleapis.com/6b/c3/21/a62eb55a0e678c/
     US7220852.pdf

29   Lerner, Sharon. March 14, 2020. "BIG PHARMA PREPARES TO PROFIT FROM THE
     CORONAVIRUS: Pharmaceutical companies view the coronavirus pandemic as
     a once-in-a-lifetime business opportunity." The Intercept. https://theintercept.
     com/2020/03/13/big-pharma-drug-pricing-coronavirus-profits

30   The United States Department of Justice, Wednesday, September 2, 2009, Justice
     News, "Justice Department Announces Largest Health Care Fraud Settlement in Its
     History: Pfizer to Pay $2.3 Billion for Fraudulent Marketing." Washington. Accessed
     June 21 2021, https://www.justice.gov/opa/pr/justice-department-announces-largest-
     health-care-fraud-settlement-its-history
     Hotten, Russell, BBC New York. Business and Human Right Resource Centre, 28
     August 2019, "US court rules drugmaker Johnson & Johnson must pay $572m for its
     role in opioid crisis in Oklahoma." Accessed June 21, 2021. https://www.business-
     humanrights.org/en/latest-news/us-court-rules-drugmaker-johnson-johnson-must-
     pay-572m-for-its-role-in-opioid-crisis-in-oklahoma

31   Kallet, Arthur; F.J. Schlink, 100,000,000 Guinea Pigs: Dangers in Everyday Foods, Drugs,
     and Cosmetics, Grosset & Dunlap, New York, 1933.

32   Peterson-Withorn, Chase. Dec 16 2020. Forbes Magazine. "The World's Billionaires
     Have Gotten $1.9 Trillion Richer In 2020." https://www.forbes.com/sites/
     chasewithorn/2020/12/16/the-worlds-billionaires-have-gotten-19-trillion-richer-in-
     2020/?sh=7593e99e7386

33   Gates, Bill. "Bill Gates: The Best Investment I've Ever Made." The Wall Street
     Journal. https://www.wsj.com/articles/bill-gates-the-best-investment-ive-ever-
     made-11547683309

34   Mukulic, Matej. Statista. November 5 2020. "Global pharmaceutical industry: statistics
     & facts" accessed online June 21 2021. https://www.statista.com/topics/1764/global-
     pharmaceutical-industry

35   Hacker, Miles. Editor(s): Miles Hacker, William Messer, Kenneth Bachmann,
     Pharmacology Principles and Practice 2009, "Chapter 13: Adverse Drug Reactions"
     Academic Press, pp. 327–352. Published online via Science Direct https://www.
     sciencedirect.com/science/article/pii/B9780123695215000130

36   National Institute on Drug Abuse (NIH). (n.d) "Opioid Overdose Crisis." https://www.
     drugabuse.gov/drug-topics/opioids/opioid-overdose-crisis

37   Ibid.

38   Sigalos, MacKenzie. CNBC, December 23 2020. "You can't sue Pfizer or Moderna if
     you have severe Covid vaccine side effects. The government likely won't compensate

you for damages either." https://www.cnbc.com/2020/12/16/covid-vaccine-side-effects-compensation-lawsuit.html

39   Endocrine Society. "Endocrine Disrupting Chemicals." https://www.endocrine.org/topics/edc

40   Whiteman, Honor. February 4 2015. *Medical News Today*. '1 in 2 people will develop cancer in their lifetime' – online article https://www.medicalnewstoday.com/articles/288916

41   Taylor, Roy. "Calorie restriction for long-term remission of type 2 diabetes." *Clinical medicine (London, England)* vol. 19,1 (2019): 37–42. doi:10.7861/clinmedicine.19-1-37

42   Environmental News Network, 13 September 2017. "Type 2 Diabetes is a Reversible Condition." https://www.enn.com/articles/52481-type-2-diabetes-is-a-reversible-condition

43   Ibid.

44   Ibid.

45   NCD Risk Factor Collaboration (NCD-RisC) (2016). "Worldwide trends in diabetes since 1980: a pooled analysis of 751 population-based studies with 4.4 million participants." *Lancet (London, England)*, 387(10027), 1513–1530. https://doi.org/10.1016/S0140-6736(16)00618-8

46   Rosenthal E. "When High Prices Mean Needless Death." *JAMA Intern Med.* 2019;179(1):114–115. doi:10.1001/jamainternmed.2018.5007

47   Belluz, Julia. "The absurdly high cost of insulin, explained: Why Americans ration a drug discovered in the 1920s." Vox [online] November 17, 2109. https://www.vox.com/2019/4/3/18293950/why-is-insulin-so-expensive

48   Ibid.

12 TECHNOLOGY

1   http://www.basilleaftech.com/dxter

2   Ostler, Blair. "Technology Is Nature." http://www.blaireostler.com/journal/2018/2/13/technology-is-nature

3   Ibid.

4   Ibid.

5   Ibid.

6   Flatt, Molly. "Nature and Technology: friends or enemies?" *Earth*. BBC. Published online 16 July 2015. http://www.bbc.com/earth/story/20150703-can-nature-and-technology-be-friends

7   Laulicht, Bryan et al. "Quick-release medical tape." *Proceedings of the National Academy of Sciences of the United States of America* vol. 109,46 (2012): 18803-8. doi:10.1073/pnas.1216071109

8   Tarasov, Sergey & Gaponenko, Vadim & Howard, O. M. & Chen, Yuhong & Oppenheim, Joost & Dyba, Marzena & Subramaniam, Sriram & Lee, Youngshim

& Michejda, Christopher & Tarasova, Nadya. (2011). "Structural plasticity of a transmembrane peptide allows self-assembly into biologically active nanoparticles." *Proceedings of the National Academy of Sciences of the United States of America*. 108. 9798-803. 10.1073/pnas.1014598108.

9   Plattner Luca, "Optical properties of the scales of *Morpho rhetenor* butterflies: theoretical and experimental investigation of the back-scattering of light in the visible spectrum." *J. R. Soc. Interface*. 22 November 2004, 149–59

10 PEARY, Brett & Shaw, Rajib & TAKEUCHI, Yukiko. (2012). "Utilization of Social Media in the East Japan Earthquake and Tsunami and its Effectiveness." *Journal of Natural Disaster Science*. 34. 3–18. 10.2328/jnds.34.3.

11 FEMA, Disaster Reporter. https://www.fema.gov/disaster-reporter

12 Cash, Hilarie et al. "Internet Addiction: A Brief Summary of Research and Practice." *Current psychiatry reviews* vol. 8,4 (2012): 292–298. doi:10.2174/157340012803520513

13 F, Carolyn. "Elon Musk's vision for the world's transition to sustainable energy." Teslarati. Feb 17, 2017. https://www.teslarati.com/elon-musk-vision-worlds-transition-to-sustainable-energy

14 https://neuralink.com

15 Ibid.

16 Freeman, D., Lister, R., Waite, F. et al. "Automated psychological therapy using virtual reality (VR) for patients with persecutory delusions: study protocol for a single-blind parallel-group randomised controlled trial." (THRIVE). *Trials* 20, 87 (2019). https://doi.org/10.1186/s13063-019-3198-6

17 http://www.iflytek.com/en

18 Institute of Medicine (US) Committee on Quality of Health Care in America; Kohn LT, Corrigan JM, Donaldson MS, editors. *To Err is Human: Building a Safer Health System*. Washington (DC): National Academies Press (US); 2000. 2, Errors in Health Care: A Leading Cause of Death and Injury. Available from: https://www.ncbi.nlm.nih.gov/books/NBK225187

19 Goyal, Manu & Knackstedt, Thomas & Yan, Shaofeng & Oakley, Amanda & Hassanpour, Saeed. (2019). "Artificial Intelligence for Diagnosis of Skin Cancer: Challenges and Opportunities." Recently, there has been great interest in developing Artificial Intelligence (AI) enabled computer-aided diagnostics solutions for the diagnosis of skin cancer. With the increasing incidence of skin cancers, low awareness among a growing population, and a lack of adequate clinical expertise and services, there is an immediate need for AI systems to assist clinicians in this domain. A large number of skin lesion datasets are available publicly, and researchers have developed AI solutions, particularly deep learning algorithms, to distinguish malignant skin lesions from benign lesions in different image modalities such as dermoscopic, clinical, and histopathology images. Despite the various claims of AI systems achieving higher accuracy than dermatologists in the classification

of different skin lesions, these AI systems are still in the very early stages of clinical application in terms of being ready to aid clinicians in the diagnosis of skin cancers. In this review, we discuss advancements in the digital image-based AI solutions for the diagnosis of skin cancer, along with some challenges and future opportunities to improve these AI systems to support dermatologists and enhance their ability to diagnose skin cancer.

THE 12 MEDICINES AND BEYOND

1   Planck, Max K. (1950). *Scientific Autobiography and Other Papers*. New York: Philosophical library.

www.ingramcontent.com/pod-product-compliance
Lightning Source LLC
Chambersburg PA
CBHW062112020426

42335CB00013B/931